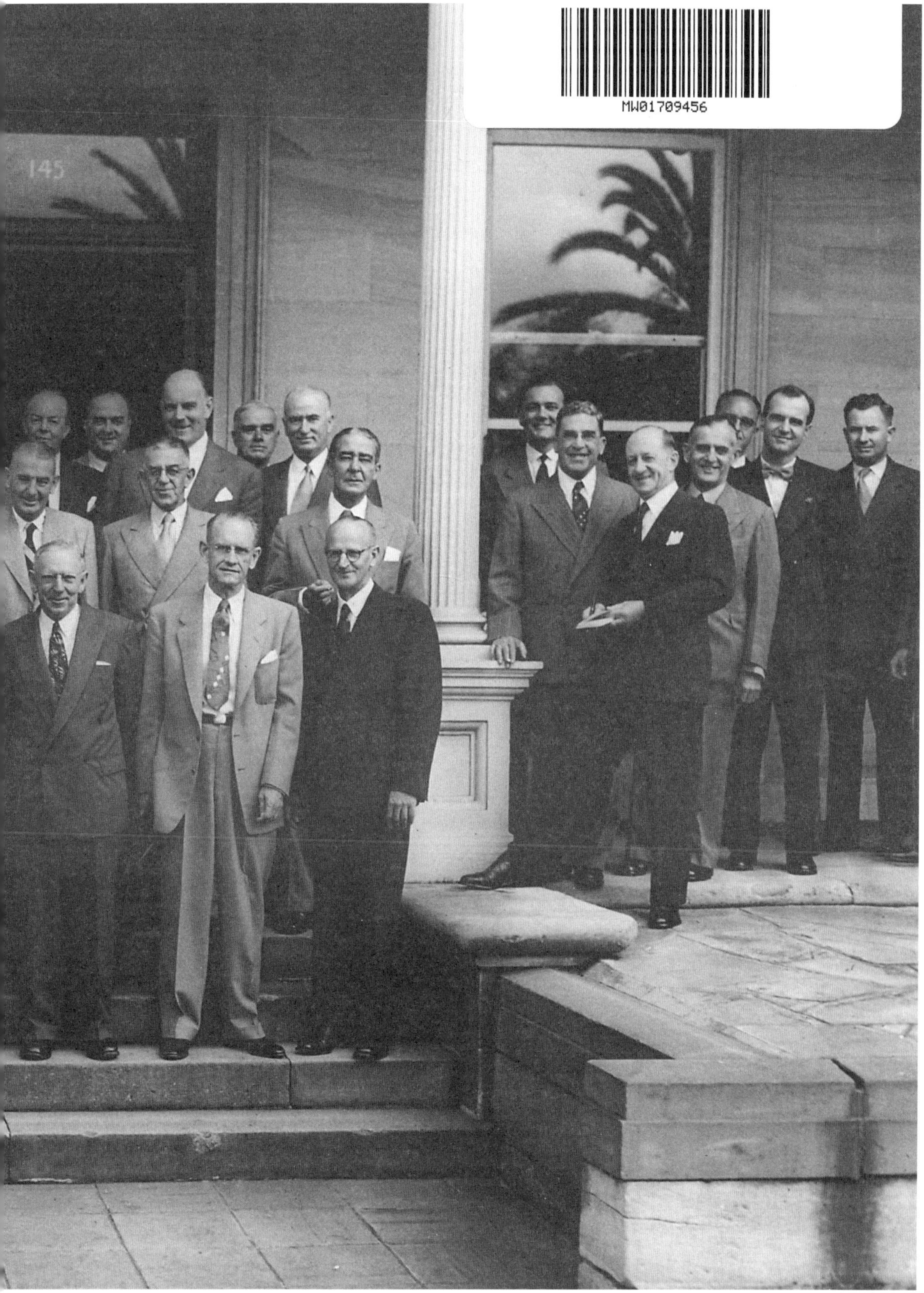
145

Joined Across *the* Water

~

A History of the Urological Society of Australasia

Arms of the Urological Society of Australasia

The Arms comprise a shield, helmet, crest and supporters along with a motto which, strictly speaking, is not part of the arms. The shield, divided down the middle, bears the colours of Australia, green and gold on the right side, and on the left side the colours of New Zealand, black and silver. These four colours were those of the College of Barber surgeons who received a grant to arms in 1569. In the centre of the shield is the badge of the Society. This represents the view seen through a cystoscope of the bladder neck with the lobes of the prostate in red and the urine portrayed in gold.

On top of the shield sits a steel helmet, visored and turned to the right. The mantling originally used to protect the head within the helmet from the heat of the sun is secured to the helmet by a wreath, in turn surmounted by the flowers of the yellow wattle of Australia with the red pohutukawa of New Zealand.

The crest is a lynx, an animal with exceptional vision. The ancients believed such keen vision could not have been provided by two eyes alone and attributed this to some other unknown method - hence the supernumerary eyes scattered throughout its body as coloured circles or roundelles. It holds aloft in its forepaws an ancient instrument called an exploratorium used in the Marian operation for stone first described by Marianus, Sanctus de Bartella in his second book *Libellus aureus* 1543, a landmark in the history of urology. Around its neck it wears a crown with the seven pointed stars of Australia and the five pointed stars of New Zealand.

On either side of the shield which they support stand St. Cosmos and St. Damian, two early exponents of uroscopy. Twin brothers, Christian doctors, martyred under the Roman emperor, Diocletian, (243-313) they have been the patron saints of barbers and surgeons throughout Europe from the time of the emperor, Justinian (482–565).

The motto – Juncta per aquam – joined across the water, emphasises in a humourous way the union of two countries separated by an ocean working together within their 'watery' medium.

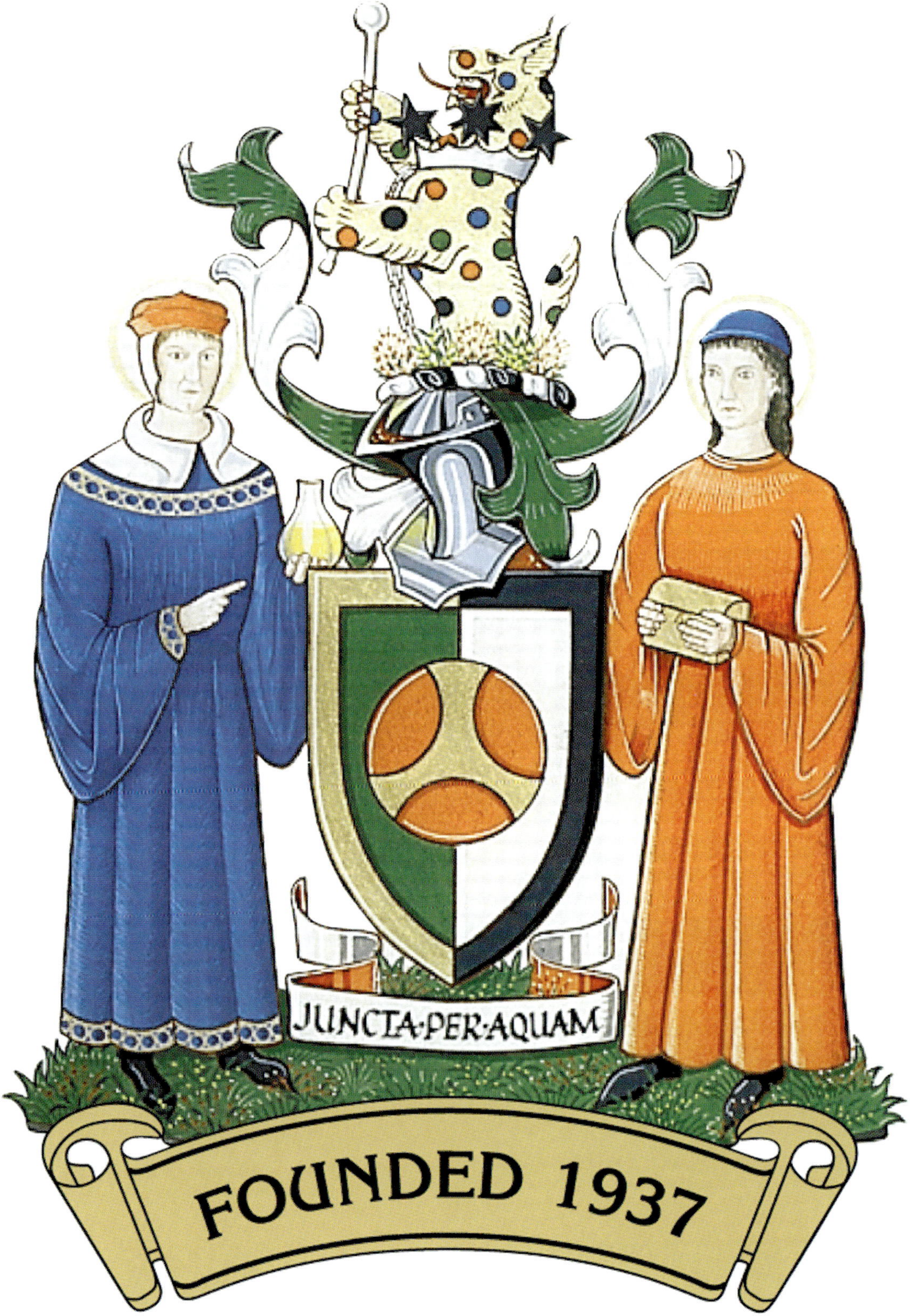
JUNCTA·PER·AQUAM
FOUNDED 1937

JOINED ACROSS *the* WATER

~

A History of the Urological Society of Australasia

~

SALLY WILDE

HYLAND HOUSE

First published in Australia in 1999 by
Hyland House Publishing Pty Ltd
Hyland House
387-389 Clarendon Street
South Melbourne
Victoria 3205

National Library of Australia
Cataloguing-in-publication data:

Wilde, Sally, 1949-.
Joined across the water: a history of the Urological Society of Australasia

Includes index.
ISBN 1 86447 058 5.

1. Urological Society of Australasia - History. 2. Urology - Australia - History. 3. Urology - New Zealand - History. I. Title.

616.600601

Typeset in Bembo 11½ on 12½ pt
Designed by Rob Cowpe
Printed by Brown Prior Anderson, Melbourne, Australia

Foreword

~

Today Urology is a high profile surgical specialty with the Urological Society leading public debate about topics as diverse as prostate cancer and impotence. However, when the inaugural meeting of the Urological Society was held in Sydney in 1937 there were only eleven members throughout Australia and New Zealand. Specialisation within surgery was in its infancy.

The Urological Society of Australasia is justifiably proud of its record, not only as the oldest Urology Society in the English-speaking world after the United States, but also for its contributions to international urological practice.

Unlike most similar societies commisioning a history, the Urology group was sufficiently confident of its standing and integrity to select as author a professional historian without a background of medical training, believing this would broaden the book's perspective and allow examination of the changing political and social times during which the Society developed.

The Society's strong endorsement of the project at the Annual General Meeting in 1996 was no surprise given the long tradition of oral and written historical presentations by Society members.

The sixty-year span has meant there are interviews with urologists who actually knew the founders of the Society.

Medical and community values have changed over time. Some strongly held views noted in the book will now be seen in an historical perspective, just as the scientific basis of disease has moved forward.

Peter Lawson (Chairman)
Frank Breslin
Tony Low
Russell McIlroy
Don Urquhart-Hay
DECEMBER 1998

To Saad

With our very best wishes

Don Moss

27.3.2001.

The idea for this history is largely that of Peter Lawson. It was he who planted the 'seed' of this book in the minds of the members of the Urological Society. Once germinated, he watered it, fertilised it, and generally nurtured it to fruition.

No doubt he was both a great help to Sally Wilde, as well as a nagging enthusiast as he pursued leads and details to help in her research.

The Urological Society of Australasia is immensely grateful to him, and to the members of his committee for their contributions. The history is that of many enthusiasts for the specialty of Urology, but would never have been completed without his particular interest.

Donald Moss,
President, Urological Society of Australasia
JANUARY 1999

Contents

~

List of Illustrations

~

Acknowledgements

A large number of the current members of the Urological Society assisted in the writing of this book, but the project owes most to Peter Lawson. He was involved at every stage, persuading the Society to commission the history, making available the results of his own research, providing further research assistance and reading and commenting on drafts. The other members of the History Sub-committee of the Urological Society, Frank Breslin, Tony Low, Russell McIlroy and Don Urquhart-Hay, were also of particular assistance, as was historian Weston Bate. Russell McIlroy, Kerry Maher and Don and Pamela Urquhart-Hay provided particular help during the research in New Zealand and Frank and Gabrielle Breslin played a similar role in Sydney.

The staff of the Royal Australasian College of Surgeons in Melbourne also offered considerable assistance. Catherine Green provided substantial research support and Colin Smith, Jane Oliver and Jennifer Jolley were unfailingly helpful. Thanks must also go to Jill Wright-Neville, Harold Story, Gail Hill, Nada Gergich, Dennis Arnold, Ted Arnold, Pat Bary, Jack Blackman, Gwynne Brockis, Ron Brown, Peter Bruce, Geof Burfield, Alex Cato, Roger Chambers, Ray Chapman, Laurence Cleeve, Glen Coorey, Alan Crosthwaite, Ernie England, Chris Farrell, Frank Gardiner, David Golovsky, Stuart Gowland, Jim Gray, Peter Harbison, Laurence Harewood, Geof Hirst, Graham Holmes, Lionel Jacobs, Patricia Jacobsen, Warren Johnson, John Jose, Gerry Joyce, Keith Kaye, Doug Keller, Mohamed Khadra, Harry Learoyd, Tony Low, Bill Lucas, Warwick Macky, John Maddern, Peter Maher, Peter Meffan, Richard Millard, Peter Mortensen, Don Moss, Joe Murnaghan, Betty Murphy, Don Murphy, Philip McDougall, Colin McRae, Helen O'Connell, Jim Peters, John Phillips, Adrian Porter, Michael Rice, D. I. Roberts, Michael Rochford, John Rogers, Lorna Sisely, Robin Smart, Durham Smith, Stephen Stening, Douglas Stephens, Stuart Taylor, Tony Taylor, Roy Towers, Alastair Tulloch, Bill Utley, Ken Vaux, Jeff Watson, David Webb, Llew Wheeler, Stan Wisniewski and David Yoffa. All provided information or photographs or both or commented on drafts. Any remaining errors are, of course, the responsibility of the author.

Abbreviations

AAS	Australian Association of Surgeons
AMA	Australian Medical Association
ANZAUS	Australia and New Zealand Association of Urological Surgeons
BAUS	British Association of Urological Surgeons
BMA	British Medical Association
FRCS Eng	Fellow Royal College of Surgeons of England
FRCS Ed	Fellow Royal College of Surgeons of Edinburgh
FRACS	Fellow Royal Australasian College of Surgeons
SIU	Société Internationale d'Urologie
SUA	Sydney Urological Association
RACS	Royal Australasian College of Surgeons
USA	Urological Society of Australasia

PART 1

~

Urology in Australasia 1914–1948

~

Chapter 1
The International Context

~

At some stage during the final decades of the nineteenth century, surgery became respectable. Anaesthesia helped reduce the degree of terror and pain experienced by patients, but it also reduced the premium on extreme speed that had previously been the hallmark of a top surgeon. Understanding of the principles of post-operative infection subsequently dramatically increased patient survival rates. Together, these developments made possible an enormous increase in the number and variety of surgical procedures. With this growth came surgical specialisation and the first step in this lengthy and continuing process was for surgery itself to become a specialty, as opposed to something practised at will by general practitioners and physicians.

One of the most interesting primary sources for this increase in surgical variety is held in the archives of the Royal Australasian College of Surgeons (RACS). Archibald Watson was Professor of Anatomy at the University of Adelaide and from the 1880s until just after World War I he travelled the world carefully recording surgical procedures. Most of his notebooks relate to Australia where he was born and where he lived and worked for most of his long life.[1]

Watson recorded many examples of urological procedures performed, of course, by general surgeons. Two extracts from his notebooks are reproduced in the following pages, including a record of Watson himself participating in an operation to repair an earlier perineal prostatectomy performed at Adelaide Hospital. He also recorded Hugh Devine's treatment for chronic gonococcal urethritis in a patient at St Vincent's Hospital, Melbourne in 1909: 'Fill bladder with solution 1 in 4000 Permanganate (about 10oz in a man)—Inject into ant. urethra with No 2 irrigator 1 in 7 peroxyd.'[2] Such strictures were much more common than later in the century, as W. G. D. Upjohn recalled in 1948, looking back over the history of the Royal Melbourne Hospital:

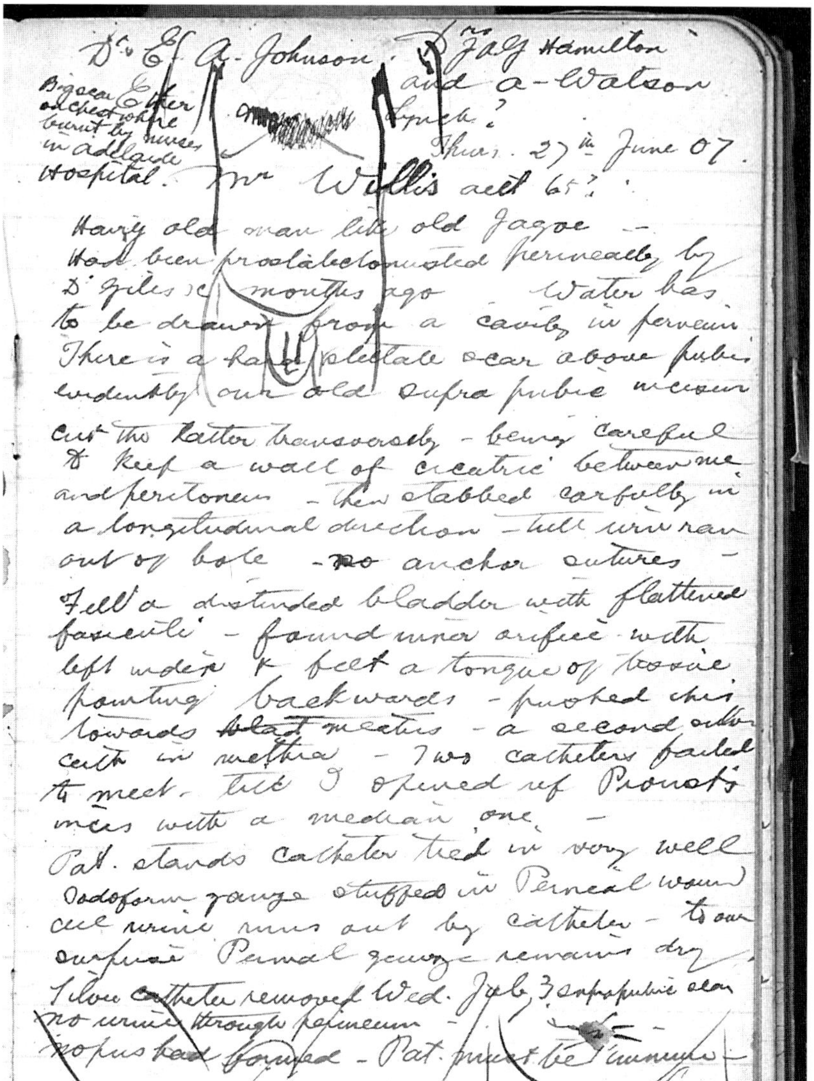
Drs E A Johnson, Drs J A G Hamilton and A Watson
Thurs. 27th June 07.
Mr Willis aet 65?
Hairy old man like old Jagoe —
Had been prostatectomised perineally by
Dr Giles ... months ago — Water has
to be drawn from a cavity in perineum
There is a hard stretchable scar above pubis
evidently our old supra pubic incision
Cut thro latter transversely — being careful
to keep a wall of cicatrix between me
and peritoneum — then stabbed carefully in
a longitudinal direction — till urine ran
out of hole — no anchor sutures —
Felt a distended bladder with flattened
fasciculi — found urinary orifice with
left index & felt a tongue of tissue
pointing backwards — pushed this
towards meatus — a second ... catheter
in urethra — Two catheters failed
to meet. Till I opened up Prostate
incis with a median one. —
Pat. stands catheter tied in very well
Iodoform gauze stuffed in Perineal wound
all urine runs out by catheter — to our
surprise Perineal gauze remains dry.
Silver catheter removed Wed. July 3 suprapubic clean
no urine through perineum
no pus had formed — Pat. must be immune

Source: Archibald Watson's notebooks, P1/2/17, Thursday, 27 June 1907, Adelaide Hospital, RACS archives

Stricture of the urethra enjoyed much greater hospital attention than it does now. The main reason for this is that the treatment of gonorrhoea throughout Australia was done badly. Most patients did not attend hospital or even private medical practitioners, but received treatment from chemists and quacks, generally in the form of sandalwood oil, copaiba or cubebs. The treatment in the Out Patient Surgical Department of the hospital was not much better and the prevailing odour in the old Melbourne Hospital Out-Patient Department was of sandalwood oil …

Emergency operations for stricture and extravasation of urine were common. The most common operation was blind internal urethrotomy by

the Wheelhouse technique. Hamilton Russell had already devised his operation of excision of the stricture after converting the urethra into a ribbon and then suturing the gap ...[3]

A number of the early urology departments in Australasia and elsewhere were combined with a venereal disease clinic and as a consequence pioneer urologists had to put up with a great many obvious jokes. But specialisation proceeded and has been a major feature of medicine as a whole in the twentieth century. The process accelerated during the 1920s and 1930s with sustained rapid increases in general medical knowledge. X-rays, blood transfusions, developments in anaesthetics and pathology all played a role.

By the end of the 1930s it was no longer possible, as it had been the at the end of the nineteenth century, for the same person to be 'an outstanding honorary physician on the staff of one hospital and an equally outstanding honorary surgeon on another'.[4]

The pattern of development of specialisation within surgery varied from country to country. Most pioneering Australasian urologists travelled to Britain for at least some of their training, but British hospitals were not generally ahead of their Australasian counterparts in setting up specialised urology departments. The outstanding exception was St Peter's Hospital for Stone, founded in 1860. A survey of British hospital histories reveals few other specialist urology departments before World War II. Typically, English hospitals appointed ophthalmic, ENT, orthopaedic, plastic, thoracic and even neurosurgeons before urologists.

Guy's Hospital appointed a genito-urinary surgeon in1910 but although Alec Badenoch at St Bartholomew's practised mainly as a urologist, the Department of Urological Surgery did not open until his retirement in 1967. In 1938 a Department of Prostatic Surgery opened at Newcastle General Hospital, under W. E. M. Wardill and Salford Royal Infirmary had an early Urology Department under J. B. McAlpine. Ireland had a pioneer in T. J. D. Lane at the Meath Hospital. By 1930 he was practising exclusively as a urologist. The earliest urology department in Scotland seems to have been at the Glasgow Royal Infirmary, from 1936, despite the distinguished work of Sir Henry Wade at the Edinburgh Royal Infirmary. Wade's work in urology was internationally acknowledged, but he was a general surgeon.

Despite the enthusiasm of solitary experts such as Lane, Wardill and Hamilton Stewart, the end of World War II saw renewed opposition to the idea of specialising in urology. A 'proper surgeon' was supposed to do anything. If general surgeons still thought they could cope with orthopaedics, what hope was there for urology? Before and during the War at St Mary's the Professor of Surgery, whose interest was the upper G-I tract, insisted that any fractured femur that came in on his take should be admitted to his ward, there to be put into traction or operated on by him. In the same hospital Dickson Wright's lists embraced all specialties: urology, plastic surgery, orthopaedics and brain surgery. It was difficult for fully trained general surgeons, even though their prime interest was in urology, to give up

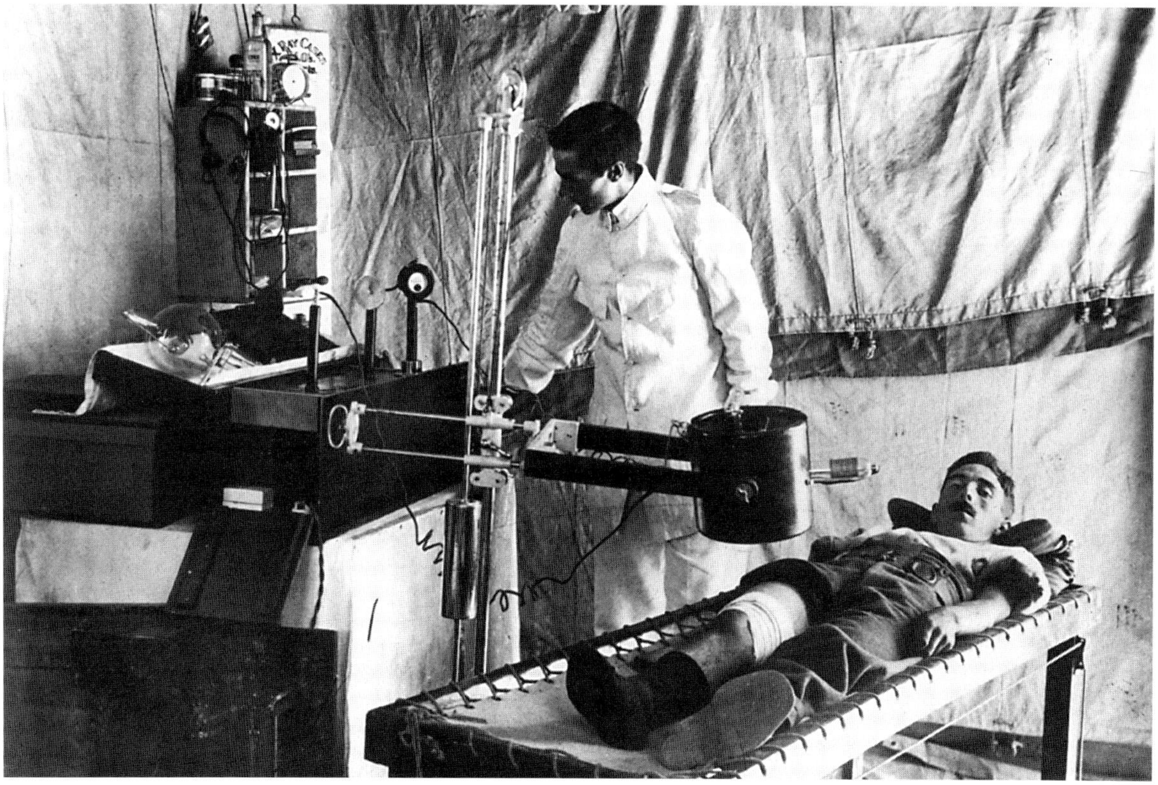

X-ray room, 1st Australian Stationary Hospital, Lemnos, 1915. On the back of the photograph is written: 'Dear Muriel, This is Les Coates at work. I was there last night and had a look at different ones under X-ray. This picture is one of a photo being taken of a bullet in position in a man's leg. It is a marvellous invention alright. Farewell, Edgar' (*Source:* Q92/003 Se 31/316, RACS archives)

their general surgery; it was equally difficult for the then general surgeon to forfeit the urological element of his private practice.[5]

In the light of this pattern of relatively late development of the specialty of urology, we should perhaps not be surprised that the British Association of Urological Surgeons (BAUS) was not formed until 1945. The exclusive American Association of Genito-Urinary Surgeons, however, was formed in 1886 and the more broadly based American Urological Association (AUA) in 1902. This was associated with the earlier development of the specialty in American hospitals, in both Canada and the United States.

By World War I, notable American urology units included the James Brady Urological Institute at Johns Hopkins Hospital, Baltimore, the urological service at the Bellevue Hospital, New York, the Urological Service of the Massachusetts General Hospital and the urology unit at the Royal Victoria Hospital, Montreal. The technology of cystoscopy featured prominently in these units. In this era, instruments were often imported from Europe. The first intravesically lit cystoscope was developed in 1877 as the result of co-operation between the Berliner Max Nitze and Beneche, the Viennese optical instrument maker, although Americans were soon to make further advances. Cystoscopy rooms and dedicated urological operating theatres were a feature of several early-American urology units.[6]

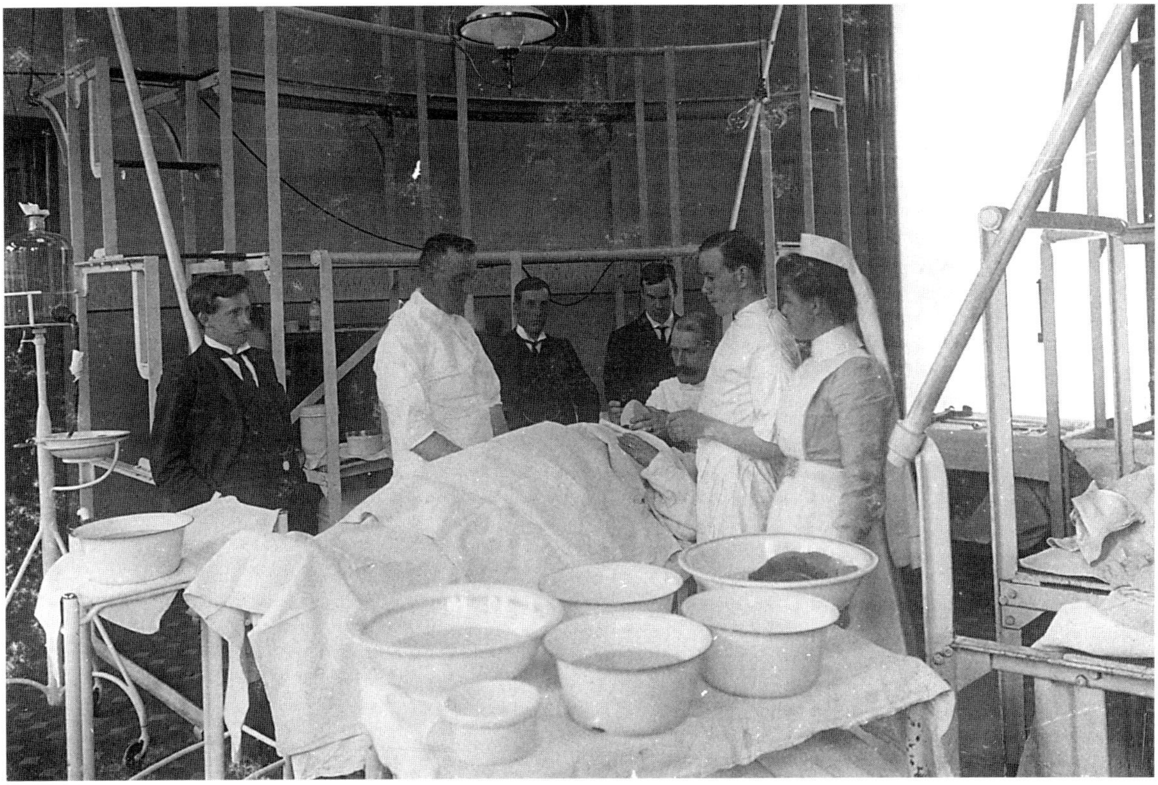

Operating theatre, Melbourne Hospital, c. 1903. Dr William 'Jerry' Moore, father of William Harold Moore one of Melbourne's pioneering urologists, is standing second from left. (*Source:* Royal Melbourne Hospital Archives)

The North Americans led the English-speaking world in the development of the specialty of urology, but the Europeans were not far behind. The Deutsche Gesellschaft für Urologie was formed in 1907 and the Dutch association, the Nederlandse Vereniging voor Urologie, a year later. The Association Française d'Urologie was founded even earlier, in 1896, and the Société Internationale d'Urologie (SIU) first met in Paris in 1908.[7]

In this context, the formation of the Urological Society of Australasia in 1937 is not particularly early. However, it was the first urological society in the British Commonwealth. The Canadian Urological Association was not formed until 1942, despite the early developments in Montreal.

In the early twentieth century there were a number of factors driving the emergence of urology as a specialty, but probably the single most important was the improvement in cystoscopes.

In January 1920 the *Medical Journal of Australia* published an article by A. S. Roe, Honorary Assistant Surgeon and Genito-Urinary Surgeon at Mater Misericordiae Public Hospital in Brisbane. It was entitled 'The value of the cystoscope as a means of diagnosis in urology'. Roe proposed that 'The ordinary cystoscopic examination of bladder and ureters can be done quite simply in one's consulting-room under local anaesthesia'. He preferred to hospitalise patients when catheterising the ureter. Roe discussed the value of cystoscopy

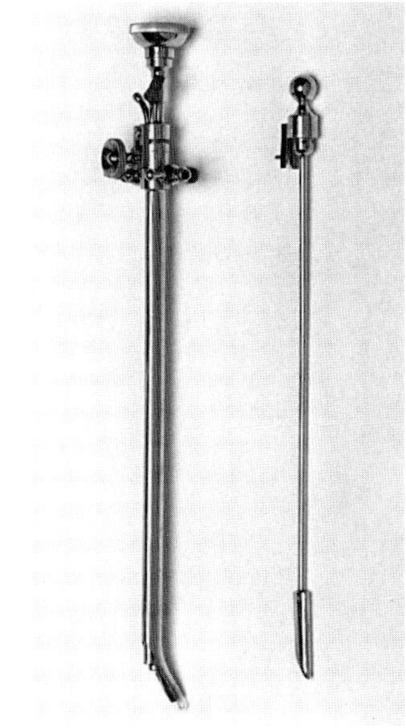

Tilden Brown double catheterising cystoscope with direct vision telescope, c. 1920s. (*Source:* Urological collection, RACS)

in determining the nature of vesical growths, kidney infections and, in conjunction with X-rays, in diagnosing stone in the ureter. Roe himself put this enormous development in cystoscopy in context for us in a paper published in the same journal forty-one years later:

> *Kidney and bladder pathology belonged in the Dark Ages. Many times, in my medical school days [in England before World War I] I had listened to learned discourses about the nature of some kidney condition, and later, at the post-mortem examination, been shown some entirely different pathology. During the period from 1908 to 1913 at a big London teaching hospital, I can remember seeing or hearing of only one cystoscopy - and that was a failure, as the lamp would not work ... However, soon after that the cystoscope was perfected and urology developed with great rapidity.*[8]

Later urologists, who struggled with the vagaries of cystoscopes in the days before fibreoptics might raise an eyebrow at the use of the word 'perfected' but there was certainly a dramatic improvement.

Cystoscopy was a specialised art and, over time, it became the prime distinguishing skill of the urologist; or as Stuart Gowland put it, the: 'main urological skill was looking down the tube, the main thing to keep the general surgeons at bay.'[9] However, general surgeons frequently regarded urologists with their cystoscopes as principally diagnosticians. Pioneer urologists at a number of Australasian hospitals had to deal with general surgeons who wanted to refer cases to them for diagnosis only.

Technical improvements in the cystoscope not only took some of the guesswork out of diagnosis. They made possible the development of other instruments. In January 1992 Bruce Pearson sent some notes on the history of urology to Frank Gardiner. They included the following:

Brown-Buerger operating cystoscope, c.1908. (*Source:* Urological collection, RACS)

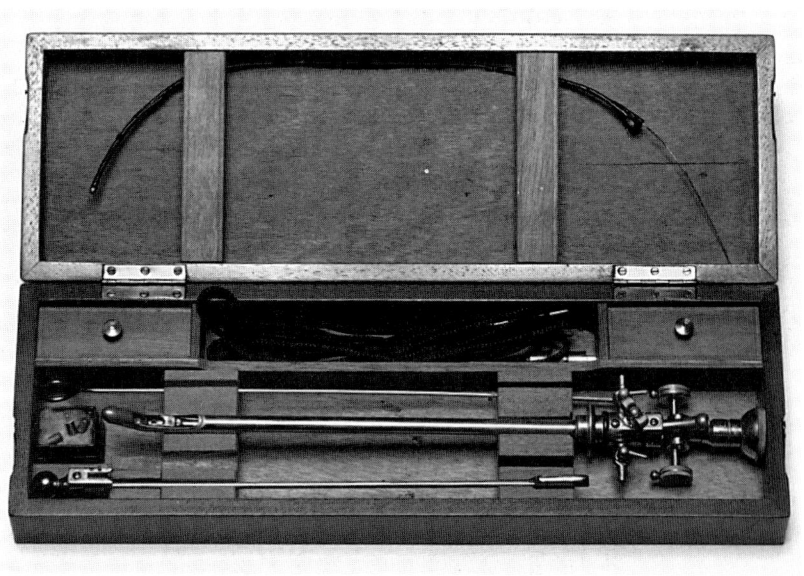

In 1909 Hugh Young designed a punch [Baltimore]
1914 George Luy's coagulated prostatic tissue
1926 Bumpus controlled haemorrhage before cutting away the prostate
1926 Stern invented the resectoscope
1931 The resectoscope was improved as the Stern-McCarthy resectoscope.[10]

This chain of events made possible enormous improvements in the treatment of prostatic obstruction, but it was many years before transurethral resection of the prostate (TUR, or TURP) was widely adopted in Australasia. In 1925 and 1926, John Tait, the father of John Thomson Tait, the first Urologist appointed to Melbourne Hospital, kept a record of his treatment for prostatic obstruction. For seven weeks his son passed a catheter morning and night and then, in consultation with senior general surgeon Basil Kilvington, performed an operation. 'They considered the tube the best and I, not knowing about it, agreed.' He was probably given a suprapubic cystotomy. The after effects were painful and embarrassing, including regular catheter changes, but he survived and died six years later aged eighty-nine.[11]

In 1925, the options for treating 83-year-old Mr Tait were very limited but at about this time there were a number of developments in the techniques for dealing with prostatic obstruction. Perineal prostatectomy had been in favour in the United States since the turn of the century and was popularised by Hugh Young in Baltimore. Leonard Murphy has argued that it remained the favoured method in America until the development of TUR in the 1930s.[12] Suprapubic prostatectomy was also pioneered in the United States but became particularly associated with Peter Freyer at St Peter's Hospital for Stone in London. A version of this operation performed by Mr Sherren was recorded by Archibald Watson. As can be seen from the illustration, the bladder wall was closed up around a tube or tubes. The resulting smell was famous and remained a noted characteristic of St Peter's Hospital for Stone for more than a generation.

The development of prostatectomy of whatever kind was particularly associated with the development of urology as a specialty. Mortality rates were high, particularly in the hands of surgeons who did not perform many prostatectomies. Specialisation and improved results were the way to 'keep the general surgeons at bay' and the first surgeon in Australasia to specialise in urology on a systematic basis was Harry Harris. From 1914, he worked as a full time urologist at Lewisham Hospital in Sydney and in 1927 he published the remarkable results of his version of suprapubic prostatectomy with complete closure of the bladder. Frank Macky of Auckland learned the operation from Harry Harris, and A. Eisdell Moore, a senior general surgeon at Auckland Hospital, soon noticed the improved progress of Mr Macky's patients:

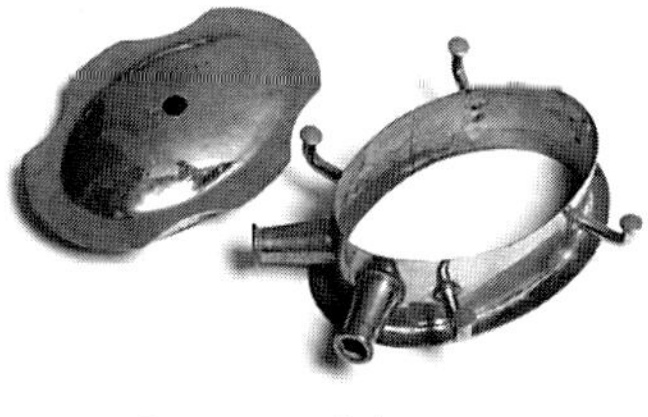

Hamilton Irvine's box or cup. This device was in use in conjunction with operations for suprapubic prostatectomy from the turn of the century until as late as the 1950s. (*Source:* Urological collection, RACS)

In the late 1930s ward 14 was shared by Kenneth Mackenzie, Frank Macky and myself [A. Eisdell Moore], each with about ten beds. It just happened that a prostatectomy of mine was next door to a patient with similar trouble and under Frank Macky's care. Both patients were operated on in the same

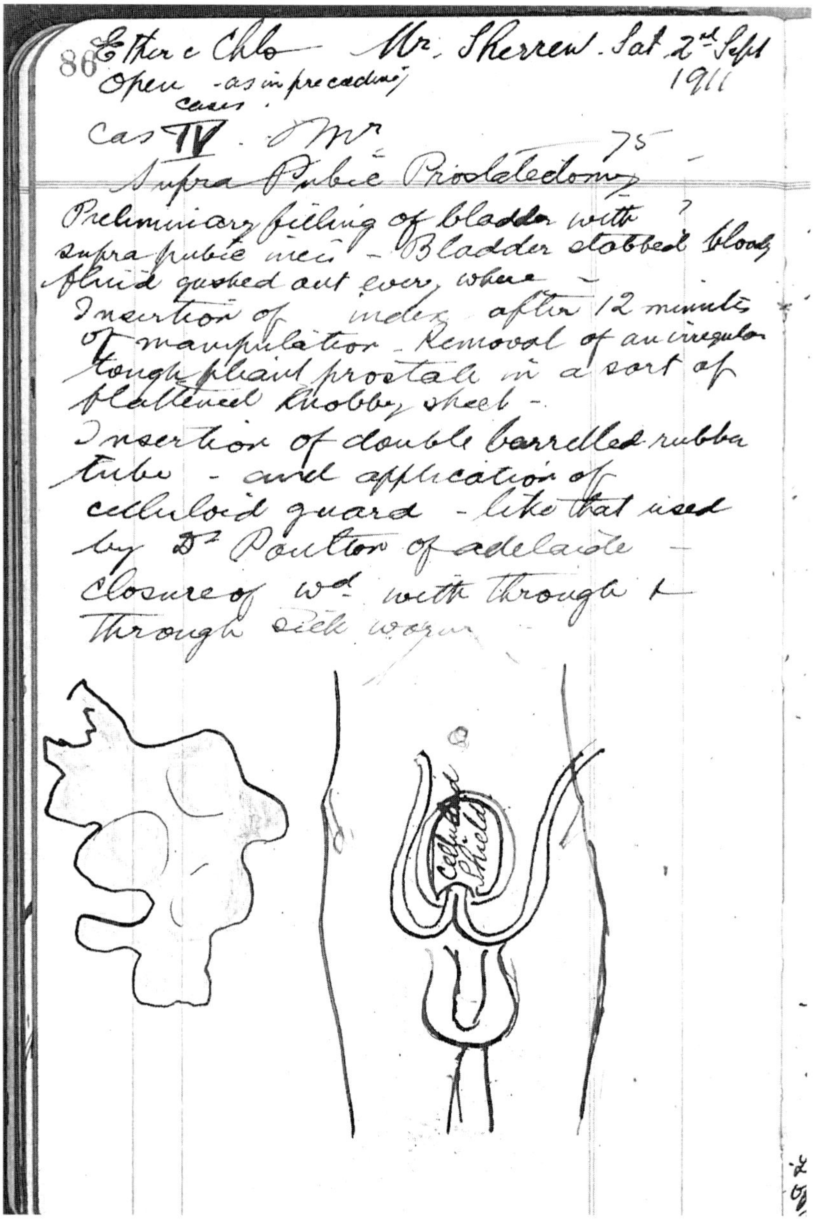

On another page Watson notes 'Rubber gloves Mr Sherren but no mask' (his emphasis) 'Ether and Chloroform when surgeon became impatient.' (*Source:* Archibald Watson's notebooks, P1/2/23, Saturday, 2 September 1911, London Hospital, RACS archives)

week. About a fortnight after, I came into the ward and noticed that the bed where Mr. Macky's patient had been was empty. I said nothing at the time. I rather feared the worst. As we left the ward I said to the sister 'What happened to Mr. Macky's patient?' and she said 'Oh, he went home yesterday, perfectly dry, a complete success.' Frank had been over in Australia, doing urological work there for a short time, and had come back with the very latest method of supra-pubic prostatectomy, and I thought it was just wonderful that the patient should be able to go out dry in two to three weeks. I always felt that prostate patients would be something like a month or five weeks in hospital. There and then I decided I would do no more urological work, and I said to the sister, 'If I have admitted into any of my beds a patient for prostatectomy, tell my house surgeon that he is to arrange transfer to Mr. Macky's care.'[13]

CHAPTER 2

The Pioneers of Urology in Australasia, 1914–1936

~

Introduction

This chapter provides some information on the careers and training of the twelve founding members of the Urological Society of Australasia, plus a number of other urologists who together made up the pioneers of the specialty in Australasia.

Like most university graduates of that era, all came from relatively comfortable backgrounds and attended private schools. All but two (Campbell-Begg from New Zealand who went to Edinburgh and Roe from Brisbane who went to Oxford) graduated from one of three medical schools. At the time, there were four medical schools in Australasia, at the University of Adelaide, the University of Melbourne, the University of Otago in Dunedin and Sydney University. However, none of the pioneer urologists graduated from Adelaide.

Of the total of twenty-four men with public hospital appointments as urologists before the foundation of the Urological Society in 1937, at least fifteen were graduates of Sydney Medical School, at least three of the five New Zealanders had spent their medical school days at the south of the South Island in Dunedin, as had Wishart, who moved to Melbourne, and the two other Melbourne urologists were graduates of the Melbourne Medical School.

The dominance of Sydney is clear. Not only were there more urologists in Sydney than in any other city (eleven), but four of the five Brisbane urologists were also graduates of Sydney Medical School. The other experience that more than half of them shared was a period of training in Britain.

The British colonial background was very strong in this era, particularly for the generation who served in World War I. Five of the twelve founding members of the Society (Roe, Silverton, Tait,

TABLE 2.1 AUSTRALASIA'S 24 PIONEERING UROLOGISTS WITH PUBLIC HOSPITAL APPOINTMENTS AS UROLOGISTS BEFORE 1937.

Date of first	Hospital of first appointment; Medical School Attended; Date of Graduation; Location of Training in Urology
1914	*Harry Harris,* Lewisham Hospital, Sydney; Sydney University, 1906
1918	*Robert Gordon Craig,* Royal Alexandra Hospital for Children, Sydney; Sydney University, 1894; Mayo Clinic Minnesota
1919	*Stanley Roe,* Mater Misericordiae Hospitals, Brisbane; Oxford University, 1911; Guy's Hospital, London
1921	*Bobby Silverton,* Royal North Shore Hospital, Sydney; Sydney University, 1915; St Peter's Hospital for Stone, London
1924	*Richard Harris,* Lewisham Hospital; Sydney University, 1923; Lewisham Hospital
1924	*R. Campbell-Begg,* Wellington Hospital; Edinburgh University, 1913; Mayo Clinic
1926	*Bobby Lee-Brown,* Royal Alexandra Hospital for Children;Sydney University, 1920; Royal Prince Alfred Hospital Sydney
1927	*John Thomson Tait,* Royal Melbourne Hospital; Melbourne University, 1911; St Peter's Hospital for Stone
1928	*Harold Moore,* Royal Melbourne Hospital; Melbourne University, 1917
1929	*Jack Power,* Brisbane General Hospital; Sydney University, 1914; Mayo Clinic
1930	*Reginald Bridge,* Sydney Hospital; Sydney University, 1912; Middlesex Hospital, London
1930	*John Laidley,* Royal Prince Alfred Hospital, Sydney; Sydney University, 1924; Royal Prince Alfred Hospital
1930	*Malcolm Earlam,* Royal Prince Alfred Hospital; Sydney University, 1924; Royal Prince Alfred Hospital
1930	*Edgar Reay,* Christchurch Hospital; University of Otago, 1923; St Peter's Hospital for Stone
1930	*Patrick Treahy,* Wellington Hospital; University of Otago, 1924; St Peter's Hospital for Stone
1930	*Mordo Sutton,* Brisbane General Hospital; Sydney University, 1914
1932	*Keith Kirkland,* Sydney Hospital; Sydney University, 1925; St Peter's Hospital for Stone
1932	*Colin Edwards,* Royal North Shore Hospital; Sydney University, 1924; St Peter's Hospital for Stone
1932	*Bruce Rennie,* Wellington Hospital; University of Otago, 1925; All Saints Hospital, London
1932	*Pip Lukin,* Mater Misericordiae Hospitals, Brisbane; Sydney University, 1923
1933	*William Wishart,* Homeopathic Hospital/Prince Henry's (Melbourne); University of Otago, 1911
1934	*Angus Walker-Smith,* Royal Prince Alfred Hospital; Sydney University, 1922; St Peter's Hospital for Stone
1934	*Alex Inglis,* Mater Misericordiae Hospitals, Brisbane; Sydney University, 1926; Mater Misericordiae Hospitals
1935	*Joseph Brownlee,* Christchurch Hospital; University of Otago, 1926

Power and Bridge) were old enough to serve in World War I and all did so. Bridge actually served in the Royal Army Medical Corps and this would not have been considered at all odd. The biographies of this generation of Australasian surgeons reveal two major patterns. If they were already in Britain at the outbreak of war (generally because they were studying for a fellowship of one of the British colleges of surgeons), they joined the British armed forces. If they were recent medical graduates in Australasia they joined the (joint) Australasian forces and then stayed on in Britain after the war to study for a fellowship. Jack Power, for instance, followed this latter pattern.

The College of Surgeons of Australasia, later the Royal Australasian College of Surgeons (RACS) was founded in 1927. The foundation fellows were soon augmented by the awarding of more fellowships but it was many years before the FRACS had suitable status to allow ambitious surgeons to dispense with a trip to Britain to sit for their FRCSEng or FRCSEd. Not all passed, of course, but it was quite common to practise as a surgeon without a senior surgical qualification.

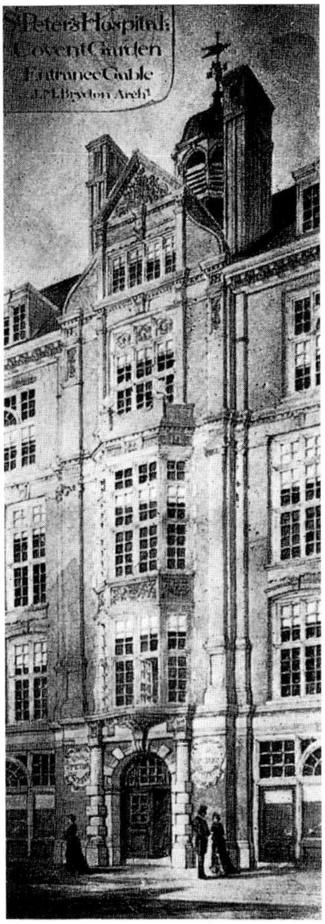

St Peter's Hospital for Stone, London, 1882

Of our group of pioneers, Alex Inglis went to England and sat for a fellowship, but failed the primary and came back still MBBS(Sydney). He thought he could never be a specialist without a FRCS and joined Dr Morgan Lane in partnership in Brisbane. He had been there some weeks when he saw an advertisement in a journal for an Assistant Honorary Urologist at the Mater Misericordiae Hospitals. Inglis applied, with some trepidation, because he had no experience. When he was interviewed by Stanley Roe, he explained that he knew little, but Roe said that Inglis could assist him at operations and with his rounds and outpatients and acquire some knowledge of urology in the process—which he duly did.[1]

Whilst in Britain, most Australasian doctors tried to get temporary work in the local hospitals. What vacancies became available where, of course, was largely a matter of luck and it is to be suspected that few, if any, of our pioneering urologists had decided on their specialty at this stage. It has already been noted that there were few urological departments in Britain before World War II, but St Peter's Hospital for Stone was an entire hospital devoted to the specialty. Rather than train large numbers of British urologists for whom there would be insufficient specialist vacancies, the hospital was quite happy to take Australasian resident medical officers and clinical assistants. At least seven of our pioneer urologists spent some time at St Peter's and six of them went on to form half of the foundation membership of the Urological Society: Bobby Silverton and John Thomson Tait, of the generation old enough to serve in World War I, plus Edgar Reay, Keith Kirkland, Colin Edwards and Angus Buchanan Walker-Smith.

However, in the 1920s and 1930s, Britain was not the centre for the most exciting developments in urology. The Americans were leading the way in many areas of surgery. Robert Gordon Craig was the first Australasian urologist to realise just how much could be learnt from visiting the Mayo Clinic. By the 1920s, the Mayo brothers had made such a success of the clinic started with their father that it had come to dominate the economy of the town of Rochester in Minnesota.

In 1924, William Mayo and Franklin Martin of the American College of Surgeons visited the Otago Medical School, as a part of the historic visit to Australasia that helped foster the foundation of the Royal Australasian College of Surgeons. This visit also seems to have inspired a number of New Zealand urologists to visit the Mayo Clinic, including Campbell-Begg and Howard Gaudin.[2]

Jack Power from Brisbane returned from the Mayo Clinic in 1928 inspired not only with new ideas about surgical technique but also with the idea of a private medical clinic based on group practice. He joined a group of doctors, including John Bostock and L. J. J. Nye, who had also spent time at the Mayo Clinic, and in 1930 they opened a group practice in Brisbane. The timing, at the height of the Depression, was unfortunate and Power felt that the concept of a clinic was unpopular with doctors who had previously referred him patients. He left the group later in the year.[3]

Australasian urologists of this era, before the introduction of the New Zealand national health service, made their living from private practice but also worked as (unpaid) honorary surgeons in public hospitals. The private system was where they made their money, but the public system also had its rewards, including status, contact with peers and the stimulus of teaching. As Peter Lawson pointed out:

> *Honorary medical staff would preferentially divert from their private rooms patients with 'interesting' medical conditions so that such a patient went to the public (or teaching) hospital and could be examined by 'the students'. The reputation of Honorary Staff so involved was quietly enhanced by nurses and junior doctors who whispered 'must be highly regarded by his peers in general practice'. 'Has the welfare of the students at heart'.*[4]

In most Australian States, this relationship between private practice and public hospitals was facilitated by the development of a system of private and intermediate beds within the public hospitals.

The Australian Hospital System 1914–1947

During the inter-war period, the Australian hospital system underwent something of a revolution and it did so at the same time and for some of the same reasons as the rapid development in medical specialisation. By the 1940s, the major charitable hospitals, most of which were founded in the nineteenth century, had come to be regarded as public utilities.

Among the factors driving this change were the rapid developments in medical science which required new and expensive equip-

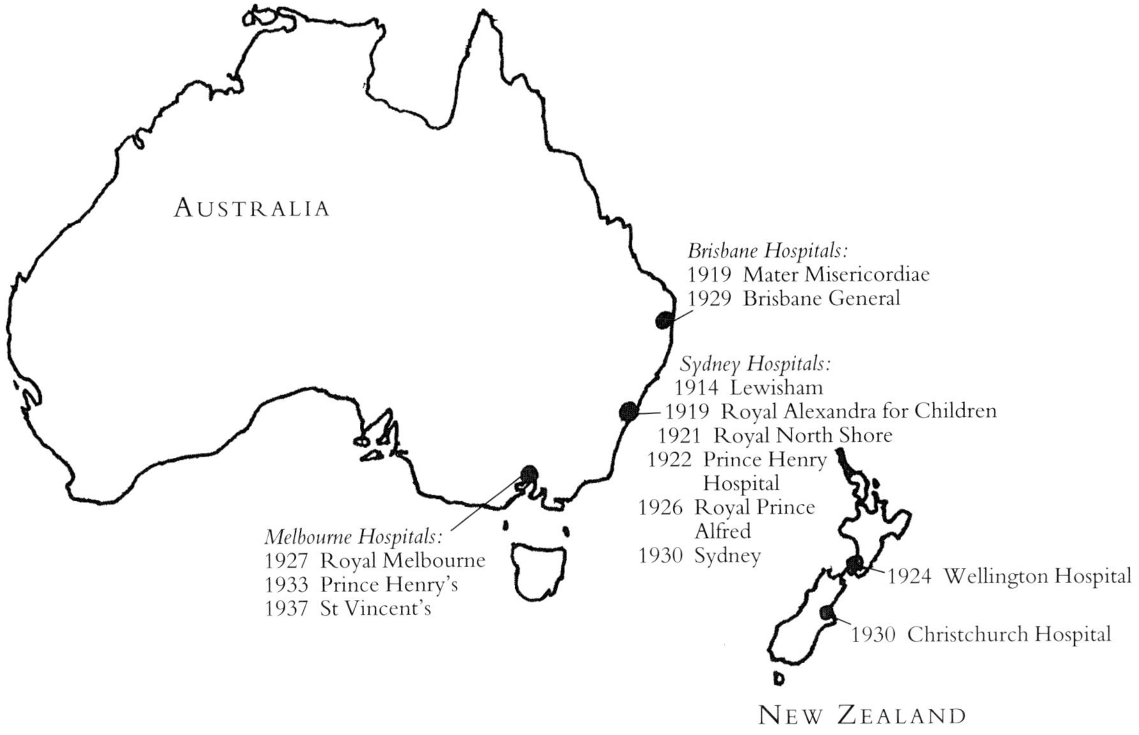

Map of early Urology Departments in Australasia

ment. The public and charitable hospitals, partly because they tended to be larger and partly because of the absence of the profit motive in funding arrangements, were more likely than the private hospitals to buy the latest equipment. In Victoria, for instance, in 1932, the Charities Board was in the process of organising standardisation and collective buying of hospital equipment for Victoria's major hospitals to take advantage of economies of scale.[5]

Over time, the perceptions of doctors and patients changed. The public and charitable hospitals had begun as basic institutions for the poor and destitute, but by the end of World War II, they had emerged as almost universally the best equipped and best staffed hospitals in every State. The private hospitals, in contrast, had come to be seen as much more comfortable, but not necessarily up-to-date. The revolutionary result was that people who were not destitute, or even struggling financially, preferred to attend the public and charitable hospitals, on the grounds that not only their pockets but also their health might benefit.

This led to considerable controversy at the time. There were frequent complaints of patients 'abusing charity'. Surgeons and physicians who gave their time for free as honorary members of the staff of these hospitals objected to treating (for free) people who could afford to pay. Each such patient was seen as a double burden–using up time and resources in the free system and removing a potential paying patient from the private system. As a result, the rights and

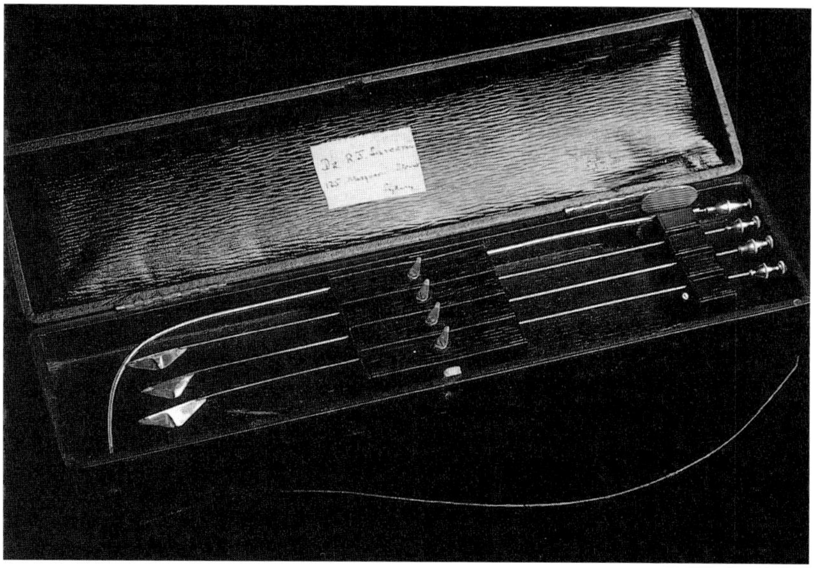

Bobby Silverton's urethrotome set, c. 1925. (*Source:* USA archives)

wrongs of this revolution in the Australian hospital system were hotly debated.

On the whole, those who objected to the admittance of patients who were not poor lost the argument. In Victoria by 1932 four of the hospitals under the auspices of the Charities Board were authorised to admit private patients and no less than forty-one hospitals were authorised to admit intermediate patients who paid a proportion of the costs of their care.

> *The introduction of intermediate and private patients' services into Country Hospitals, though necessarily limited in many cases, has amply demonstrated the soundness of the policy. Apart from very valuable financial results, the tendency of a certain section of the community to seek charitable aid has lessened in some centres now that moderate payments are possible; moreover, where there was a tendency towards subterfuge to obtain the special services which many Public Hospitals render, this has been removed. Many difficulties with medical practitioners have also disappeared.*[6]

By 1947 there was some provision for private and intermediate patients in most public and charitable hospitals in most States. Meanwhile, hospitals of this kind were more often called public than charitable and by the end of World War II the latter term had more or less dropped out of use. The system of honorary appointments to the medical staff continued to operate in all States except Queensland, but an increasing proportion of hospital funding was raised under Government auspices.

In all States except South Australia, where gambling was seriously frowned on, and Victoria, where it was frowned on unless it was on horses at the track, the hospitals were largely funded by the proceeds of lotteries and sweepstakes. As of 1943, three-quarters of hospital beds were in the 'government' sector, containing 571 hospitals.

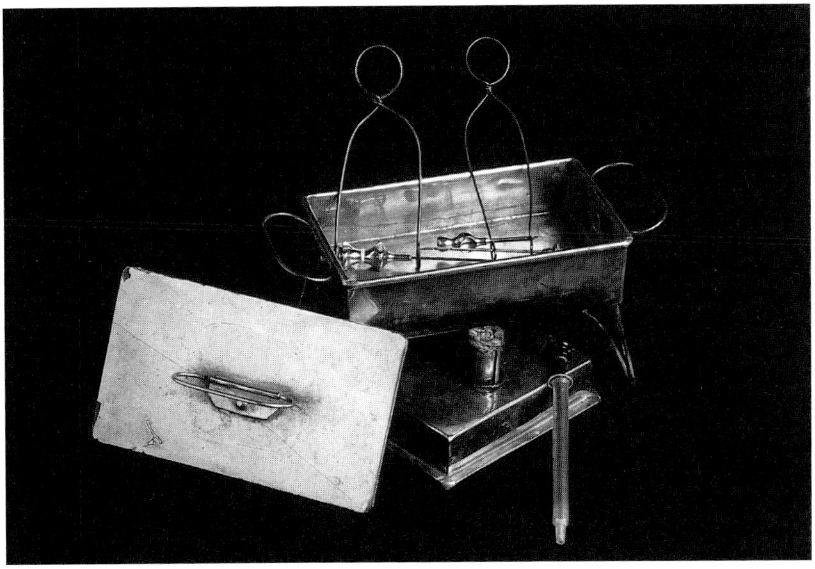

'Bobby Silverton carried this self-contained spinal needle set with him from hospital to hospital. Spindly wire legs folded out so the tray sat about five centimetres above the small spirit burner. Glass syringes and reusable steel needles were boiled in the covered tray.'—Peter Lawson. (*Source:* Gerry Joyce)

There were just over twice as many private hospitals but they accounted for only about one quarter of the total number of beds.[7]

This change took place in an international context of debate over welfare provision. Initially, concern was for the fate of returned soldiers, but from 1929 there was also much debate about provision for the poor and unemployed. Both Australia and New Zealand were heavily influenced by the debates current in Britain at the time.

In 1938, the Australian Commonwealth Government passed the National Insurance Act, which among other things gave the Government control of doctors' incomes through a system of capitation payments. Australian doctors did not extend their admiration of things British to ideas on social insurance. Resistance, particularly through the Australian Branch of the BMA, was such that the Act was never implemented. New Zealand doctors had less success in resisting their Social Security Act of the same year.

The New Zealand Hospital System, 1914–1947

From 1885, New Zealand hospitals were run by a system of elected regional hospital boards with the power to raise rates. Over the years, the number of boards and the areas they covered varied. In 1941 there were 42 hospital boards, covering populations varying from 2000 to 300 000.

Between 1914 and the passing of the Social Security Act in 1938, New Zealand experienced a growth in the number and popularity of public hospitals similar to that in Australia. Private hospitals, as a consequence, experienced relative decline and this accelerated after

1941. As in Australia in this period, the perception was that the public hospitals were better equipped and better staffed.

The expense of providing the benefits of highly trained staff and constantly changing and progressively more expensive medical technology made it extremely difficult for private hospitals to keep up to date. An obvious, but paradoxical consequence of this was that during the early years of this century the standard of medical care received by poorer patients treated at minimal or no cost in public hospitals was better than that received by those who could afford to pay for their own private treatment.[8]

This was particularly the case with the new and larger public hospitals opening on the North Island. However, the South Island, with its earlier pattern of more scattered settlement, underwent a relative decline in hospital facilities. In 1915 New Zealand had sixty-five general hospitals providing 3531 beds, or 3.22 per 1000 population, a figure very similar to the Australian average at the same date.

As in Australia, the increased use of public hospitals by those who could afford to pay led to heated debate. But in New Zealand, the system of funding hospitals partly from rates led:

to growing feelings that public hospitals ought to be available free (or at little charge) to all. This feeling, and its observable consequences, emerged in the form of conflict between honorary doctors—who worked for no payment in public hospitals–-and hospital boards. The 'honoraries', finding that they were treating many people who could well afford private care, demanded that income limitations be placed on public hospital patients by hospital boards. Supported in their stand by the Department of Health, the boards did not concede to the doctors' demands and eventually many hospital boards resolved to employ only full-time salaried officers—that is, they 'closed' their hospitals to honorary practitioners.[9]

The doctors carried on their fight through the New Zealand branch of the BMA and had some success, at least partly because those hospitals which employed full-time salaried staff could not afford to employ the full range of specialist skills. Both a revival of the honorary system and discussion of private patients in public hospitals followed. However, in 1935 New Zealanders elected a Labour Government. Opposition from the medical profession managed to delay implementation of the Social Security Act, 1938, but only until 1941.

In 1941, New Zealand introduced the world's first comprehensive government health care system in a free-market economy. This was despite considerable opposition from the New Zealand branch of the BMA including pioneering urologists such as Frank Macky. Over the years, the provision of general practitioner services was progressively modified to include an increasing proportion of direct payments by the patient, but the hospital system remained free at point of use for many years.[10]

The Pioneers

In 1842, Carlyle wrote that 'The history of the world is but the biography of great men.'[11] This is a view that generally became unfashionable among historians quite early in the twentieth century, but it continued to thrive in the art of biography, particularly political biography, and among medical historians. When Australasian urologists began to look back over the history of the specialty, most began by collecting the curriculum vitae and obituaries of their predecessors. What follows is a tribute to their work, but it is also an acknowledgement of the relevance of this pattern of thinking in this context.[12]

SAMUEL HENRY HARRIS (1881–1936)

The major university teaching hospitals were the crucibles of change in Australasian surgery. However, urology as a specialty in Australasia did not begin in any of these high-profile hospitals. In 1914, Harry Harris was appointed as Urologist to Lewisham, a Catholic hospital run by the nuns of the Little Company of Mary in a southern Sydney suburb. Although Harry Harris died before the first meeting of the Urological Society of Australasia, he was a vital figure in the events leading to its formation. Harris was the first full-time specialist urologist in Australasia and he was also the first Australasian urologist to achieve an international reputation for his work.

It is difficult through all the added information provided by hindsight to assess the significance of Harris's example. He was not only a

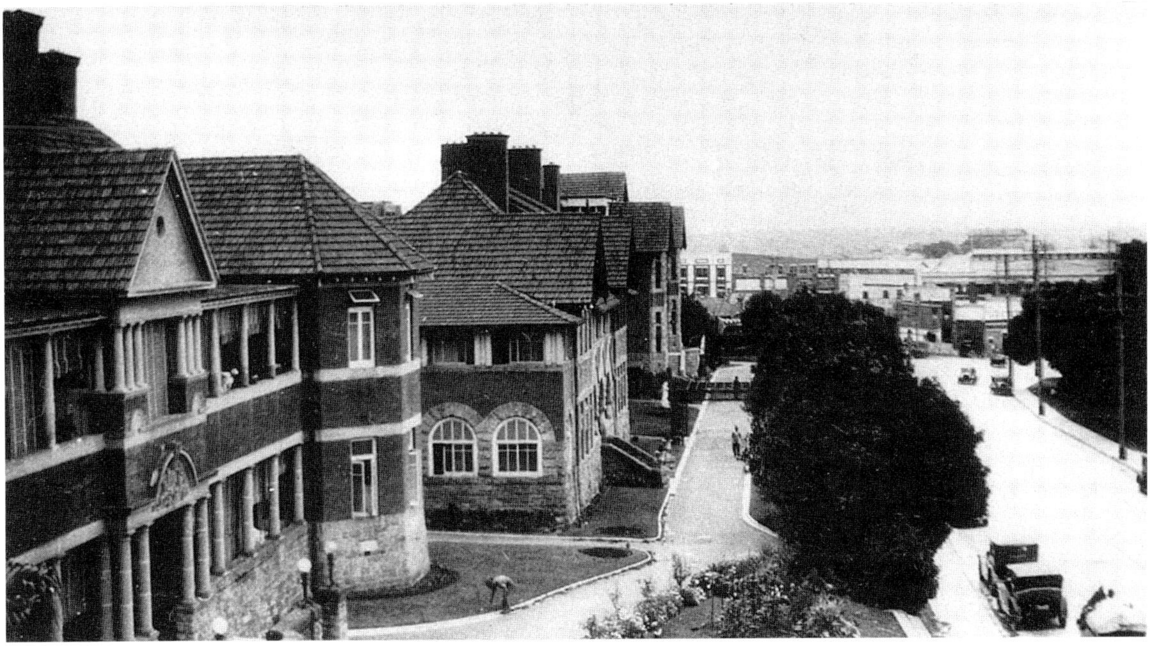

Lewisham Hospital, Sydney, run by the nuns of the Little Company of Mary. It was here, in 1914, that Harry Harris was appointed to the first urology unit in Australasia.

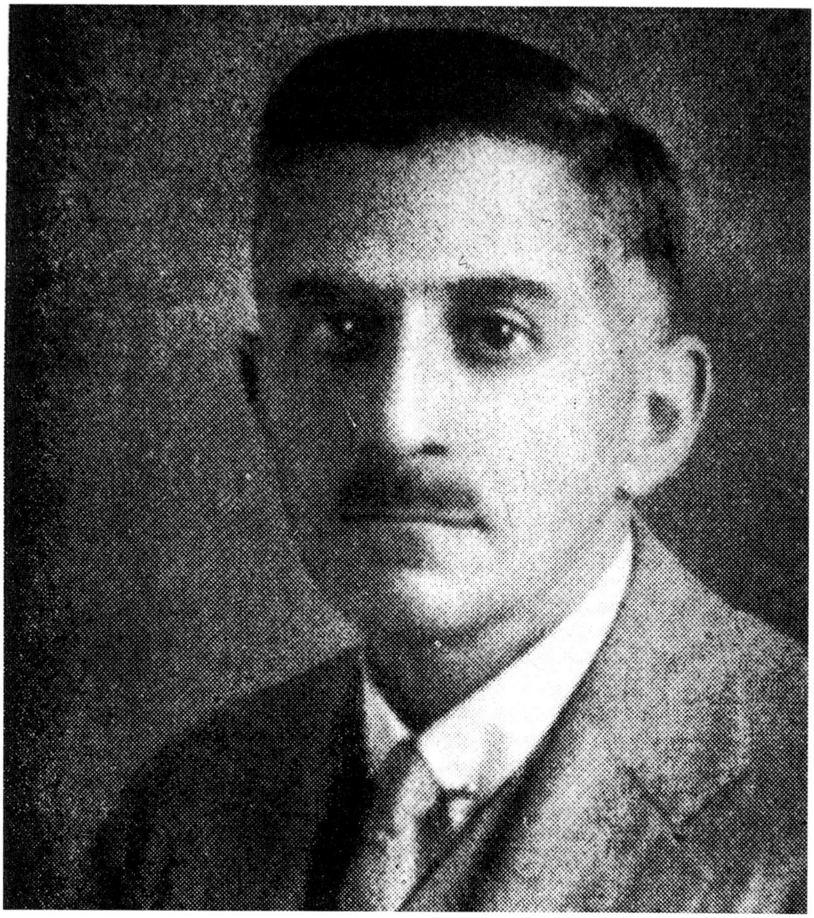

Harry Harris. In 1928 he first published results of his suprapubic prostatectomy with complete closure. Harris' mortality rate for his own operation was 2.8 per cent, the lowest at the time, and for many years afterwards, for any method of open prostatectomy.

pioneer in the specialty of urology but also a highly creative surgeon. Sydney, the city in which he worked all his life, became the most important centre in the early development of Australasian urology. At least a part of the early dominance of Sydney must be attributed to the example set by Harry Harris.

Harry Harris was born and educated in Sydney and after graduation as Bachelor of Medicine and Master of Surgery in 1906 he spent a year as resident medical officer at Sydney Hospital. Harris then went into general practice in the Sydney suburb of Enmore.

Harris came to urology via gynaecology and bought his first cystoscopes to study pyelitis and hydronephrosis and hydroureter of pregnancy. His thesis for Doctor of Medicine in 1914 was on 'Ureteral catheterisation in obstetrics'.

In 1914 Harry Harris was appointed Honorary Urologist to the new department of urology at Lewisham Hospital. Almost at once he turned his attention from female urology to the prostate, publishing on the subject in 1916, 1917 and 1921. In 1922 he published a series of 146 operations using the Freyer technique of suprapubic prostatectomy with a mortality rate of 3.4 per cent. This was lower

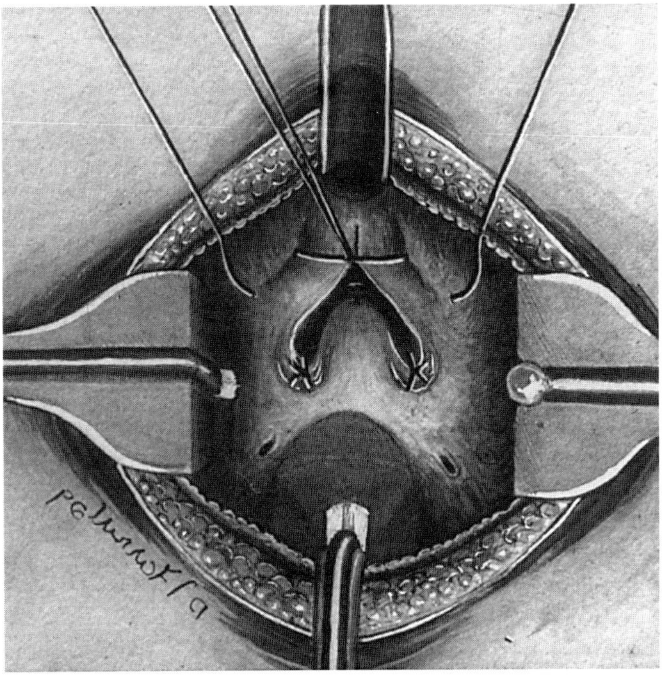

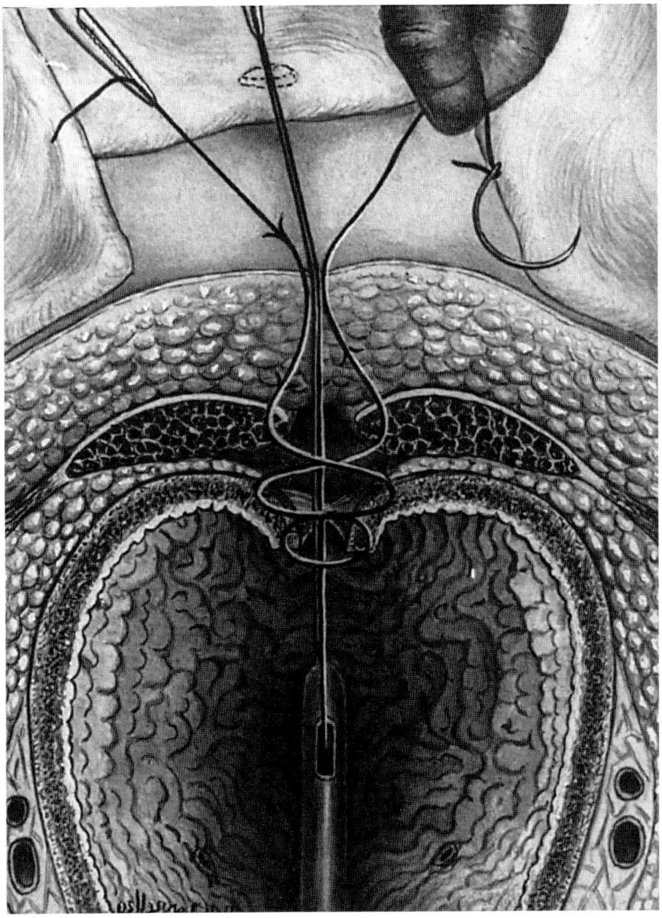

Illustrations from a lecture given by Harry Harris on his suprapubic prostatectomy, c. 1930. (*Source:* Archives of the Little Company of Mary)

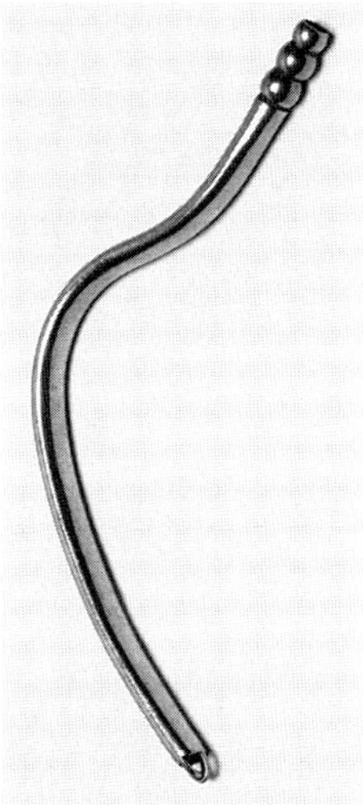

Suction tube as used in Harris prostatectomy, c. 1930, donated by Richard Harris to the RACS.

than the 5.4 per cent reported by Freyer in 1920 on a series of 1625 operations. Elsewhere, versions of the Freyer technique were reported to have mortality rates of 9.9 per cent at St Peter's Hospital for Stone and sometimes mortality rates in excess of 20 per cent when performed by general surgeons.

In 1927 Harris published his revised version of the Freyer technique and in 1928 he described his 'Prostatectomy with complete closure'. Harris's mortality rate for his own operation was 2.8 per cent, the lowest at the time, and for many years afterwards, for any method of open prostatectomy. Possibly surgeons elsewhere disbelieved the figures. Certainly the technique was slow to be adopted outside Australasia until Harris's trip to Britain and Europe in 1935–36. On that tour he demonstrated his operation in London, Edinburgh and Vienna and during the following few years the technique was adopted in Britain and Europe as well as in Australasia.

There has been some speculation as to the reasons for Harris's low mortality rates, especially as other surgeons were not always so successful with the Harris prostatectomy. In his obituary of Harris in the *British Medical Journal,* Clifford Morson described him as a 'brilliant craftsman'. In a speech at the RACS Sir Gordon Gordon-Taylor recalled 'the gentle touch of his fingers coaxing the prostate from its bed'. Besides being a skilled and gentle surgeon, Harris was strict in his adherence to asepsis.

> *Any visiting surgeon, who was seen to put his hands in the pockets of his street clothes underneath his gown, had his gown pinned together at the back to prevent any repetition of this possible source of contamination.*

Leonard Murphy, who made a particular study of Harris, also noted that he

> *was a specialist urologist working almost exclusively in one hospital with a very experienced and unchanging staff. Such favourable conditions were very rare at a time when prostatectomy was still regarded as part of the repertoire of a general surgeon.*[13]

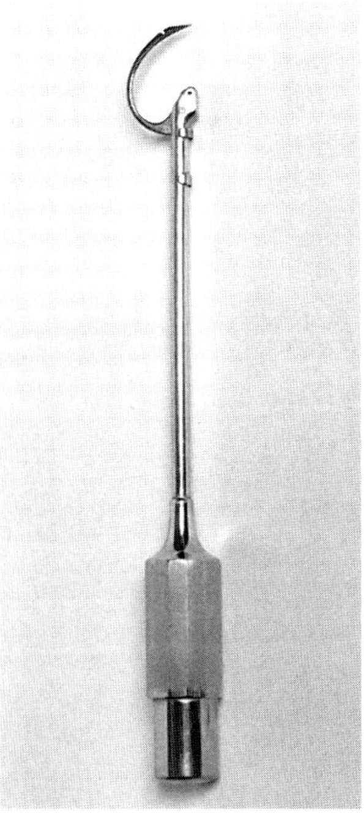

Harry Harris' modification of the Young boomerang needle, in use from the 1930s to the 1960s. (*Source:* Urological collection, RACS)

Harry Harris published thirty-seven papers on urology and was on the editorial boards of not only the *Australia and New Zealand Journal of Surgery* but also the *British Journal of Surgery*. He was a foundation fellow of the RACS, a member of the International Society of Urology and would have been foundation president of the Urological Society of Australasia if he had not died in December 1936. The inaugural meeting of the Society took place the following month.

ROBERT GORDON CRAIG (1870–1931)

Robert Gordon Craig was born in Scotland, the oldest son of a sea captain. His father did well out of a merchant shipping business, trading in, among other things, guns, brandy and tea. In 1878, when Gordon was eight, the family moved to Sydney.

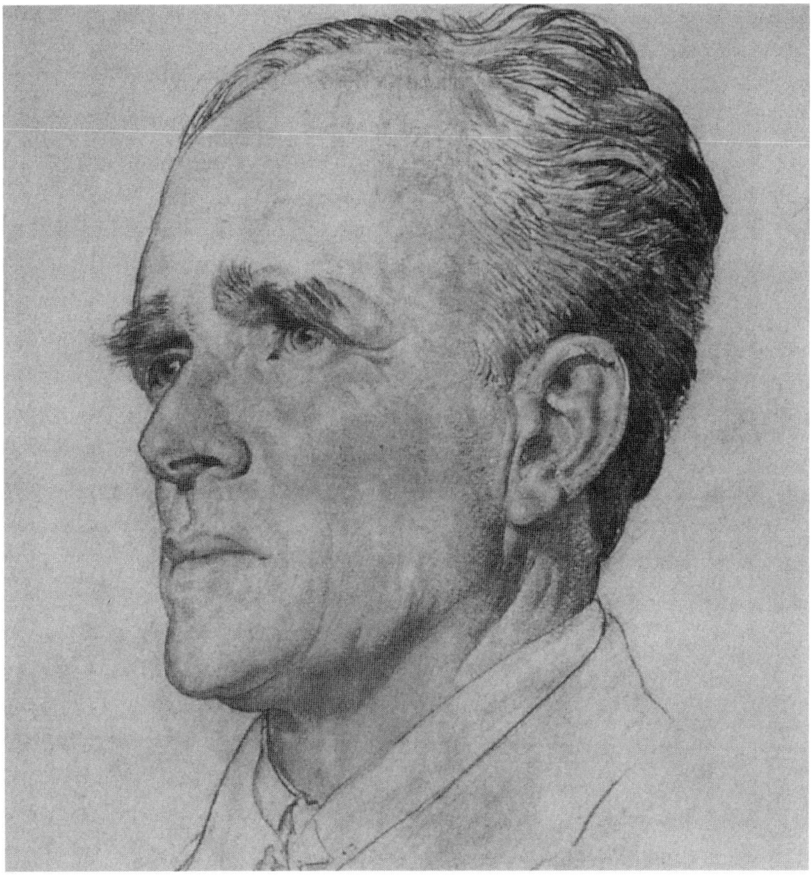

Robert Gordon Craig, from the portrait in the Robert Gordon Craig Library, Royal Australasian College of Surgeons, Melbourne. He was the second urologist in Australasia and founded the units at the Royal Alexandra Hospital for Children, Sydney, in 1918, and at Royal Prince Alfred Hospital, in1926. He made a considerable fortune from investments in Malaysian tin mines and used some of the money to set up the Gordon Craig Fellowship, as a pioneer training scheme for urologists.

Gordon Craig attended the University of Sydney and was then RMO for 12 months at Royal Prince Alfred Hospital (RPAH). In 1901, he set up in general practice with a surgical appointment at RPAH. In 1908 Gordon Craig went on a study tour of England and the United States, including a visit to the Mayo Clinic. There he learned the technique of open ether administration and introduced it to RPAH on his return. Gordon Craig was most impressed with the Mayo brothers and returned to their clinic about every five years. He was also impressed with Critchley Hinder and his technique of cystoscopy. After a period of service in the hospital ship *Karoola* during World War I, he returned to Sydney and his specialist practice in urology.

The first urological unit established by Gordon Craig was at the Royal Alexandra Hospital for Children, in 1918, but his name is principally associated with RPAH. The Department of Urology there was set up under his leadership in 1925-26 and played a vital role in the development of urology in Australasia.

In 1926 Gordon Craig donated the huge sum of £20 000 to the University of Sydney to establish the Fellowship in Urology. The holders of the fellowship were to be trained in urology and conduct research at RPAH. Gordon Craig's generosity provided for the first professional specialist training of urologists in Australasia and the list of Gordon Craig Fellows testifies to the enormous benefits that flowed from his gift.

Gordon Craig was also an active player in the events leading to the foundation of the RACS and was one of the ten elected members of the first Council of 1927. He died in 1931, leaving the sum of £60 000 to the RACS, money which made possible, among other things, the foundation of the Gordon Craig Library.[14]

Arthur Stanley Roe (1885–1966), Founding Member of the Urological Society

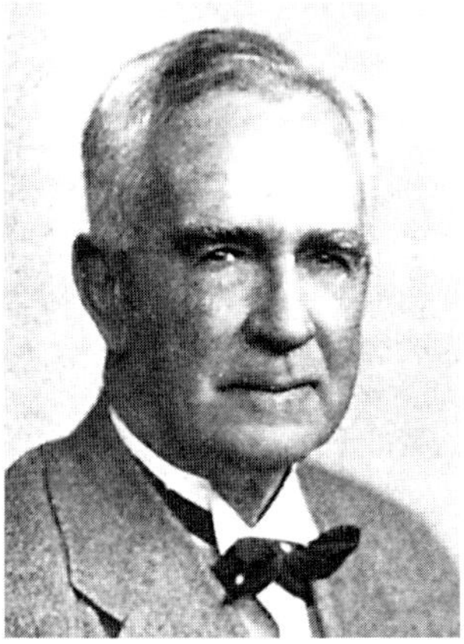

Stanley Roe. The third urologist in Australasia was a Queenslander. In 1919, he was appointed Honorary Urologist to the Mater Misericordiae Hospital, Brisbane.

Arthur Stanley Roe was born in Brisbane in 1885, the fourth child of Reginald Heber Roe. Roe senior was an Oxford graduate, and headmaster of Brisbane Grammar School for thirty years before becoming Director of Education for Queensland and the first Vice-Chancellor of the new University of Queensland.

Against this distinguished educational background, A. S. Roe was Queensland's first Rhodes scholar and went to his father's old college at Oxford to study medicine. He graduated in 1911 and then held a series of house surgeon appointments at Guy's Hospital, London, obtaining his FRCSEd in 1913. His son Charles, who was also a urologist, believed:

> *His orientation changed when the intravenous urogram, the direct-vision cystoscope and ureteric catheters appeared on the scene just before World War I permitting complete imaging of the urinary tract, including both kidneys.*[15]

There was also the question of the standard of urology as performed by general surgeons. From 1917 to 1919, Stanley Roe held an appointment as Surgeon-Gynaecologist at the Mater Misericordiae Hospitals, Brisbane. Charles Roe wrote that 'soon after he got back from World War I, Dad assisted at a nephrectomy, and thought it was done so badly he decided to specialise in urology.'[16]

In 1919, Roe was appointed Honorary Urologist at the Mater Misericordiae Hospitals. Like Harry Harris, he seems to have come to urology via gynaecology. The campus of the Mater Hospitals, Brisbane, includes a women's, a children's and an adult hospital and at various stages Stanley Roe worked at all of them. The urology clinic he founded there in 1919 was only the third in Australasia. In the 1990s it remained an active clinic, while in Sydney, the Lewisham Hospital had closed and the Royal Alexandra Hospital had become the New Children's Hospital, Westmead.

Stanley Roe was a great nature lover and maintained the tradition started by his father of Roe's Kamp on Stradbroke Island, Moreton

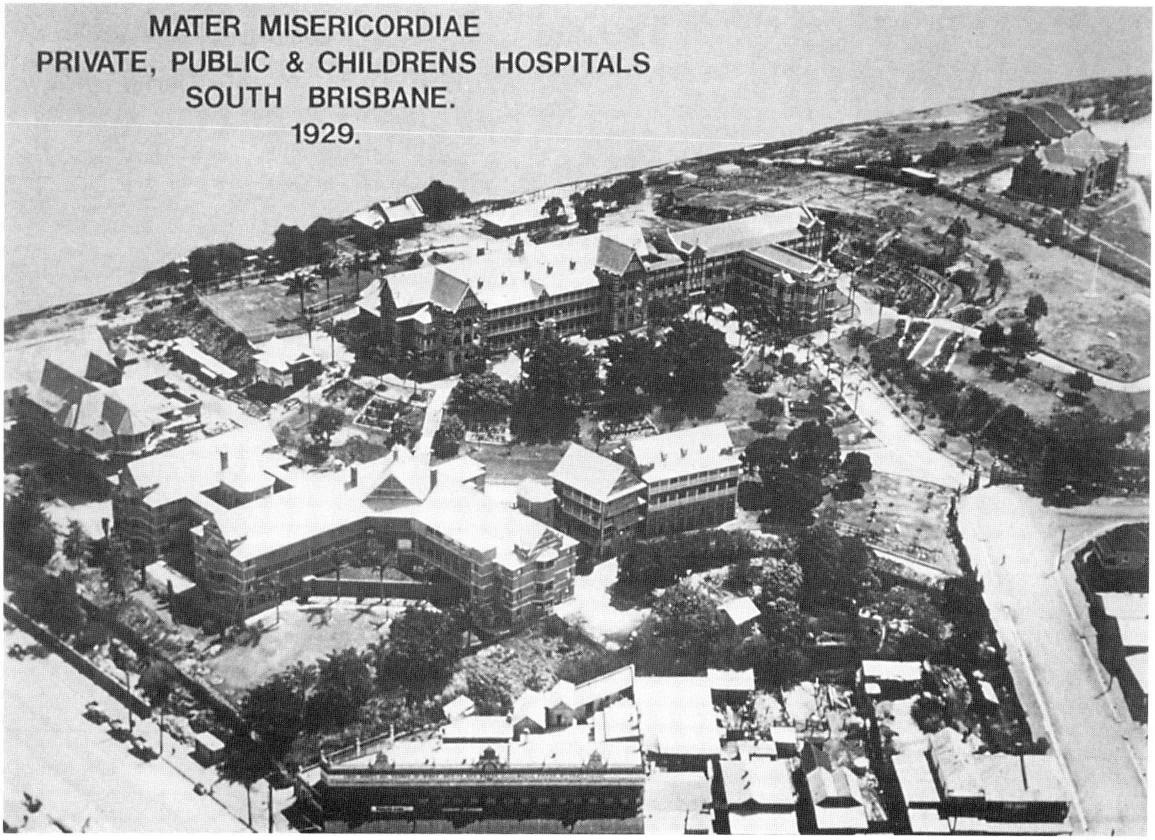

Source: Mater Misericordiae Hospitals, Brisbane

Bay. He was a foundation fellow of the RACS and a foundation member of the Urological Society of Australasia, becoming president in 1941.

Bobby Silverton and Colin Edwards, Founding Members of the Urological Society

In1921, according to the annual report, Royal North Shore Hospital, Sydney, appointed Dr R. J. Silverton to the new post of Honorary Urologist. This was only the fourth urology unit in Australasia and in 1921 it was not very busy, with only twelve cystoscopies, fourteen suprapubic cystostomies and one suprapubic lithotomy. It appears from other records of the hospital that Silverton actually began work in 1922. The hospital was founded in 1888, but Silverton was only the fourth appointee with a college of surgeons fellowship. The hospital had one each from Ireland, England and Edinburgh. Silverton obtained his FRCSEd in 1920.[17]

In 1922, a Mr Ross of Wagga Wagga made a donation to the hospital, through Dr Silverton, for the purchase of X-ray equipment. The work of the department grew rapidly and the annual report of 1923 noted 108 operations on the kidney and urinary tract.

Bobby Silverton studied at Sydney University and graduated MB,

TABLE 2.2 OPERATIONS ON KIDNEY AND URINARY TRACT, ROYAL NORTH SHORE HOSPITAL, SYDNEY, 1923

Cystoscopy	26
Cystoscopy and ureteral catheterisation	23
Suprapubic cystostomy	9
Suprapubic cystotomy	2
Suprapubic prostatectomy	14
Suprapubic wound, repair of	5
External urethrotomy	1
External urethrotomy and suprapubic cystostomy	1
Internal urethrotomy	1
Urethroscopy	1
Passing sounds	6
Urethral caruncle, excision of	1
Perineal fistula, excision of	1
Perineal sinus, curettage of	1
Diathermy to median bar of prostate	3
Diathermy of papilloma of bladder	1
Nephrolithotomy	1
Nephrotomy	1
Nephrectomy	5
Peri-nephritic abscess, draining of	2
Decapsulation of kidney	1
Vesical diverticulum, excision of	1
Litholapaxy	1
Total	108

Source: Royal North Shore Hospital, Annual Report, 1923, Lawson collection

ChM. In 1915 he was RMO at Fremantle General Hospital, WA, and in 1916 he returned to Sydney and was RMO and Registrar at Sydney Hospital before going to Egypt as a Captain in the Army Medical Corps.

While in Cairo, Silverton was impressed with the results of spinal analgesia 'which is used almost as a routine for operations below the ribs in the large Egyptian Hospital of that city'. Silverton began to make a study of the subject and often carried out the lumbar puncture himself, as he noted in a paper on the subject published in 1921: 'Through the kindness of the honorary surgeons under whom I worked I was allowed to give spinal injections in most of the 106 cases I am reporting.'[18] The study took place while he was resident at St Peter's Hospital for Stone.

In 1932, Colin Munro Edwards was appointed Assistant Urologist at Royal North Shore Hospital. He was later Honorary Urologist at Royal North Shore and held honorary appointments at a number of other hospitals. A Sydney graduate of 1924, he was RSO at St Peter's Hospital for Stone in 1929-30, a decade after Silverton. He, too, was

TABLE 2.3 PRINCE HENRY HOSPITAL, SYDNEY
OPERATIONS OF THE GENITO-URINARY SYSTEM, 1935

	Recovered*		Died		Total
	Male	Female	Male	Female	
Circumcision	32				32
Cystoscopy	54	55			109
Cystotomy	4	1			5
Dilation of urethra	4	4			8
Nephrectomy	2	3		1	6
Nephro-lithotomy	3	2			5
Other operations of the kidney	2	1			3
Operations for:					
Hydrococele	5				5
Varicocele	11				11
Vesical calculus	1				1
Urethral calculus	1				1
Orchidectomy	3				3
Perinephric abscess	1	3	1		5
Plastic operations					
Hypospadias	2				2
Closure of sinus	1				1
External urethrotomy	2				2
Prostatectomy	11		1		12
Prostate, endoscopic resection	6				6
Total	**145**	69	2	1	217

Source: Report of the Director General of Public Health, New South Wales, for the Year 1935, Section III; Report upon the State Hospitals under the Control of the Director-General of Public Health, p. 132.
* Recovered = survived for at least ten days after the operation

a foundation member of the Urological Society of Australasia and president in 1953-54.[19]

'Bobby's interest in urology was always paramount' wrote Colin Edwards in his obituary, but he also found time for singing and was fluent in French and German. Douglas Anderson wrote that 'Few medical men in Sydney were the subject of as many anecdotes as Bobby Silverton' and not all were to his advantage. Douglas Keller remembered that although he could be egotistical, he was an acknowledged master of lumbar puncture.

> *Many a time the anaesthetic department were struggling to get a needle in. He would arrive, put his Homburg hat on the end of the theatre trolley, and insert the needle with one deft, swift movement of his hand.*[20]

In 1922, Bobby Silverton was appointed as the first head of the fifth urology department in Australasia at Prince Henry Hospital. The *Report of the Director-General of Public Health, New South Wales, for the Year 1935* provides a snapshot of what was happening there that year. Prince Henry was a Government-run hospital and in 1935 it had fifteen hon-

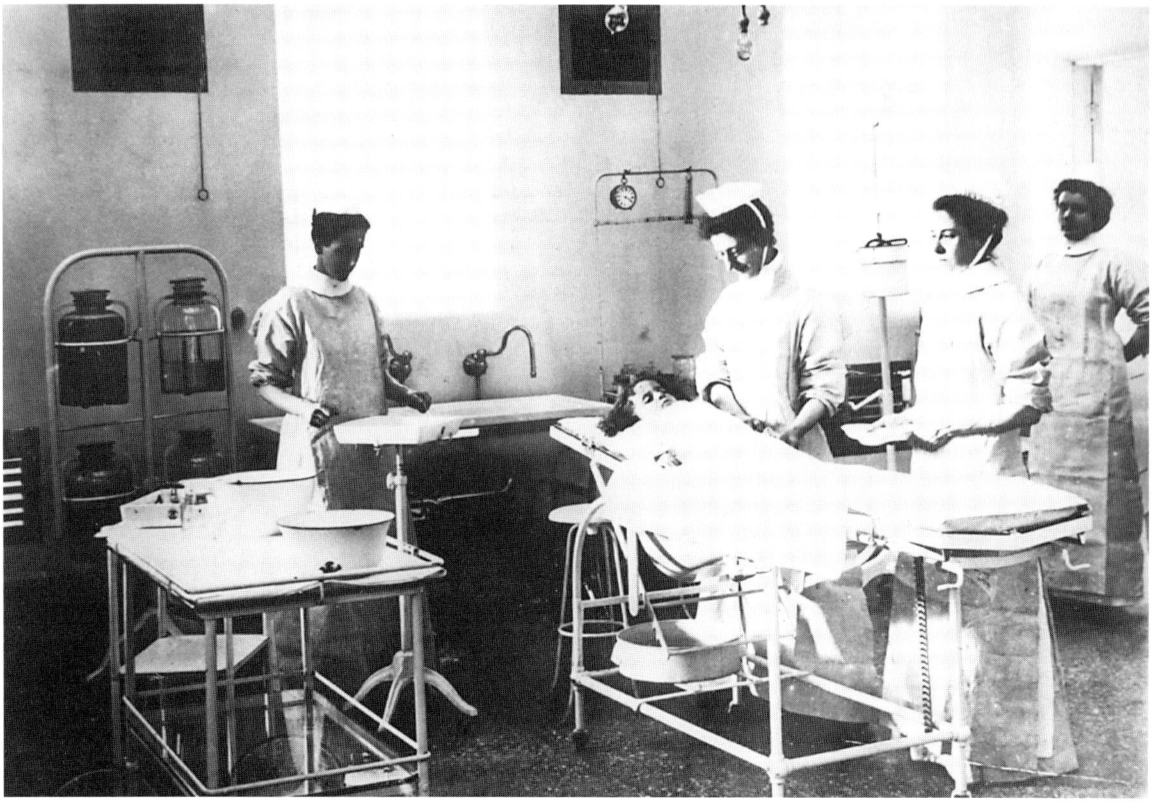

Operating theatre, Wellington Hospital, 1903

orary surgeons, including Robert Joseph Silverton, Urologist, and Angus Buchanan Walker-Smith, Honorary Assistant Urologist.

The hospital specialised in infectious disease and there was an Auxiliary Hospital at Randwick providing 120 beds for tuberculosis cases. In 1935 the hospital treated 458 cases of TB, only eight of whom were recorded as cures. 'Tuberculosis of Respiratory System' resulted in 180 deaths. The prognosis was better for those with 'Tuberculosis of Genito Urinary System'. Of nine cases during the year none died, one was 'cured' and five were 'relieved'.

Urology was a growing area and a new urological block was under construction, to include a theatre and an X-ray plant. During the year, 699 patients were admitted for 'diseases of the genito-urinary system' and 217 of these were operated on. This makes an average of about four procedures per week, of which half were cystoscopies.[21] Interestingly, during 1935 either Silverton or Walker-Smith carried out six resections of the prostate in addition to eleven open prostatectomies.

RICHARD HARRIS (1902-1962), FOUNDING MEMBER OF THE UROLOGICAL SOCIETY

Lewisham Hospital, Sydney, will always be associated in the history of urology with Harry Harris and his operation for suprapubic prostatectomy. Harris was head of the urology department from 1914 till his death on Christmas Day, 1936. During that time he trained his brother Richard, twenty-two years his junior. After Harry Harris's death, Richard succeeded him as head of the department and continued to perform his operation for prostatectomy.

At Lewisham Hospital, Harry Harris developed a strong and stable team, with Harry Daly as his anaesthetist and the excellent post-operative care of the Sisters of the Little Company of Mary. After 1924, Richard Harris joined the team as his assistant.

Like his brother, Richard graduated in medicine from the University of Sydney. In 1923 he was RMO at Lewisham and in 1924 he was appointed Honorary Assistant Urologist. In 1933 he opened the urological department at the Hornsby and District Hospital and in 1935 he was made Honorary Urologist at Lewisham, the year Harry Harris and Harry Daly went to Britain to demonstrate the Harris suprapubic prostatectomy.

Richard Harris ran the urology department at Lewisham in the tradition set by his brother. Alban Gee, who was his assistant at Lewisham and later his partner in private practice, remembered that he often 'remarked there was only one standard for the patients—the best.'[22]

Sister M. Jeanne Hyland of the Little Company of Mary remembers she once had 'a slap on the gloved hand for not releasing an artery forceps in good time. But all was quickly forgiven.'[23]

Richard Harris was Senior Urologist at Lewisham Hospital from his brother's death in 1936 until his own in 1962. He was a foundation member of the Urological Society of Australasia and President in 1949-50.

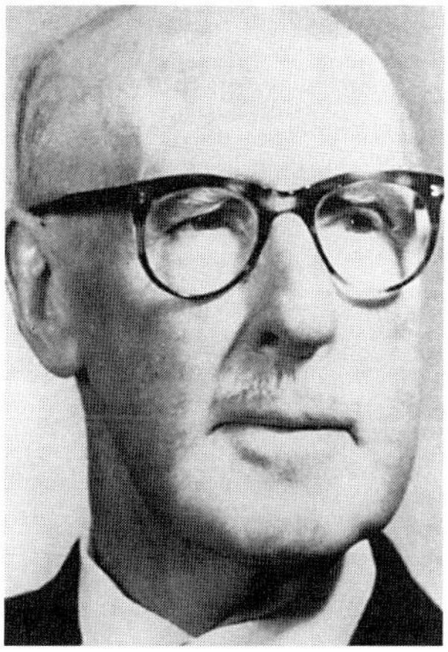

The first urologist in New Zealand was R. Campbell-Begg. From about 1924, he held an appointment as urologist at Wellington Hospital. If his autobiography is to be believed, he led an exciting life and Wellington Hospital could not hold him for long. Early in 1937, he left for South Africa.

R. Campbell-Begg (1886-c.1970)

R. Campbell-Begg was born in Dunedin, the son of a minister of the church and trained for the same calling himself before deciding to become a surgeon. In 1907 he left New Zealand for the Edinburgh medical school, following in the footsteps of two of his brothers. At that date, one brother was already a surgeon practising in Wellington.

Campbell-Begg had a varied career, to say the least, with a stint as a medical officer in the gold mines of South Africa before spending World War I as a medical officer in France, Cairo and Mesopotamia. He returned to New Zealand via Ceylon and Sydney and set up as a GP on Willis Street, Wellington.

This did not mean the end of his travels and he returned to Britain for further study, obtaining his FRCS Edinburgh in 1923, by which time he was 36 years old. He returned to Wellington in about 1924 and at some stage was involved in founding an extreme right wing political party. He continued to live a varied life with frequent travel to Europe and the United States, becoming a FACS in 1926. In 1927 he was in the United States, spending time at the Mayo Clinic, Rochester, because he believed that the Americans were leading the way in urology.

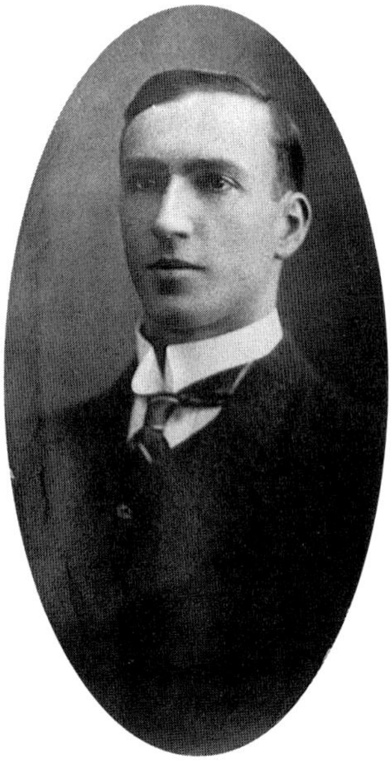

John Thomson Tait, the first urologist in Melbourne, at the time of his graduation MBBS in 1911.

In about 1924 Campbell-Begg was appointed as Urologist at Wellington Hospital. In 1936, he was invited to become a foundation member of the Urological Society of Australasia, but declined because he had decided to leave New Zealand for good and return to South Africa.[24]

JOHN THOMSON TAIT (1888-1962), FOUNDING MEMBER OF THE UROLOGICAL SOCIETY

John Thomson Tait served in France during World War I and was resident at St Peter's Hospital for Stone in 1922-23.

In 1927, Tait was appointed to head the new urology department at the Royal Melbourne Hospital. He was the third urologist (after Gordon Craig and Campbell-Begg) to be admitted to the Fellowship of the RACS, pre-dating Roe and Silverton by some months, and he was the pioneer urologist in Melbourne. As was the case with many of the pioneers, he encountered problems with the general surgeons. The Melbourne Hospital unit was only allocated four beds and they were generally occupied by the cases that other surgeons were not anxious to tackle.

In 1928 he was joined by William Harold Moore, son of the distinguished Melbourne surgeon 'Jerry' Moore. Tait and Moore 'were rather shy retiring and slow-moving men. Their practice reflected this and they were sometimes referred to as Potter and Moore.'[25]

Tait was not present at the inaugural meeting of the Urological Society of Australasia, but he was one of the twelve foundation members (the only Victorian) and was elected the third president, in 1939.

JACK POWER (1889-1966), FOUNDING MEMBER OF THE UROLOGICAL SOCIETY

In 1914, J. J. Power graduated in medicine from Sydney and joined the resident medical staff at St Vincent's Hospital. During World War I he served as Regimental Medical officer to the 25th (Queensland) battalion in France and, as has already been noted, took the opportunity to study in Britain after the war. He obtained his FRCSEd and in 1919 returned to Queensland with the new technique of blood transfusion.

In 1928 he went to the United States and studied urology at the Mayo Clinic, returning to open the Urology Clinic at the Brisbane General Hospital in 1929.

Jack Power managed to combine a busy urological practice with a lifelong interest in the breeding and racing of horses. He was a foundation member of the Urological Society of Australasia and president three times, in 1938, 1946-47 and 1952-53. In later life the horses were allowed to take more of his time. He was Chairman of the Queensland Turf Club from 1947 until his death in 1966 and in 1961 was awarded the CBE.

At the inaugural meeting of the Urological Society of Australasia,

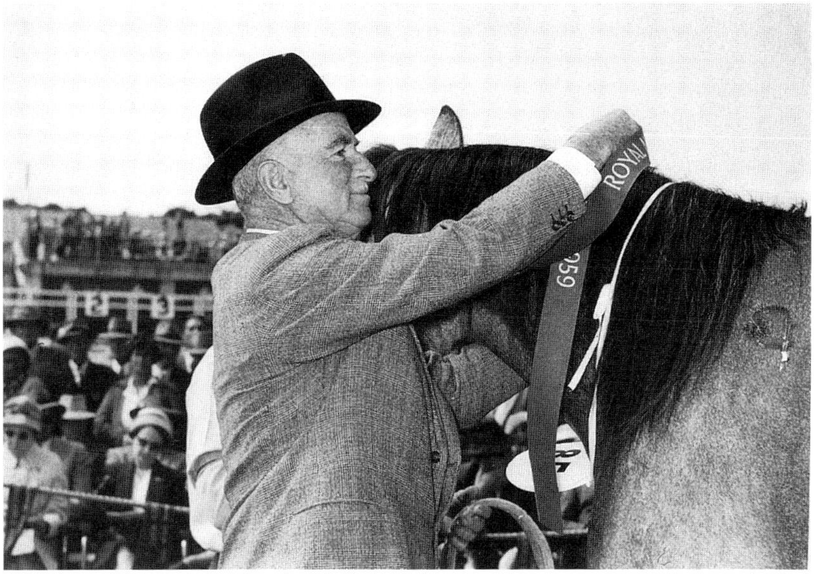

Jack Power, Chairman of the Queensland Turf Club, 1947-66, and from 1929 Queensland's second urologist.

Jack Power was elected the first vice president and thus became the second president of the Society, in 1938.[26]

Reginald Bridge (1888–1944) and Keith Kirkland (1901–1971), Founding Members of the Urological Society

In 1937, R. H. Bridge was elected the first president of the Urological Society of Australasia. Bridge was the first ever graduate with first class honours from the Sydney Hospital Clinical School and maintained his association with the hospital until his death. In 1920, he was appointed Honorary Assistant Surgeon. Ten years later he resigned to become the first Honorary Urologist at the hospital, a position he held until his death in 1944. The new urology department had the benefit of an operating theatre with a special urological operating table and the latest in X-ray equipment.

In 1932, Keith Kirkland was appointed as Assistant Urological Surgeon. He is the towering figure in the early years of the Urological Society and his successors tell many stories about him. In his youth, he was a champion swimmer and represented Australia in the seventh Olympic Games in Antwerp in 1920. He was big, self-confident and outgoing and there is a popular anecdote that highlights the qualities that allowed him to take urology out of the hands of the general surgeons without generating too much ill will. During World War II, Sir Gordon Gordon-Taylor visited Sydney Hospital. He had the reputation of having helped many young Australasian urologists while they were in London and was a noted British general surgeon. At the time, he was Surgeon Rear Admiral with the British Fleet. 'At one time watching Keith doing a nephrectomy, he said "there does not appear

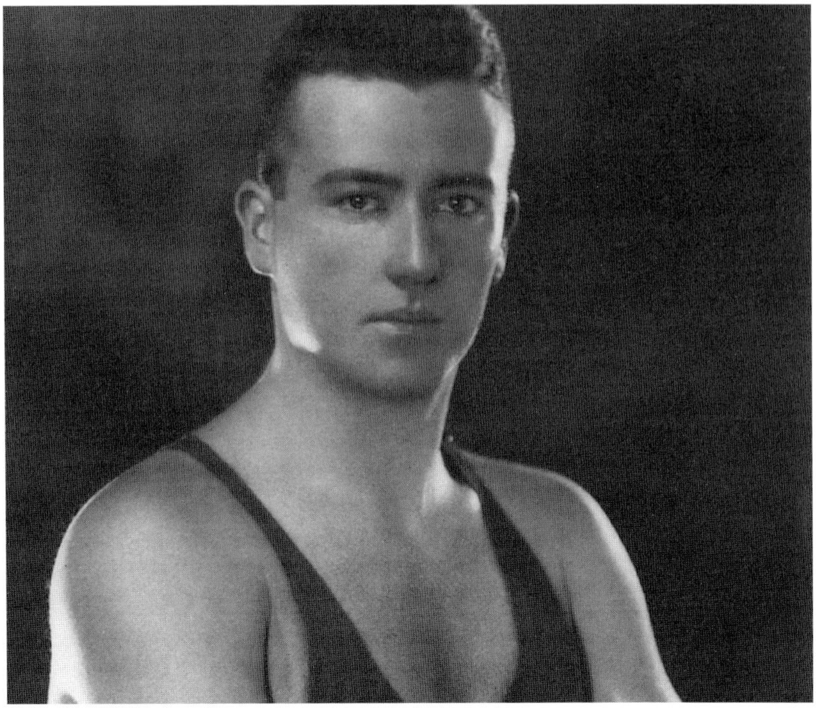

Keith Kirkland, olympic swimmer and the driving force behind the formation of the Urological Society of Australasia. He was New South Wales Champion and reserve for the Olympic 4x200 metres freestyle relay team in Antwerp in 1920, when the Australian team won the silver medal. (*Source:* Mrs Janet Cullen)

to be much bleeding Kirkland" at which Keith replied "It is a matter of knowing your anatomy Sir Gordon".'[27]

The Sydney Hospital team was particularly active in the events leading to the foundation of the Urological Society of Australasia. Keith Kirkland was the foundation secretary and treasurer and more or less ran the organisation from 1937 to 1946. His boss, R. H. Bridge, was appointed as the first president in 1937 and Kirkland himself was president in 1947-48 and treasurer again during 1950-53.

JOHN LAIDLEY (1900–1955), **MALCOLM EARLAM** (1901–1981) **AND ANGUS BUCHANAN WALKER-SMITH, FOUNDING MEMBERS OF THE UROLOGICAL SOCIETY, AND BOBBY LEE-BROWN** (1894–1934)

The Department of Urology at Royal Prince Alfred Hospital, Sydney, was set up in 1925-26 under Robert Gordon Craig with twelve male and six female beds. His gift to the University of Sydney ensured that RPAH was to have the benefit of the Gordon Craig Fellows, each for three years. John Laidley was the first and Malcolm Earlam the second. They had been contemporaries at Sydney University, passing out second and first respectively in their year. However, Laidley was slightly older, born in 1900, and came from an old Sydney family, whereas Earlam was born in 1901 in England. Whatever the reason, Gordon Craig thought it appropriate that Laidley should be awarded his first fellowship.

Gordon Craig appointed Dr Adolph Bolliger as Director of Research to the Department of Urology and both Laidley and Earlam worked with him during their fellowships.

On completing their fellowships, Laidley and Earlam were appointed to the staff of RPAH. They also worked together in private practice, taking over from Robert Gordon Craig and his son-in-law, Bobby Lee-Brown. They were the two most notable early examples of Australian-trained urologists but both subsequently travelled the world to see what urologists were doing elsewhere. In 1936, for instance, Malcolm Earlam visited the Mayo Clinic:

> *Did ward rounds with Thompson who in common with other men at the Mayo turned out to look suprisingly young ... I got the very definite impression that Thompson's technical ability in resection is probably a long way ahead of his general urological ability, and he resects everything he can get hold of irrespective. I have seen nothing to support the criticism, so often made, that resectionists resect cases that do not require operation at all.*
>
> *Gaudin from Auckland, N.Z.—fellow in Urology in his third year. Is very keen on urinary tract ... and has done a great deal of original work. A very decent bloke.*

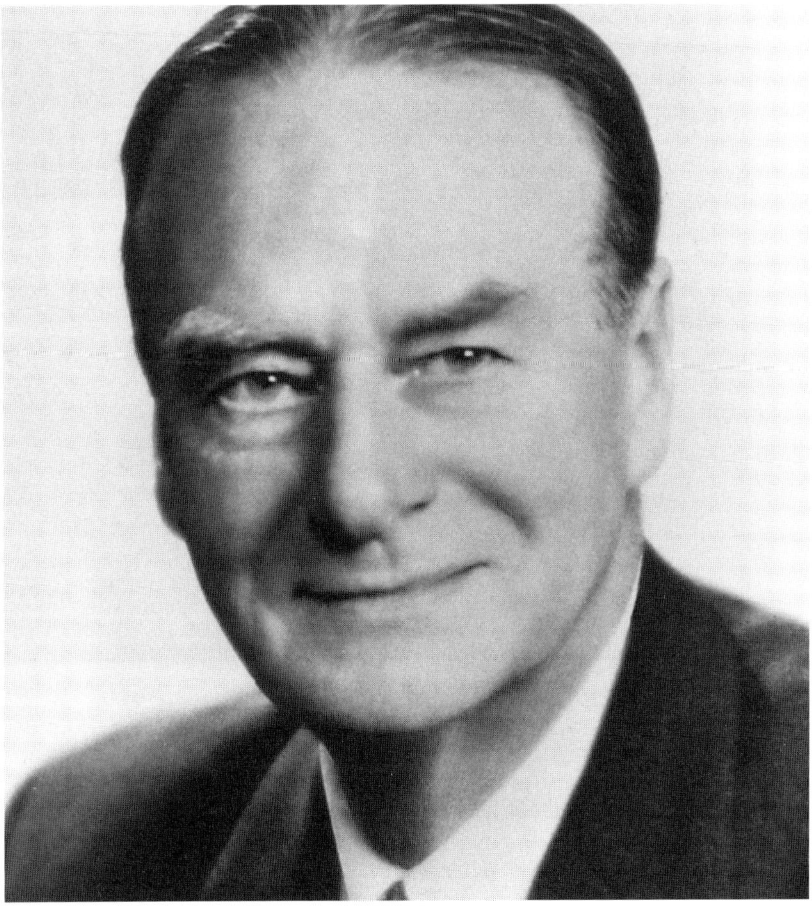

Malcolm Earlam, the second Gordon Craig Fellow in Urology at Royal Prince Alfred Hospital, Sydney

In 1938, John Laidley was in London and visited Terrence Millin at his rooms on Harley Street:

> *Very pleasant Irish type in early 40s. Enquired ... for M.S.S.E. [Earlam] Spent 2 hours with him in his rooms. Has consulting room, X-ray room & cystoscopy room. Trained nurse in attendance. Sends pts after cystoscopy to nursing home a few doors away where they spend the night. He talked a great deal about resection & prostatitis in general. He is now resecting about 40%.*[28]

Bobby Lee-Brown was initially mainly responsible for the out patients' work in urology at RPAH. After Gordon Craig's retirement in 1930, he became head of the Department of Urology. Bobby Lee-Brown died in 1934 in a plane crash and John Laidley took over as head of department.

In 1934 the vacancy left by Bobby Lee-Brown's death was filled by the arrival of Angus Buchanan Walker-Smith. Walker-Smith graduated from Sydney two years before Laidley and Earlam, but went into general practice for some years before going to England. He trained at St Peter's Hospital for Stone and obtained his FRCS Edinburgh, returning to Sydney in 1934.

John Laidley, Malcolm Earlam and Angus Walker-Smith were all foundation members of the Urological Society of Australasia. John Laidley was treasurer of the Society in 1953-55. In his obituary, Malcolm Earlam notes that Laidley would have been president of the Society in 1956, had he survived. Malcolm Earlam was president in 1945-46 and again in 1956-57 and was made a Fellow of the Society in 1967. He was co-editor of the *Australia and New Zealand Journal of Surgery* with Robert Lawson, and later editor in 1968-76. He died in 1981 aged 80.

Edgar Reay (1898–1969), Founding Member of the Urological Society

Edgar Reay was the sole New Zealand urologist present at the foundation meeting of the Urological Society of Australasia. Edgar Reay graduated from Otago in 1923 and went to Edinburgh, obtaining his FRCSEd in 1924, before completing his MD in New Zealand. In 1925 he preceded Treahy as a New Zealand urologist in London and worked at the Royal Sussex Hospital and the London Temperance Hospital, besides working as a clinical assistant at St Peter's Hospital for Stone.

Reay returned to New Zealand in 1926 and was appointed as Assistant Surgeon at Christchurch Hospital. He remained at the hospital until his retirement in 1960.

It is not clear exactly when Reay's title was formally changed to that of Urologist, but it was probably about 1930 and by 1935 Joseph Brownlee had joined him in the role of Assistant Urologist. Edgar Reay was an advocate of the Harris technique for prostatectomy and was responsible for making Christchurch one of the strongholds of the operation. From the early years his anaesthetist was Charles

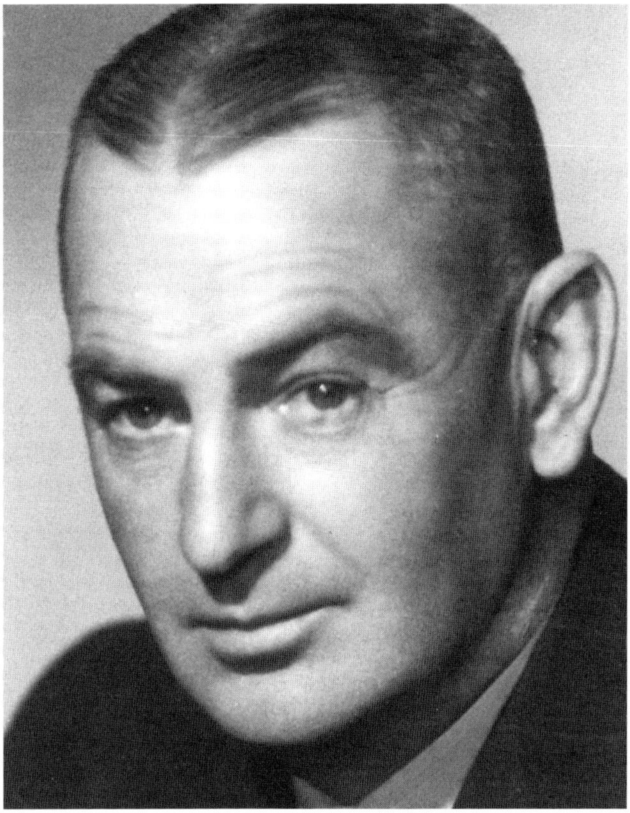

Edgar Reay, the only New Zealander to be a founding member of the Urological Society and the first New Zealand President. He was appointed as Urologist to Christchurch Hospital in 1930.

Markane and together they provided another instance of the value of teamwork, particularly in difficult operations.[29]

FRANK MACKY (1891-1975)

Frank Macky was a New Zealander who trained in Melbourne, graduating in 1914. Macky served in the Middle East, was invalided home and then returned to work in various military hospitals, including one at Le Havre. After the war, he remained in London for further study before returning to New Zealand. In 1922 he was appointed as Assistant Surgeon at Auckland Hospital and promoted to Senior Surgeon in 1926. Again, the date at which the urology unit began is unclear, but Warwick Macky believes it was in about 1940.

In 1929 Macky went to Sydney to watch Harry Harris perform his prostatectomy technique and returned to New Zealand a convert to the new operation. He introduced the Harris prostatectomy to New Zealand and his son Warwick, also a urologist, remembers the significance of the operation in establishing the specialty in Auckland.

> *After the Harris operation was adopted in Auckland about 1929 the average post-operative stay dropped from 42 to 16 days with mortality of about 5.5%. These results steadily improved and were a key factor in the setting*

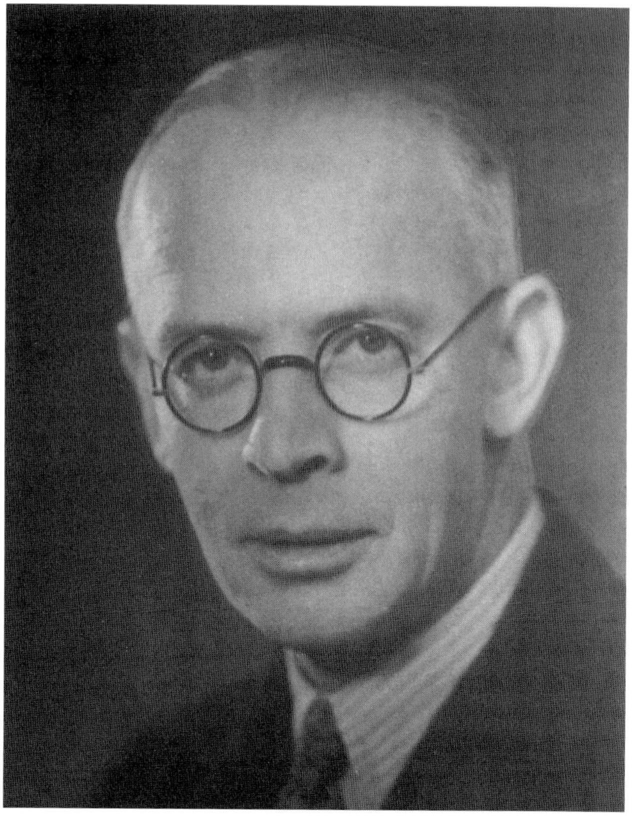

Frank Macky, the pioneer urologist in Auckland who introduced Harry Harris' operation for suprapubic prostatectomy to New Zealand. During the 1940s, Frank Macky became an Associate Member of the Urological Society, but he did not play a leading role in its affairs. His son Warwick, however, was the second New Zealander to become President of the Society.

up of the Department of Urology at Auckland Hospital after years of implacable opposition from the surgical staff.[30]

Frank Macky became a Fellow of the RACS in 1931, only the tenth urologist to do so, and must be considered one of the pioneers of Australasian urology. He was one of those invited to the March 1936 meeting of the Sydney Urological Association, the first occasion on which urologists from outside Sydney were invited to discuss the formation of an Australasian organisation. He did not attend. He was home in Auckland and may even have been hosting Harry Harris, who spent a brief period with the Mackys in March 1936, on his way back from Europe via San Francisco. Macky was not invited to be a foundation member of the Urological Society of Australasia and only became an Associate Member in 1946, by which date he had retired from his Auckland Hospital appointment.[31]

Henry Newman Mortensen (1898–1977)

Henry Mortensen trained at Melbourne University and subsequently went into general practice at Yarrawonga, on the Murray River. His wife, Lorna Bray, was an anaesthetist and in 1930 she returned to Melbourne to the position of Honorary Anaesthetist at St Vincent's. From 1929 to 1931 Henry Mortensen was in England as RSO at St

Paul's. In 1930 he obtained his FRCSEd and in 1931 he obtained his MS at Melbourne. From 1937 to 1955 he was head of the Urology Clinic at St Vincent's Hospital, Melbourne.

In 1931, Mortensen published an article on 'Modern methods in urological surgery' in the *Medical Journal of Australia*. He discussed the various methods of prostatectomy that he had seen in London and noted the high mortality rates. He did not mention Harris' work in Sydney but he did describe Luy's operation or forage of the prostate. 'It consists in a tunnelling *per urethram* of a channel through the prostate, and the operation is performed at the present time with a diathermy electrode or a diathermy punch.'[32] He noted the extremely low mortality rate.

Fred Colahan, a colleague at St Vincent's, spent some time in Ann Arbor, Michigan and returned with the information that Reed Nesbit was reporting a mortality rate of 2 per cent with the McCarthy resectoscope. At that time, the Mayo Clinic was reporting a mortality rate of 9 per cent with Thompson's cold punch. Mortensen 'caught the next boat' and learnt the use of the resectoscope from Nesbit.[33]

Henry Mortensen was not a foundation member of the Urological Society of Australasia, because the Urology Clinic at St Vincent's was opened after the inaugural meeting of the Society. However, he was one of the next three members elected, in 1938, and quickly made his mark on the Society. During the 1940s and 1950s he was almost as important a figure in the Society as Keith Kirkland and they worked together very well. Both were inveterate travellers and attended many international meetings, together and separately, in their determination to keep up to date with the latest developments in urology.

Like Jack Power, Henry Mortensen was president of the Urological Society three times, in 1942, 1944-45 and 1948-49. In 1963 he was made a Fellow of the Society.

James Alfred Jenkins

In this era there was no full-time urologist at Dunedin Hospital. However, there was a urology department, which must have played a significant role as a model for urology departments elsewhere in New Zealand, given the position of Dunedin as the Dominion's only medical school. In 1922 James Alfred Jenkins was appointed Assistant Lecturer and Tutor in Clinical Surgery. He had the benefit of a theatre for cystoscopy and a small number of beds for urological cases. By the time he retired in 1951 he had built up a well-equipped urology department, despite having to give part of his time and energy to general surgery.[34]

George Ronald Davidson (1899–1978)

In 1923 George Ronald Davidson graduated in medicine from Melbourne University. He spent time as a house surgeon in Perth and then in England at the Middlesex Hospital, gaining his FRCSEd in 1926. In London, he spent time as a surgical clinical assistant at All Saints' Genito-urinary Hospital. On returning to Melbourne, he was surgical clinical assistant at the Royal Children's and St Vincent's.

In 1929 he opened a practice in Ballarat with a strong urology bias and in later years became an extremely active member of the Urological Society, regularly giving papers at the meetings in the late forties and early fifties. Like Jimmy Burnell from Adelaide, he was among the first group of Associate Members admitted to the Society in 1941 and it was through his influence that the first meeting of the Society ever held outside a capital city was at Ballarat in 1948.[35]

South Australia

There was no full-time specialist urologist in Adelaide before World War II but Sir Ivan Jose and Jimmy Burnell had an interest in urology with some specialist training. Both sent their apologies to the March 1936 meeting of the Sydney Urological Association. Jimmy Burnell, in particular, was a very active urologist, and Keith Kirkland consulted him over the foundation of the Urological Society of Australasia. Because he also practised general surgery he was not eligible to become a foundation member of the USA. He was, however, among the first group of Associate Members admitted in 1941.[36]

Tasmania

No Tasmanian was either a full or an associate member of the Urological Society of Austraslasia until after the incorporation of the Society in 1948. However, John Ramsay at the Launceston General Hospital began performing Freyer and then Young prostatectomies as early as 1904. By 1912, when he retired from the position of surgeon superintendent, he had performed twenty-seven Young perineal prostatectomies, all under chloroform or ether anaesthesia. One of his successors as surgeon superintendent, Clifford Craig, made attempts to reduce the size of the prostate by surgical devascularisation.[37]

Western Australia

The pioneer of urology in the West was Frank Gill. He graduated from Melbourne University Medical School in 1911, and served in France during World War I. He obtained his FRCSEd and was a foundation fellow of the RACS. Frank Gill started the Cystoscopy Club in Perth and in 1934 was appointed General Surgeon and Urologist to the Royal Perth Hospital. The urology unit there was not formally founded until after he retired in 1945.[38]

CHAPTER 3

The Sydney Urological Association and the Urological Society of Australasia, 1935–1948

~

Introduction

The Urological Society of Australasia (USA) was founded as an association of successful men. They had all been successful on many levels—as medical graduates giving them entry to the life style of professional men; as post-graduate students, taking their careers beyond those of most doctors; as Honorary Surgeons to major public hospitals, reflecting and re-inforcing their successful private practice as surgeons; and as pioneers in developing urology as a specialty in the face of considerable opposition from general surgeons.

The major tension that the pioneer urologists shared in their careers was certainly not the struggle to make a decent living, that motivated the formation of trade unions. It was not even the struggle for adequate recognition in terms of status (and pay), that motivated other professional associations, including the British Medical Association (BMA). Their shared struggle was for recognition of their specialty in the face of opposition from the general surgeons.

This struggle goes a long way to explaining the relationship between the USA (and other specialist surgical organisations) and the Royal Australasian College of Surgeons (RACS). Urologists benefited from the work of the RACS but it was also seen as the stronghold of the general surgeons, with whom they sparred in their on-going battles to set up specialist departments and ensure that urological cases were treated by urologists.

One major concern was training. The RACS was founded, among other things, to provide a bench-mark for surgical standards in Australasia. Over the years it did come to play that role but certainly in the period before the end of World War II, the College offered no bench-mark for urologists.[1]

What both the BMA and the RACS did offer was a forum for the discussion of clinical cases and matters of mutual concern. The scientific meetings of the section of surgery of the BMA were the venue for important discussions leading to the foundation of the College and on a more modest scale surgeons regularly presented cases at the scientific meetings of the State branches of the BMA. Early in 1937, for instance, Reg Bridge and Keith Kirkland demonstrated urological conditions at Sydney Hospital for a scientific meeting of the NSW branch, while at around the same time, Dr Lazarus gave a demonstration of urological conditions at St Vincent's Hospital for the Victorian branch of the BMA.[2]

The scientific meetings of the RACS provided a venue for more specialised demonstrations. The first meeting in 1928 was devoted to plastic surgery, but by the 1930 meeting, held in Melbourne, a more varied program had been established. Fellows were provided with the opportunity to view demonstrations and operations at the major Melbourne hospitals. 'Some Urological Operations will be Performed by General Surgeons', and urologists could have attended a demonstration by W. H. J. Moore at the Melbourne Hospital, or watched Julian Smith operating at St Vincent's.

At the Sydney meeting in March/April 1931 there was a more extensive program of urological work and it was carried out by urologists, but it still appeared in the RACS program under the heading of General Surgery. Harry Harris and Richard Harris provided the demonstrations at Lewisham Hospital on 31 March and Messrs Lee-Brown, Laidley and Earlam were in charge of the urological program at Royal Prince Alfred.

At the fifth AGM in Melbourne in February 1932, urology was still listed under General Surgery, but the appeal of the meeting to interstate fellows was clear. Both Bridge from Sydney and Burnell from Adelaide, for instance, were there to talk on urological procedures.

The sixth AGM in Sydney was the first where urology appeared as a separate specialty on the scientific program, but at the seventh AGM, in Adelaide, urology was back under the heading of General Surgery. This was despite the fact that the Harris prostatectomy was featured at the meeting. A film of the procedure was shown and Harry Harris gave a lecture. Meanwhile, Ivan Jose demonstrated prostatic resection.

The Harris prostatectomy was also featured at the eighth AGM, in Melbourne, in 1935, when R. St Clair Steuart demonstrated the operation at the Alfred Hospital and gave a lecture on a year's experience of the operation. At the same meeting, Tait demonstrated internal urethrotomy and Laidley came from Sydney to read a paper on diathermy for bladder papilloma, but the whole urology program was still under General Surgery.[3]

This was the state of affairs before the first meeting of the Sydney Urological Association. The RACS was not willing to recognise urology as a specialty, and even in the urological sections of its scientific programs, urological procedures were frequently demonstrated by general surgeons.

Another problem facing urologists in the early years was shortage of numbers. There were only a dozen or so of them in all of

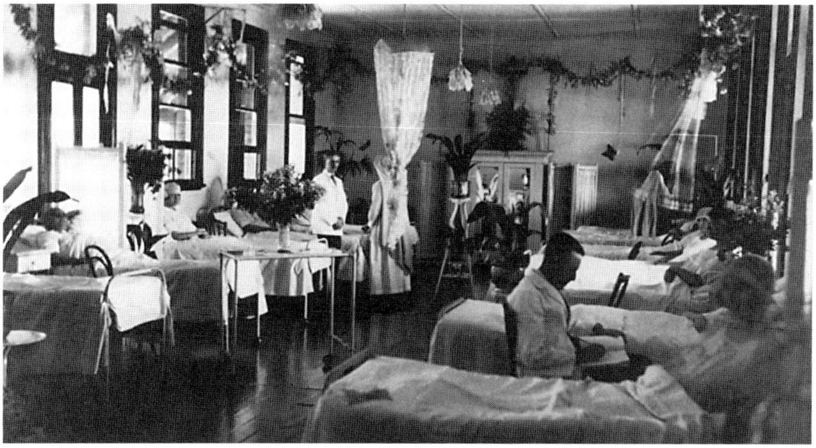

Christmas at Lewisham Hospital, c.1920. (*Source:* Archives of the Little Company of Mary)

Australasia and they were scattered around the fringes of the continent and the islands of New Zealand in ones and twos and threes. The problems of professional isolation were very real and the first attempt to overcome them was made in the only Australasian city where more than two or three urologists could easily gather together: The Urological Society of Australasia had its beginnings in Macquarie Street in Sydney.

The Sydney Urological Association

In April 1935, Keith Kirkland sent a letter to nine Sydney urologists. The only letter that had to travel very far was the one to Harry Harris, who was overseas at the time, or as they said in the 1930s using the English expression, 'abroad'.

Keith Kirkland wrote from BMA House, 137 Macquarie Street, Sydney. The eight letters went to:

R. H. Bridge	141 Macquarie Street
M. S. S. Earlam	139 Macquarie Street
C. M. Edwards	135 Macquarie Street
R. G. S. Harris	185 Macquarie Street
J. W. S. Laidley	139 Macquarie Street
G. H. Pfeiffer	135 Macquarie Street
R. J. Silverton	135 Macquarie Street
A. B. Walker-Smith	141 Macquarie Street

135 Macquarie Street was also part of BMA House. The other addresses were consulting rooms. Laidley and Earlam, it will be noted, were in practice together.

On 29 April, eight urologists met at the University Club, in Phillip Street, behind Macquarie Street. They were called together to form an 'Association of men practising urology' in which 'membership should be restricted to those who are Honorary Urologists at the Hospitals and practising the specialty or those who have special training in the subject.'[4]

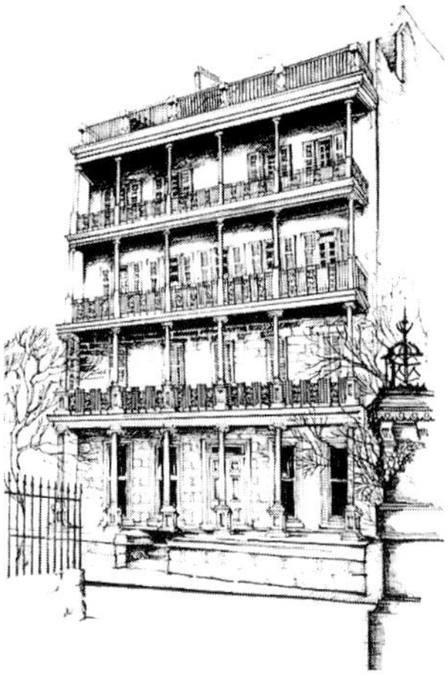

Royal Australian College of Physicians Building, 145 Macquarie Street, Sydney, venue for many early meetings of the Urological Society, including those of 1949, 1951, 1954, 1957 and 1961.

This was actually a broader definition of potential members than was later accepted. Hence the invitation to Pfeiffer, who was not a full-time urologist, but had been RSO at St Peter's Hospital for Stone in 1924-25. He did not attend any meetings of the Sydney Urological Association, presumably because he was warned of the narrowed membership.

At the first meeting it was resolved that: 'Membership be restricted to Surgeons specialising in Urology and holding Honorary appointments in that capacity.' Of those invited, only Harry Harris and Pfeiffer did not attend. The other eight Sydney urologists formed the Sydney Urological Association (SUA) and subsequently the nucleus of the Urological Society of Australasia.

The aims of the SUA were not clearly defined but Keith Kirkland noted a general aim of furthering 'the science of urology' and there was discussion of both links with visiting urologists and the possibility of an Australian association.

At the first meeting, the position of Harry Harris was made very clear and Kirkland wrote to Harris after the meeting, to keep him informed of events.

> *Eulogistic references were made to Dr Harris' contributions to Urology and it was recalled that he has not only been one of the pioneer specialists in genito-urinary work in Sydney, but is the Senior Urologist of this city.*[5]

The other senior urologists in Sydney were R. H. Bridge and R. J. Silverton. Both were regular attenders at meetings, but it appears to have been the younger men who did most of the work. Kirkland in particular, as secretary and convener of the SUA, ran the association, but Richard Harris and Colin Edwards were also very active members.

On 1 July 1935, the SUA met again at the University Club and discussed urological cases over dinner. The members decided to invite Clifford Morson to their next meeting on 6 September.[6] At least half the members would have known Morson. He was first appointed Surgeon to St Peter's Hospital for Stone in 1919, and since then Silverton, Edwards and Walker-Smith had all spent time there as RSOs and Kirkland was a clinical assistant.

In September the Sydney urologists entertained their distinguished guest at the Australia Club. Despite their training at St Peter's, the Sydney urologists did not share Morson's reservations about the value of TUR. There was a lively discussion and some amicable disagreement. Morson suggested that the Association should investigate the possibility of membership or affiliation with the Société Internationale d'Urologie and the idea was pursued at a number of subsequent meetings.

The Association met again at the University Club on 19 December and attendance was down, both Laidley and Earlam sending their apologies. The wider aims of the Association were discussed and for the first time the possibility of forming an Australasian Association appears in the minutes.

On 20 March 1936, the SUA met at the Australia Club and the minutes of this meeting are the first in the bound and embossed minute

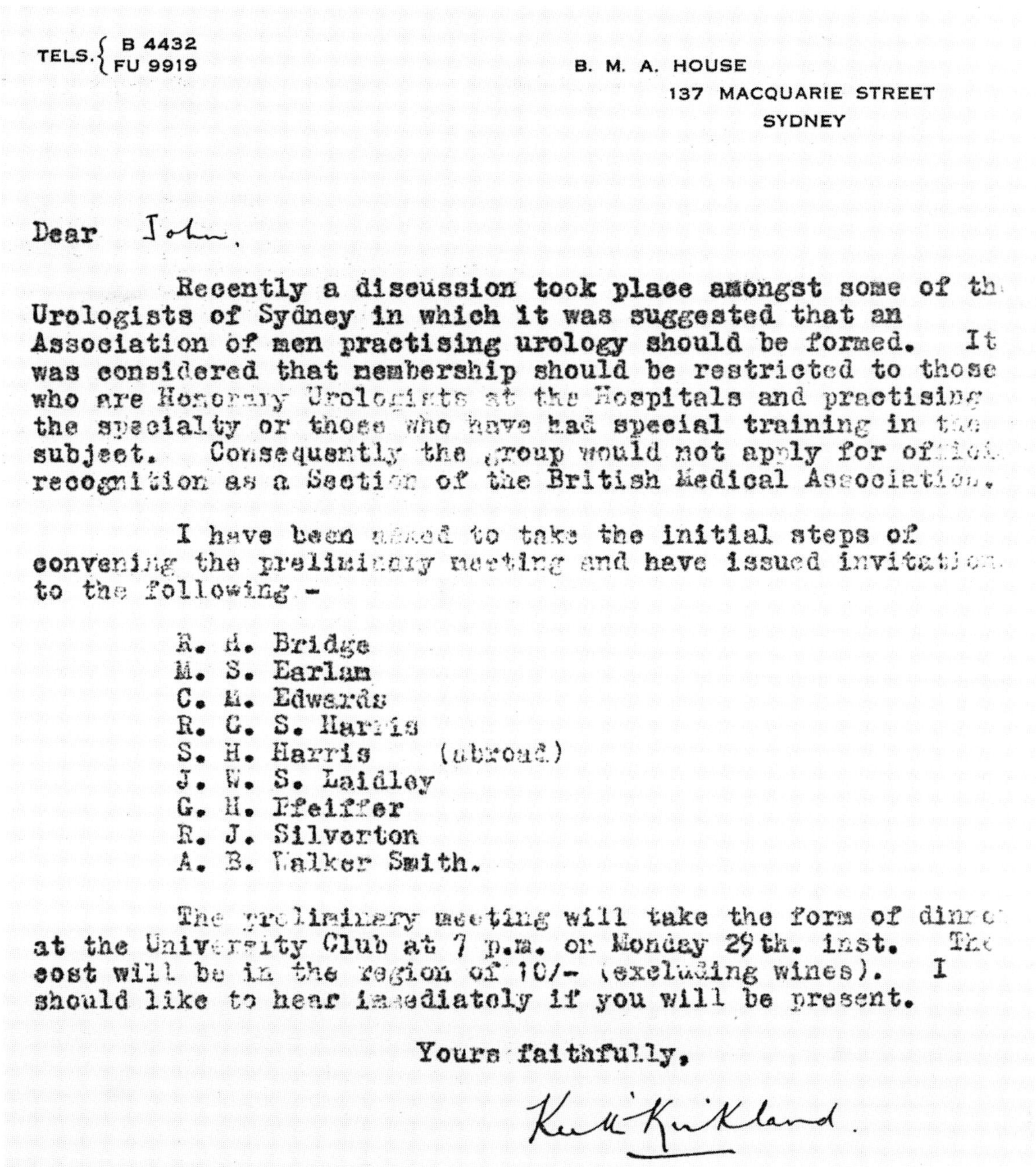

TELS. { B 4432
FU 9919

B. M. A. HOUSE
137 MACQUARIE STREET
SYDNEY

Dear John,

Recently a discussion took place amongst some of the Urologists of Sydney in which it was suggested that an Association of men practising urology should be formed. It was considered that membership should be restricted to those who are Honorary Urologists at the Hospitals and practising the specialty or those who have had special training in the subject. Consequently the group would not apply for official recognition as a Section of the British Medical Association.

I have been asked to take the initial steps of convening the preliminary meeting and have issued invitations to the following -

R. H. Bridge
M. S. Earlam
C. M. Edwards
R. G. S. Harris
S. H. Harris (abroad)
J. W. S. Laidley
G. H. Pfeiffer
R. J. Silverton
A. B. Walker Smith.

The preliminary meeting will take the form of dinner at the University Club at 7 p.m. on Monday 29th. inst. The cost will be in the region of 10/- (excluding wines). I should like to hear immediately if you will be present.

Yours faithfully,

Keith Kirkland.

The copy of the Kirkland Letter, April 1935, sent to John Laidley

book, presented by Clifford Morson. This was an enlarged and very important meeting. Besides the eight members of the SUA, there were three urologists from other cities: John Power from Brisbane and K. MacCormick and C. M. Greenslade from New Zealand. These three had not travelled to Sydney especially for the SUA meeting. They were there for the Annual Congress of the RACS.

A number of other fellows of the College 'known to be interested in urology' were invited, but declined. They were Moore, Roe, Jose,

Campbell-Begg, Jenkins, Lazarus, Collier, Mortensen, Lennon, Burnell, Sutton and Macky. The names are interesting because they include several men who were not full-time urologists. At this stage in attempting to form an Australasian association of urologists, the SUA was casting its net fairly wide.[7]

The visitors expressed themselves in favour of the formation of an Australasian Association of Urology and it was resolved that Kirkland should correspond with Power in Brisbane, Tait in Melbourne, MacCormick in Auckland and Burnell in Adelaide.

> *Inquiries were to be made also as to the number of men practising urology in the various cities and an opinion invited as to whether co-operation in the formation of an Australasian Association would be forthcoming.*[8]

It was proposed that the Association be established at the Auckland Congress of the RACS in January 1937. The perceived relationship to the College is evident in this resolution, as it was in the context of the March 1936 meeting. At the inaugural meeting of the Urological Society of Australasia it was decided that the Annual General Meetings take place during the first three months of the year, if possible contiguous with those of the RACS.

The idea of an inaugural meeting in Auckland died at the next meeting of the SUA on 23 August 1936. There it was learnt that the proposal for an Australasian Association had been positively received in Melbourne, Brisbane and Adelaide, but there was silence from Auckland.

At the August 1936 meeting, Earlam and Laidley were again absent, but Harry Harris was there, the only meeting he managed to attend. Ill health prevented him from attending the next two meetings and he died on 25 December. The meeting spent some time debating the question of membership qualification. The case of Burnell highlighted the problem because he was not a full-time urologist. There was prolonged discussion and eventually Harry Harris formally proposed the formation of the Urological Society of Australasia. Membership was to be limited to consultant urologists 'at this stage'.

The members of the SUA were clear that they wanted only senior full-time urologists. This was important for the future status of the USA, but it drastically limited the potential membership and excluded a number who would have been active members, including Burnell.

Apart from the nine members of the SUA, invitations for foundation membership of the USA were sent to Campbell-Begg of Wellington, Reay of Christchurch, Tait of Melbourne and Power and Roe of Brisbane.

The next two meetings of the SUA, on 29 October and 17 December, were devoted to preparation for the inaugural meeting of the USA, to be held in Sydney, not Auckland. This was eventually fixed for 7 January 1937, because Reay would be in Sydney then, on other business, and able to attend. Power also indicated that he would be there. The other interstate members accepted the invitation to join, but would not be at the meeting. Subsequently, Campbell-Begg declined the offer of membership because he was going to South Africa.

The inaugural meeting of the Urological Society of Australasia did not mean the end of the Sydney Urological Association. Members continued to meet once a year to discuss urological cases and there were meetings in April 1937, March 1938 and October 1939.

At the 1939 meeting 'The present unsatisfactory position of the Urological Society of Australasia was discussed.' The restricted membership had not provided sufficient numbers to be a viable organisation outside Sydney. At this meeting, the members of the SUA acted as a sort of Sydney caucus of the USA and resolved on a number of measures to try and re-invigorate the Australasian body. Kirkland and Edwards proposed a correspondence letter for members of the USA, and maybe additional 'corresponding members'. It was also proposed that the annual meetings (all so far held in Sydney) include two or three days of clinical demonstrations to make it worthwhile for interstate members to make the journey.

At this October 1939 meeting, Edwards and Kirkland were also given the go ahead to set about turning the SUA into a section of urology of the New South Wales branch of the British Medical Association. This possibility had been in the background since the very first meeting of the SUA and had been rejected more because of problems with the BMA rules than because of any desire for independence.

The last meeting of the SUA was held at BMA House in November 1939. After that it became a section of urology of the BMA under by-law 27.[9]

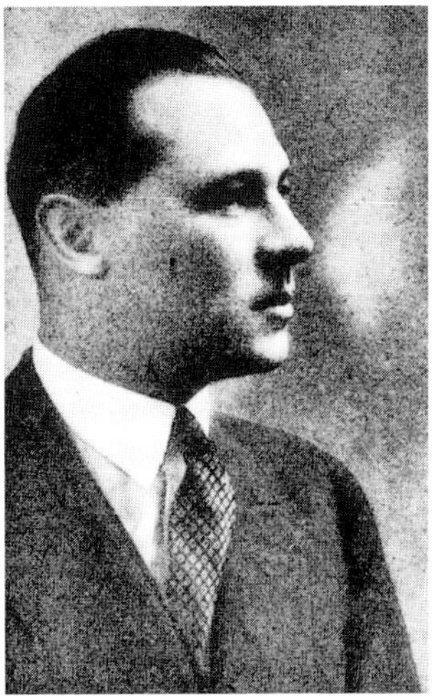

Reginald Bridge, first President of the Urological Society, 1937

Keith Lindsay Hugh Kirkland

Kirkland wrote that the Urological Society of Australasia was founded following a proposal by Harry Harris at a meeting of the Sydney Urological Association. This is true, but misleading. The USA was not founded by Harris and an Australasian society had been under discussion for months while he was overseas. If it was founded by any one person, that person was Keith Kirkland. He was the driving force behind both the Sydney Urological Association and the Urological Society of Australasia, but as a young man in his thirties at the time he was not inclined to take the credit.

Clearly Kirkland was impressed with Harris and shortly after Harris left for Europe to demonstrate his operation for suprapubic prostatectomy, Kirkland wrote the letter inviting nine men to join him in founding the SUA. The early Australasian urologists were all enormously proud of Harry Harris and perhaps the best way to sum up the foundation of the Urological Society of Australasia is that it was set in motion by Keith Kirkland in honour of Harry Harris.

Kirkland was a man of talent and energy who could carry others with him. In sport, he represented Australia as an Olympic swimmer.

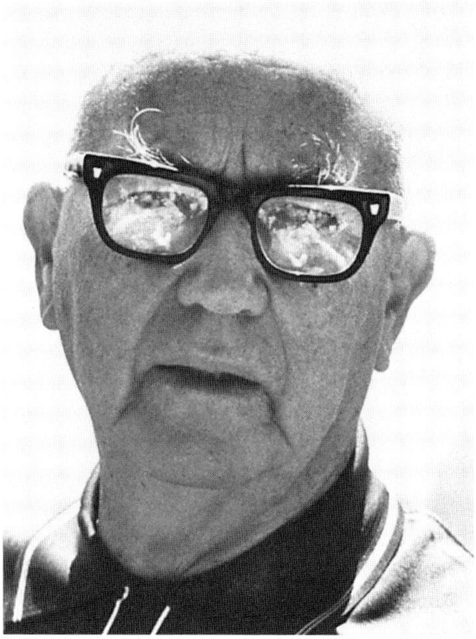

Left: Keith Kirkland, the driving force behind the founding of the Urological Society of Australasia, photographed in 1968. (*Source:* Dennis Arnold)

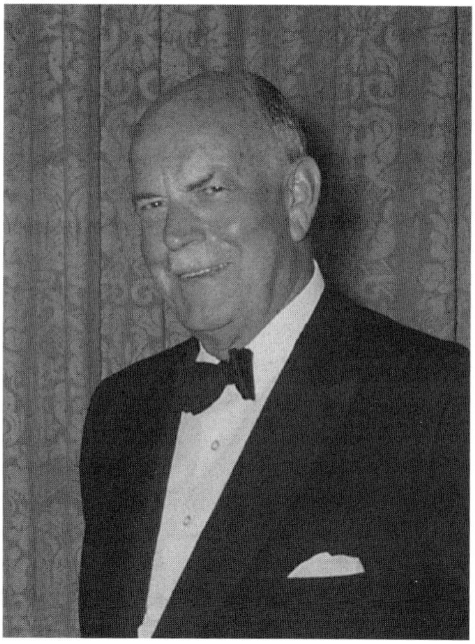

Right: Henry Mortensen, President of the Urological Society in 1942, 1944-45 and 1948-49 at the Annual General Meeting in Melbourne, 1968

In urology he also represented his country and in 1961 was elected Vice-President of the International Society of Urology. Even his hobby took him onto the international stage. He was Vice-President of the Australian Orchid Council and in 1967 presented a paper on behalf of the Australian society at the fifth World Orchid Conference, in the United States.

Kirkland's secretary, Marie Corbey, was the only woman involved in the early years of the USA. She typed the minutes, dealt with the correspondence and, when the Society was incorporated in 1948, witnessed the signatures of Keith Kirkland, Richard Harris, Arthur Carrodus and Alban Gee.

Kirkland graduated from Sydney University in 1925 and then went to England where he spent some time at St Peter's Hospital for Stone and gained his FRCSEd in 1930. He returned to Sydney and was admitted FRACS in 1932.

Besides his work at Sydney, St Vincent's and a number of other hospitals, he was involved in the installation of the first artificial kidney in Australia, at the Kanematsu Institute. The Keith Kirkland Renal Unit was named in his honour.

Kirkland died in October 1971.[10]

The Urological Society of Australasia 1937–43

Keith Kirkland was both Secretary and Treasurer of the USA from its formation until 1946. He was, as Colin Edwards pointed out in 1945, 'the moving spirit in the formation of the first urological organization in Australasia'.[11]

The early minutes of the USA were typed and bound into a

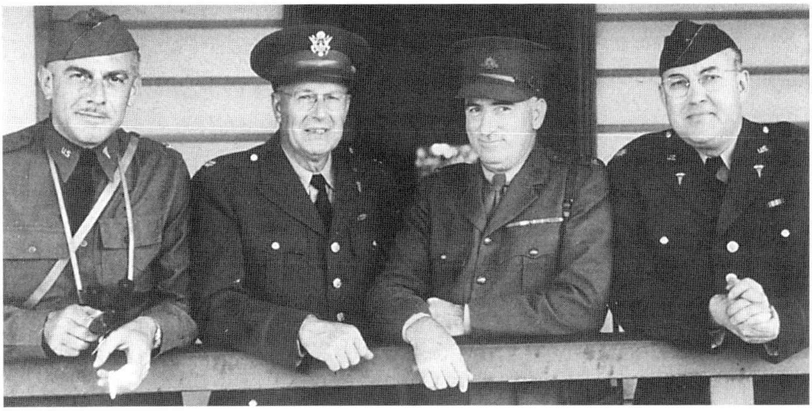

Jack Power, second President of the Urological Society, with three American doctors at a Brisbane race meeting during World War II. *Left to right:* Colonel William Blackween, Colonel Roy Brown, Jack Power, Major John Marshall. Jack Power was President of the Society in 1938, 1946-47 and 1952-53. (*Source:* William Lucas)

volume presented by R. H. Bridge, following in the tradition set by Clifford Morson. Bridge was elected the first president of the USA and his vice-president was John Power from Brisbane. The only other interstate member present at the first meeting in Sydney was E. R. Reay from Christchurch.

It was resolved that 'The object of the Society shall be to advance the science of urology.' Full membership was to be limited to surgeons practising solely the specialty of urology and provision was also made for the election of Honorary Members.

The meeting began with a silent toast to the memory of Harry Harris and references to his 'brilliant work'.

Members decided that future Annual General Meetings should if possible be held at the same time as meetings of the RACS. With this objective in mind the AGM was tied to the first three months of the year. However, the foundation meeting of January 1937 took place in Sydney while a General Meeting of Fellows of the RACS was held later the same month in Auckland.[12]

The announcement of the foundation of the Urological Society met a frosty reception. The editor of the *Medical Journal of Australia,* 8 January 1938, whilst acknowledging the specialised technical skill and clinical judgement required for what the Americans called genito-urinary surgery, argued that urologists would become too narrow if they did not first train as general surgeons and later continue to perform some general surgery. The editorial referred to a similar discussion in the *American Journal of Surgery,* but did not directly mention the Urological Society of Australasia. There were, however, scathing references to 'pure' urologists.[13]

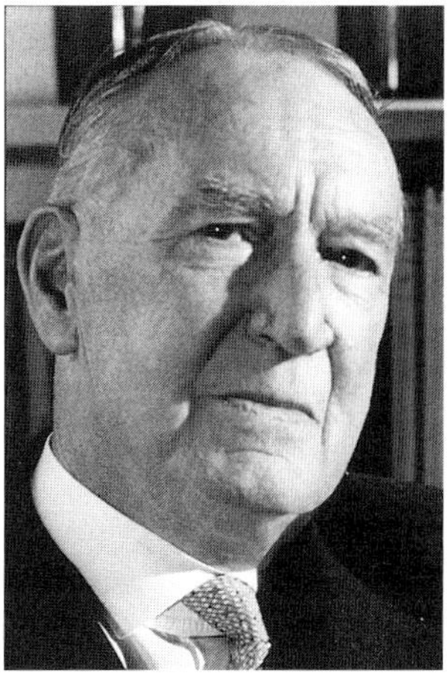

John Thomson Tait, third President of the Urological Society, 1939

The reaction from the RACS was an expanded program of urology at the next Congress. The eleventh AGM and scientific meeting, held in Sydney from 24 March 1938, included a symposium on prostatic obstruction. It featured general surgeons, including Julian Smith and Sir Henry Newland, as well as urologists, and was held under the heading of General Surgery. However, there was also a separate Urology session, featuring urologists.[14]

The first Annual Meeting of the USA took place just before the

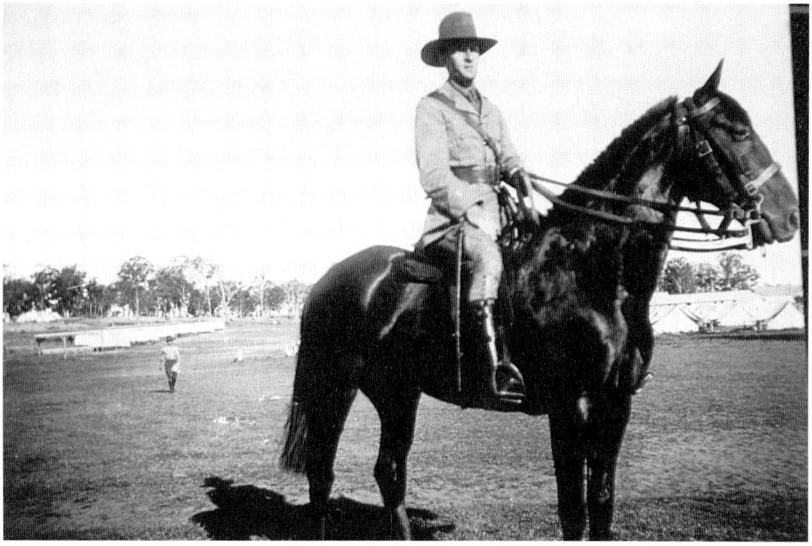

Bobby Silverton, fourth President of the Urological Society, 1940

RACS meeting, on 22 March. Three more members were elected—Mortensen from Melbourne, plus two additions to the Macquarie Street contingent—Archibald Telfer of 135 and D. Coleman Trainor of 215. Of course, Sydney was not the only city where surgeons clustered together. Both the Brisbane men had rooms on Wickham Terrace and both the Melbourne men ran their practices from Collins Street.

The minutes from the 1938 meeting were not bound into Bridge's book and no minutes have been found from the March 1939 meeting, the year Tait was elected president to succeed Power. In 1939, the RACS held its AGM in Melbourne, but the USA did not follow the College and held its AGM in Sydney.[15] Attendance may have been poor. However, ten urologists attended the third Annual Meeting of the USA in Sydney in March 1940, including Power, Tait and Mortensen from interstate. There, the thorny question of membership was raised again and Edwards proposed a category of 'Associate Members' who need not be full-time urologists. He was supported by his boss, Silverton, and the matter was to be considered by the Executive. Edwards was not on the Executive, but Silverton was elected president that year, with Roe as vice-president.

Interstate attendance at all the early USA AGMs was very low and the problem of inter-state attendance was not resolved until after the war. Then, the increase in membership, greater ease of travel and the interest generated in the programs of the annual meetings combined to persuade urologists to travel the enormous distances involved.

Because of the strict limitations on membership, the infant Society was very nearly stillborn. Only four of the twelve foundation members were not from Sydney and while Power valiantly travelled from Queensland to the Sydney meetings, Reay did not make it to another meeting until after the war. Roe, who was semi-retired, did not join

Power in the long trek south and Tait only made it to one Sydney meeting. Once Henry Mortensen was elected a member, in 1938, he joined Power in providing the energy, enthusiasm and willingness to travel that kept the USA from being Australasian in name only in these early years.

At the 1940 meeting, Mortensen and Kirkland were enthusiastic about the urological correspondence letter then in vogue in America and Edwards proposed adopting something along the same lines. The objective of both this proposal and the move to include Associate Members was the same: to put some life into a society that was in danger of being too small and scattered to survive, especially with the added problems of travel and manpower during the war.

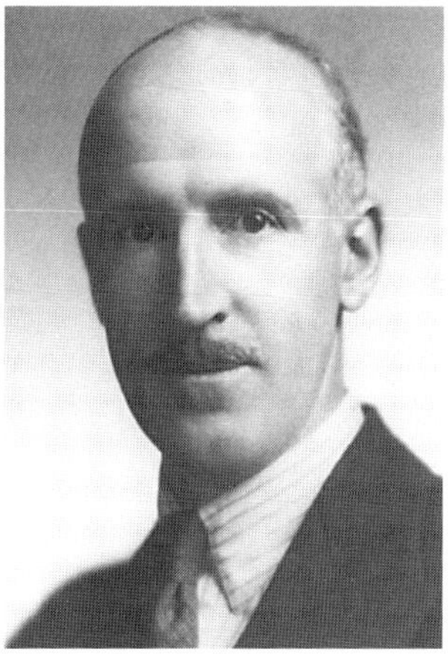

Patrick Treahy was first appointed as a urologist to Wellington Hospital in 1930 and remained for thirty years.

At the fourth Annual Meeting, in April 1941, the idea of wider membership was taken a stage further. There was to be a vote on changing the constitution to allow Associate Members, with provision for postal and proxy voting. Meanwhile Silverton and Walker-Smith proposed the other idea that had come out of the SUA—larger and more interesting annual meetings with clinical demonstrations.

On 29 May 1941 an Extraordinary General Meeting was held in Sydney, with only four members present: Kirkland, of course, who never missed a meeting, Silverton, Edwards and Telfer. However, they had postal and proxy votes to assist them and passed Edwards' motion to change the constitution and allow Associate Members. The date of the annual meeting was also freed from its constitutional chains to the first three months of the year and a Spring meeting was duly held on 2 October 1941.

The October 1941 meeting was called a General Meeting, as there had already been an Annual Meeting that year. The main business was to increase the membership of the USA. Ten urologists were present and they elected three new full members: Bruce Rennie and Patrick Treahy from Wellington and Harold Moore from Melbourne. They also elected the first nine Associate Members, thus at one meeting increasing the strength of the Society from 15 to 26.

This did not, in fact, have the desired effect of rejuvenating the Society. Stanley Roe was president in 1941 but did not attend any of the three meetings in Sydney. The war was having too much of an impact, with the younger men away in the forces and the older men carrying an increased load, in Roe's case coming out of retirement to resume his public hospital workload.

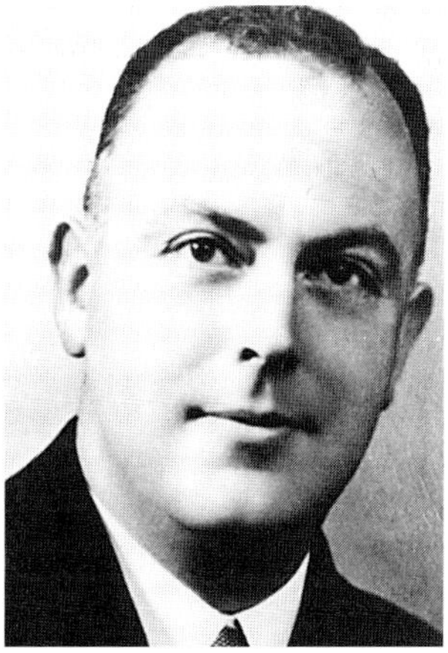

Bruce Rennie was the third urologist at Wellington Hospital, joining Treahy in 1937. He retired in 1964.

There were also severe difficulties in travelling. Petrol rationing had been introduced in 1940, but the real restrictions on interstate movement followed the Japanese entry into the war. After Christmas 1941, the Curtin Government introduced restrictions on leave and cancelled public holidays and many workers went onto a 13-day fortnight. The Federal Government took over the running of all trains and from July 1942 Priority Permits were needed to travel any distance.

The USA went into recess for the next two years. Henry Mortensen was president in 1942 and Roe again in 1943, although this last position does not appear on customary USA records. In any case, both presidencies were nominal only. The USA did nothing for two years.[16]

The Urological Society of Australasia 1944–48

The fifth Annual Meeting of the USA was held on 12-13 October 1944. Henry Mortensen was elected president at the first meeting to include a program of clinical demonstrations. Twelve members were present and the wisdom of introducing Associate Membership was visible in the persons of Burnell from Adelaide and Davidson from Ballarat. Although neither were full-time urologists, they were both to make a substantial contribution to the rejuvenation of the USA.

The RACS had not yet resumed its program of scientific meetings, so that there was no other program of demonstrations and operations to compete with that of the USA. Whether or not the absence of College scientific meetings during the war was the reason for the original 1941 proposal for a scientific program at USA meetings, the decision transformed the Society.

The war was not yet over, but the 1944 meeting took place in an atmosphere of self-confidence and building for the future. Kirkland spoke about provision for returned soldiers who were medical men, Laidley about the training of urologists and co-operation with the RACS, while Earlam and Kirkland spoke about post-graduate lectures in urology. There were clinical demonstrations at Lewisham, Royal North Shore and Sydney Hospital and the next meeting was planned for Melbourne, transport regulations permitting.

From 1944 onwards the annual meetings of the USA went from strength to strength and the whole tone of the minutes and annual reports became very much more optimistic and enthusiastic. The Urological Correspondence Club, agreed on at the 1944 meeting, began in 1945 and contributed to the atmosphere of friendship and shared experience.

At the sixth Annual Meeting in 1945, the first held outside Sydney, it was clear that the urologists attending had rather a good time, possibly somewhat to their own surprise. As the retiring president, Mortensen was the host and this was the first time a meeting was run in quite that way. The meeting began on 28 October, with Mortensen entertaining the interstate visitors at his home. There were clinical and operative demonstrations for the next three days at the Royal Melbourne, St Vincent's and Alfred Hospitals and members also found time for dinners at Menzies Hotel and the Athenaeum Club and a visit to the gardens of the Nicholas family at Burnham Beeches, in the hills east of Melbourne. As Kirkland wrote in the Annual Report:

> *The clinical and social activities combined to make the Melbourne Meeting the most successful and pleasant yet held. All arrangements for the Meeting were in the hands of Henry Mortensen who put on a magnificent show.*[17]

The seventh Annual Meeting in 1946 was held in Brisbane, again completely separate from the scientific meeting of the RACS. Earlam was the retiring president, replaced by Power. The most notable event at the 1946 meeting was that Kirkland stood down as secretary and treasurer to take up the position of vice-president. Appropriately, he was replaced by two men, Alban Gee just back from the war as secretary and Arthur Carrodus, also of Sydney, as treasurer.

This meeting also had an important impact on H. B. Devine. Later that year he wrote:

> *Of later years it has been obvious that specialist surgeons have been forming Australasian associations of their own (note they all include New Zealand), and at the last meeting in Sydney [the RACS AGM and scientific meeting of 1946] I noticed how few specialist surgeons there were ... And yet, three weeks later, in Brisbane, there was a full meeting of the urologist surgeons.*[18]

Devine was worried that the College was in danger of being weakened by the loss of specialist surgeons and had a number of suggestions, including providing more of interest for the specialists at the RACS scientific meetings. He proposed, for instance, inviting Hinman from San Francisco, as one way to tempt the urologists back to College scientific meetings—and presumably away from meetings of the Urological Society.

The eighth Annual Meeting of the USA, in April 1947, was back in Sydney and was a mammoth affair with 31 members. The previous highest attendance was 13, in Melbourne. Partly this was made possible by the steadily increasing membership since 1944. By 1947 there were 19 full members and 20 associate members.

The eighth Annual Meeting was the first to have its *Proceedings* published and the last before incorporation proceedings commenced.

Stanley Roe was the fifth President of the Urological Society in 1941 and President again in 1943. The photograph shows the adult surgical ward at his principal public hospital, the Mater Misericordiae Hospitals, Brisbane, 1914. (*Source:* Mater Misericordiae Hospitals)

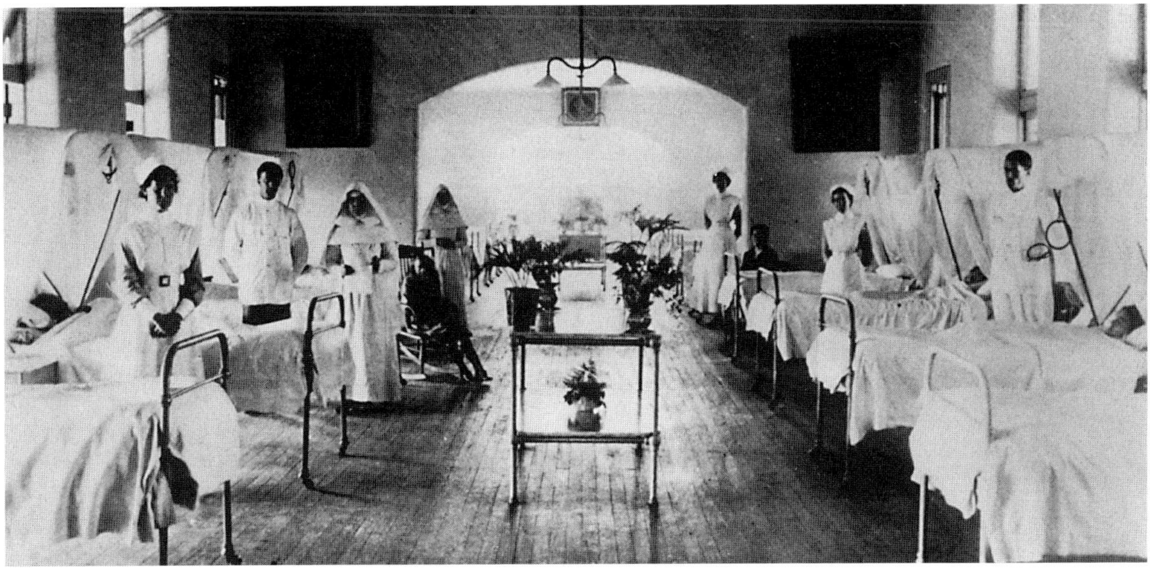

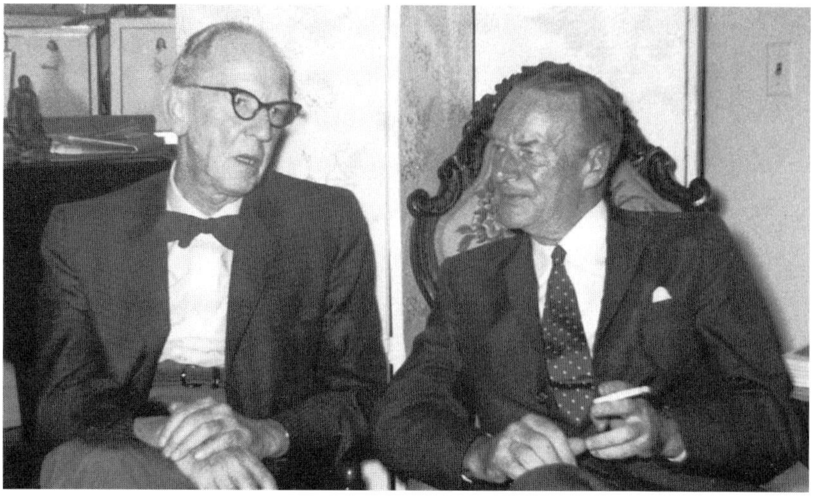

Malcolm Earlam, President of the Urological Society in 1945–46 and 1956–57. He is shown here with Frederick Foley, inventor of the Foley catheter. Earlam first met Foley in 1936. 'Thinking it would be nice to watch him at work on a Monday morning ... I phoned him from Minneapolis one Sunday. He said: "Sure, but why don't you come over for afternoon tea with myself and my wife." So I did to find that "afternoon tea" was a combination of Scotch, rye and martinis. I tried to escape after this, but no, I must stay for supper. I tried again, but no, some friends were coming in for a rubber or two of bridge ... Again I tried to escape, but no, I must stay the night ... Also remember quite vividly Bentley Squier in New York ... Driving along Park Avenue in his Rolls Royce he said: "This, Earlam, is Park Avenue ... This is where you see good dogs and bad women."—Malcolm Earlam, letter to Dick Craven, 25 September 1980. RACS archives. (*Source:* Emily Earlam)

The meeting accepted the need for a legally constituted body under the Companies Act and Harris, Earlam and Kirkland had been busy working with solicitors to draw up a constitution for the USA as a limited company.

The ninth Annual Meeting of February 1948 was noteworthy in a number of respects. It was held at Ballarat and Melbourne, with the Ballarat part of the meeting hosted by Davidson, an associate member. The days in Ballarat were the subject of a number of comments in the letters of the Urological Correspondence Club. Colin Edwards wrote:

> *This letter goes before the Melbourne portion of the Victorian Meeting but the Ballarat session exceeded all expectations. Ronald Davidson excelled himself both on social and clinical sides and was most ably supported by specialists on the staff of the Ballarat Hospital.*[19]

And Richard Harris wrote:

> *The Victorian meeting was the success that we had anticipated and considerable knowledge and other things were absorbed without untoward results. I feel that mention should be made of Ron and Mrs Davidson for their magnificent efforts at Ballarat.*

Jack Power also enjoyed himself:

> *My congratulations to the Victorians on the excellent meeting we had. I nearly made the mistake of saying Melburnians although, even if I had no one would have taken me seriously as we all agreed on Ron's excellent efforts at Ballarat.*[20]

Although work to incorporate the USA as a limited liability company began in 1947, there were a number of delays and the formal date of incorporation was 23 February 1948.[21] The ninth Annual Meeting earlier in the month was thus held under the old Executive of the unincorporated Society, fittingly under the presidency of

FULL MEMBERS OF THE UROLOGICAL SOCIETY OF AUSTRALASIA, 1948

A. L. Carrodus	Sydney	E. H. Reay*	Christchurch
M. S. S. Earlam*	Sydney	B. Rennie	Wellington
C. M. Edwards*	Sydney	A. S. Roe*	Brisbane
A. H. Gee	Sydney	R. J. Silverton*	Sydney
R. G. S. Harris*	Sydney	J. B. Somerset	Melbourne
K. L. H. Kirkland*	Sydney	J. Thomson Tait*	Melbourne
J. W. S. Laidley*	Sydney	A. C. Telfer	Sydney
F. W. R. Lukin	Brisbane	D. C. Trainor	Sydney
W. H. J. Moore	Melbourne	P. A. Treahy	Wellington
H. N. Mortensen	Melbourne	A. B. Walker-Smith*	Sydney
J. J. Power*	Brisbane		

* = Foundation member

Source: USA Membership Register, 1948; List of Members, 1958; including addresses; Minutes of AGMs 1937–1948, showing dates of election of new members and city of origin, RACS archives.

Keith Kirkland. It firmly established the tradition that the meetings were now places to have a good time.

By law, the first general meeting had to be held within three months after incorporation. A separate General Meeting of the USA was therefore held at BMA House, Sydney in March 1948, at which Kirkland stood down as the last president of the old society and Mortensen was elected the first president of the new. Only eight members were present at this procedural meeting, all from Macquarie Street.[22]

The Urological Correspondence Club

The club began, following an invitation circulated at the bottom of the report of the fifth Annual Meeting, 1944.

As president, Henry Mortensen wrote the first letter in January 1945. Mortensen stressed two points which seem to have been causing concern to urologists at the time.

The first was the relationship with general surgeons. 'It is our duty' he wrote, 'by our example, efforts and results to continually impress upon the profession the better handling of the genito-urinary case by urologists.'[23] The statement struck a chord with his colleagues and both Earlam and Silverton quoted it in their own letters later in the year.

The other matter that concerned Mortensen was the general shortage of urologists in Australasia and the need to recruit young doctors or, as he put it 'It is our duty to encourage the younger men of suitable ability to wander along these paths.'

These twin tasks of winning wider recognition for the specialty and recruiting and training more urologists were the major challenges facing the USA for many years to come. In subsequent years, the next generation of urologists was prone to comment on the kindness and helpfulness of men like Mortensen—only to remember the continu-

'The public and the profession in general are not yet entirely freed from the idea that urologists are diagnosticians only, and are not operating surgeons.'

—J. THOMSON TAIT, UCC, MAY 1945, RACS ARCHIVES

'The reference in these letters to education of Urologists leads me to report the obvious progress of what must be our youngest recruit. The wife of one of our Sydney doctors took her son aged 5 to the cinema version of the 'Citadel'. The audience were listening intently to the interviewing by the doctor of a patient when a shrill clear voice enquired "When is he going to test the urine mother?" The theatre crowd, I believe, never really settled down to a quiet viewing of the rest of the picture.'

—ARCHIBALD C. TELFER, UCC, JULY 1945, RACS ARCHIVES

'I do not know whether I should send the story of this case to you or to Ripley. However, here it is.

The patient was a man of 75 who had had a prostatectomy performed 12 years ago. He was quite well until two years ago when he commenced to get urinary discomfort. About 3 weeks before he came to hospital this became very severe, and he was admitted with his suprapubic wound broken down and discharging urine.

I put a probe into the sinus and it struck solid rock.

To cut a long story short, I opened his bladder and removed the largest vesicle calculus that I have seen. It weighed a pound!'

—D. COLEMAN TRAINOR, UCC, JULY 1945, RACS ARCHIVES

'About this time last year I circulated a questionnaire on current practice in Prostatectomy largely with the idea of assessing the influence of the late Harry Harris' work twenty years after its introduction. Fourteen replies were received from Australia and New Zealand, some of them in great detail, and all of real interest. Thanks a lot.

In the analysis these fourteen report that their combined prostates number 1739, divided into three methods—

Suprapubic	*652*
T.U.R.	*1016*
Millin	*71*

Discussing the suprapubic cases almost everyone said he did a Harris with some modification usually in the form of a resort to drainage of the bladder by one of a variety of methods.'

—FRANK MACKY, UCC, NOVEMBER 1948, RACS ARCHIVES

ing rivalry among urologists. The two things, of course, went together. Mortensen's generation fostered young urologists because they needed more urologists, but that did not mean that the struggle to win and hold a place in the specialty was not tougher with increased competition.[24]

Meanwhile, the Correspondence Club made an important contribution to the Society's aim of furthering the science of urology. Although funny stories and medical politics cropped up now and then in the letters, most were devoted to discussions of difficult or interesting cases. The senior men showed a willingness to admit their failures on paper and the junior men and especially the Associate Members were not too proud to ask for help.

As a result, the Urological Correspondence Club began strongly. There were two letters a month for the first two years, with brief breaks for the annual meetings, and three letters a month from 1947 to provide space for the increased membership.

Clinical cases in 1945 and 1946 record the novelty of penicillin and the good results that followed from its use. Kirkland, Power and Tait commented on the possible relationship between excessive consumption of tomatoes and crystalline deposits in the urine. In 1948 a number of letters reported on the use of streptomycin in cases of TB, but the letters also at times offer us glimpses of the personalities behind the foundation of the Urological Society.

'As the senior urologist at present practising in Australasia', wrote Silverton in his first letter, 'I rejoice to see the establishment of yet another link between the widely scattered workers in our fascinating specialty.'

John Power wrote on the state of urology in Brisbane where the three urologists at the Brisbane General Hospital had eighty-one occupied urological beds. There was plenty of room for a fourth man, he noted. 'Southern hopefuls please keep your seats.' Power's views on 'the south' can also be glimpsed in the story he tells of a junior general surgeon 'recently arrived from the south' who 'objected to urology and orthopaedics being special departments, considering this was part of the general surgeon's domain.'

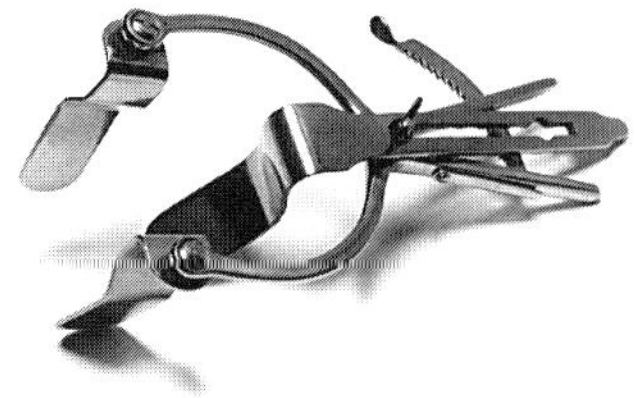

Millin retractor for retropubic prostatectomy donated by John Somerset. Millin first described his prostatectomy in 1945. (*Source:* Urological collection, RACS)

The New Zealand urologists also found the letters enjoyable. At last there was an activity of the USA in which they could participate on equal terms. Edgar Reay's first letter in June 1945 ranged from penicillin through the shortage of staff due to the war and the inspiration of Harry Harris to the trials of 'political medicine'. In August 1945 Patrick Treahy wrote straightforwardly that he was feeling remote in New Zealand and welcomed the regular exchange of ideas.[25]

The Urological Correspondence Club helped make the USA truly Australasian.

Conclusion

The isolation of Australasia's widely scattered urologists was a very real problem. Between 1937 and 1944, the Urological Society did little to relieve that isolation. It was just too difficult, expensive and time-consuming to get from Wellington, or even Melbourne, to Sydney for a brief meeting of fellow specialists. These formidable problems of geography were compounded by the restrictions on travel during the war years.

From 1944, however, with longer and more interesting annual meetings, and not always in Sydney, matters began to improve. The foundation of the Urological Corrrespondence Club and the end of the war both contributed to improved communication between the members of the Society. By 1948 the USA was beginning to play a real role in helping to bring urologists around Australasia together. Distance was no barrier to participation in the UCC and by 1948 the New Zealanders were able to think it might be their society too.

The Auckland urologists were slow to join, although Howard Gaudin was eligible from 1940. Frank Macky became an Associate Member in July 1946. However, the Society was incorporated in 1948 without a single member from either Western Australia or Tasmania.[26]

Despite the problems of small and scattered numbers, the Society was a success. Besides the growth in membership and attendance at the Annual Meetings, this success can be measured in the response of the RACS.

In 1949 the President, George Bell, and the Vice-President, Harold Dew, produced a 'Memorandum on the relationship of the College of Surgeons and various special sections of surgery'. Dew was a guest at the eighth Annual Meeting of the Urological Society. He and Bell wrote that New South Wales Fellows in particular were 'perturbed about the drift of surgical specialists away from the College.' The associations of Opthalmologists, Urologists, Orthopaedists and Neurosurgeons were specifically mentioned. All were described as having well attended and attractive scientific meetings which were tending to draw attendance away from the College meetings. This was seen as a particular problem when the specialist society did not hold its meeting in the same city as the College meeting. 'For example, the Urologists, a powerful association, has a meeting next year in Brisbane and the College has one in Adelaide, so that it is doubtful whether many will attend both meetings.'[27]

Some progress, it would seem, had been made in obtaining recognition for the specialty from the general surgeons.

PART 2

~

The Urological Society of Australasia, 1948–1996

~

CHAPTER 4

The Scientific Meetings of the Urological Society of Australasia

~

Introduction[1]

Throughout the 1950s, the Society remained firmly centred around Macquarie Street, Sydney. Five of the first ten meetings of the new, incorporated, Society were held there and that is where the Executive also met, until June 1951 when the meetings were moved to the University Club in Phillip Street, the next street back from the Domain.

This dominance by Macquarie Street is hardly surprising given the membership of the Society. In 1950, fifteen of the twenty-seven full members were from New South Wales and of those fifteen, only J. Broughton, from Newcastle, did not have an address in Macquarie Street. Over the years, the proportion of the membership from New South Wales gradually declined, but the Executive continued to meet in Sydney and until 1957, all the members of the Executive were from Sydney with the possible exceptions of the president, past president and vice-president. In any one year, one of these three would be from Melbourne and one from Brisbane. But these 'interstate' members of the Executive, as they were revealingly called, seldom attended meetings. The cost was too high. They did, however, receive copies of the minutes.

At Henry Mortensen's suggestion, major decisions of the Executive were reserved for two meetings, one just before the Annual Scientific Meeting, when the 'interstate' members were generally present, and the other in about December. In practice, interstate past presidents and vice presidents seldom attended executive meetings and even interstate presidents varied in attendance, and hence in influence on the Executive. This gave the Sydney presidents greater influence than their interstate colleagues.[2]

Keith Kirkland was Secretary and Treasurer in 1937-46, President in 1947-48, Treasurer again in 1950-53 and never off the Executive from the foundation of the Society until 1956. His large personality and boundless self-confidence dominated the first twenty years of the Society. This was despite the counterbalancing force of Henry Mortensen's equally impressive presence in Melbourne. If they had been antagonists, the Society might have turned out very differently, but they were friends. They attended so many overseas meetings together that Warwick Macky recalls that in the United States they were known as the heavenly twins.[3]

Mortensen contributed ideas and energy to a show that was run from Sydney and the interplay of those two personalities and Power in Brisbane laid the foundations for the good-natured rivalry between States that moulded the annual meetings. Although the dominance of Sydney declined over time, it remained an important factor in the development and thinking of the Society.

Rivalry between urologists was always important, but it was tempered by the need for more urologists, particularly in the early years and particularly outside Sydney. There was also rivalry between the States and hence an emotional investment in the annual meetings. The scientific program of the annual meetings provided a stage for individuals to shine and the social program provided a stage for the States to show what they could do.

Scientific Meetings 1948–1957—Establishing Rituals

The rivalries within urology, both personal and between the States, were partly contained and channelled by the rituals established at the annual meetings. The framework for this was largely set by the Executive in Sydney.

In later years, the work of the Society grew to encompass a broad role, representing Australasian urologists to the AMA, the RACS, Governments, both State and Federal, hospitals, other specialist organisations, overseas urologists and the general public. During the 1950s, however, although recognised as the representative body for urologists, the amount of work of the Society was limited. In May 1959, for instance, the Secretary reported receiving only four letters since the previous Executive meeting in April. Most of the time and energy of the Executive went into planning the annual scientific meetings.

Meetings rotated between Sydney, Brisbane and Melbourne. Each meeting had a local secretary who assisted the president in arranging the social side of the meeting. The Executive in Sydney played a much greater role in drawing up the program for the scientific side of the meeting.

Keith Kirkland in particular put a great deal of effort into trying to persuade distinguished overseas urologists to attend the meetings. In 1949 and 1950 he succeeded, but for the next three years he suffered

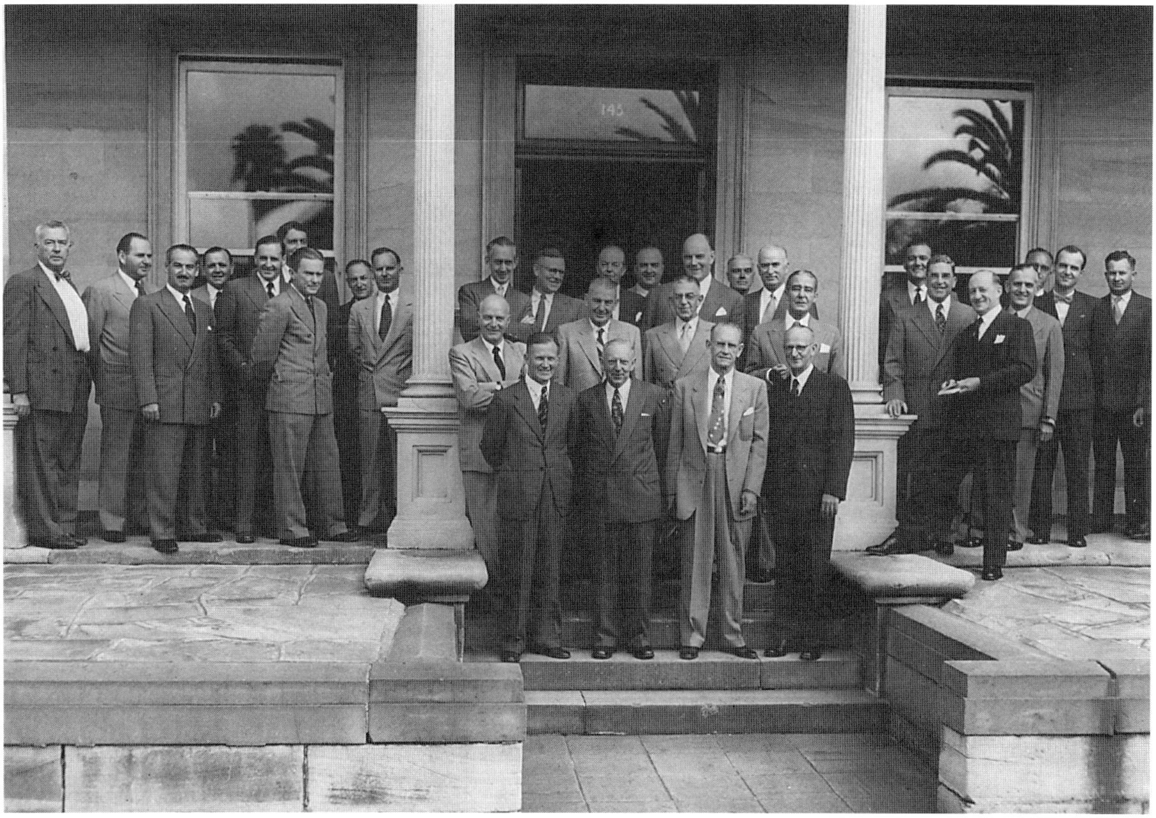

Delegates to the 1954 meeting in Sydney outside 145 Macquarie Street. The group of nine on the left is: Keith Kirkland, Errold Maloney, Lionel Jacobs, Hugh Pearson, Jim Peters, Noel Bonnin half hidden at the back, Gordon Pfeiffer and Alban Gee. The central group includes Colin Edwards, who was President that year, on the right of the front row. Beside him is the principal guest, Roger Barnes from the United States. The other two in the front are Des Trainor and Peter Row. Behind them on the steps are, from the left, Bernays Melville, Edgar Reay (the only New Zealander present), Richard Harris and Malcolm Earlam. At the back are Leonard Murphy, Ron Davidson, John Laidley, Mick Hogg, Henry Mortensen, Harold Moore peering over his shoulder and Jack Power. The group on the right is Ian Potts, Eric Kyle, Bobby Silverton, Paul Hopkins, Arthur Carrodus, Charles Roe and Llew Wheeler. (Information and copies of photos supplied by Moira Peters, Gwen Pearson and Harold Story)

repeated disappointments. Millin might attend—Millin was not coming; Flock was invited—Flock would only attend if the Society could pay his fares; Huggins was invited—Huggins couldn't come; and so it went on. The Society only managed to persuade O'Conor and Scholl to attend the 1950 meeting, because they were coming to Australia anyway. This was also the case with Roger Barnes in 1954. When the Executive heard he was coming to Australia, the Secretary wrote back offering to set the date of the 1954 meeting to suit Barnes' itinerary.

During the 1950s the position of 'program arranger' evolved. This mainly involved doing what Kirkland had always done anyway, and he held the position from 1953, when he stepped down as Treasurer, until 1956, when he resigned from the Executive. Supposedly, the program arranger was appointed by the incoming Executive, at the annual meeting. The position triggered a rare glimpse of conflict on the Executive. In April 1955, while Keith Kirkland was away overseas, Hugh Pearson was appointed to take over as program arranger. There was something of a row at the September meeting, Pearson stepped down, saying he had misunderstood Kirkland's wishes and Kirkland was reinstated.

After Kirkland's retirement, Lionel Jacobs arranged the

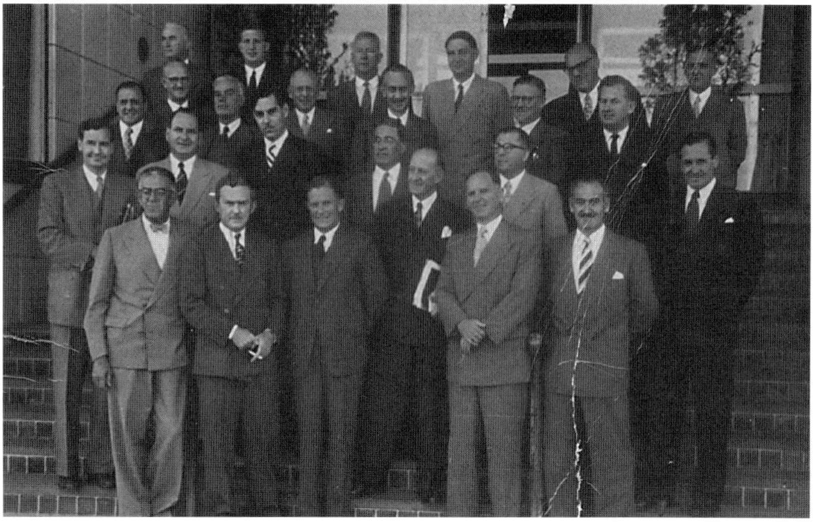

Delegates to the 1955 meeting in Melbourne, photographed on the Grattan Street steps of the Royal Melbourne Hospital. In the front row, from the left, are Richard Harris, John Somerset, cigarette in hand, who was President that year, Peter Row, who succeeded him, Bobby Silverton, Alban Gee and Lionel Jacobs. Behind Richard Harris are Doug Duffy, Hugh Pearson, Errold Maloney, Colin Edwards and, at the top of the steps, Jack Power. Behind Somerset are Jim Mortensen, Harold Moore and, at the top of the steps, Bill Utley. On his left are Des Trainor and Keith Kirkland. Behind Silverton are Eric Kyle, Leonard Murphy and Noel Bonnin. O. J.Ellis and Ron Davidson are standing behind Alban Gee and the group of four at the top right are Henry Mortensen, Llew Wheeler, Paul Hopkins and Jim Peters. (*Source:* Muriel Gee)

scientific programs for a couple of years, but the general pattern was for the president and a few members of the Executive to arrange the program between them.

The interstate presidents in this era—Lukin, Moore, Power, Somerset and Row, may have had only a limited say in the scientific program, but they had more room to make their mark on the social program. The meeting began with a Sunday outing, at first wholly and later partly paid for by the local members and the other key rituals were a formal dinner (men only, dinner jacket) and the President's At Home. In this era, this was often held in the President's own house, hosted by his wife.

These early meetings were relatively inexpensive and run on a tight budget. There was no money, for instance, for a tape recorder at the 1950 meeting in Surfers Paradise, so a stenographer was employed instead. The registration fee was £4, and this covered the cost of the annual dinner plus tea and coffee breaks. The Scientific Meeting itself cost very little. At that 3rd Meeting, both Mortensen and Lukin were in favour of a trade exhibition in 1951, but nothing seems to have come of it. The first recorded trade stand was Watson Victor, in 1954.

At the 1950 meeting, the Society decided to break with any idea of holding the meetings in conjunction with the College of Surgeons. This seems to have been the result of a row over a meeting held on 12 July in Sydney. In an attempt to take full benefit from the visit of Dr V. J. O'Conor, a joint meeting was arranged with the RACS. At the AGM in Brisbane, 12 days later, Keith Kirkland moved that the 1951 meeting 'not be held concurrently with the College of Surgeons meeting in Sydney as lecture room facilities would be overcrowded, previous co-operation with the College had not always been happy, and June was an indifferent month in Sydney.' Henry Mortensen seconded the motion and the date of the meeting was changed to April.

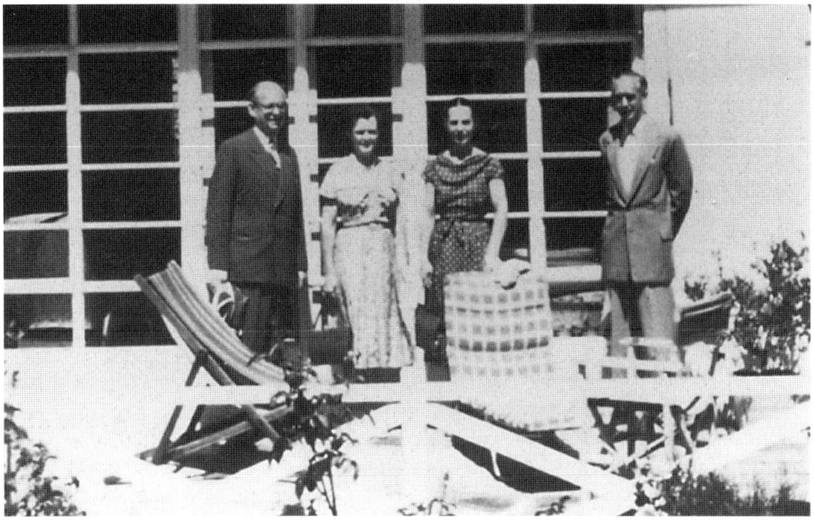

Professor Ljunggren and Mrs Blackman, at the home of Betty and Leonard Murphy, Hawthorn, March 1959. That year, Murphy was the President and Betty Murphy was again involved in entertaining on behalf of the Urological Society. Einar Ljunggren from Sweden was the international guest and he stayed with the Murphys. 'He was a very easy guest. He would click his heels and bow and say goodnight. On the days when Leonard had to go out, he would go for a walk. He was never any trouble.' (*Source:* Betty Murphy)

In 1952, Leonard Murphy was the local secretary for the meeting in Melbourne and his wife, Betty, remembers that in those days the wives were not allowed to attend the Annual Dinner. Instead, she entertained them, all thirteen of them, at her home. In April 1953, at the sixth meeting, Power (who found the time and money to attend every meeting of the Executive in 1952-53), managed to replace the formal dinner with a dinner dance—dress informal and ladies, of course, welcome. In July the Executive resolved firmly to return to the formal dinner, men only.

Scientific Meetings 1958–1967—Making Money

Every three years, the rotation of meetings between New South Wales, Victoria and Queensland gave members in those States a chance to be president. By 1955, this was becoming a problem. Laidley, the last of the Australian foundation members yet to be president was vice-president. Victoria and Queensland had already had second generation members as presidents (Lukin, Moore, Somerset, Row). With the aid of a few extra meetings in Sydney, all the foundation NSW members had had a turn, plus Telfer. It really was Edgar Reay, and New Zealand's, turn.

In 1956, Edgar Reay was elected vice President. The choice of Christchurch for the 1958 meeting was not, initially, unanimous. Eric Kyle, from Western Australia, had joined the Society and he wanted the 1958 meeting there. WA was the venue for the 1958 RACS meeting, but the Society had long broken free from any link between the two meetings.

Henry Mortensen and Keith Kirkland both backed the move away from the three-State rotation and at Mortensen's instigation this was reinforced by a change in the membership of the Executive. From the 1957 meeting onwards, there was a representative of each State

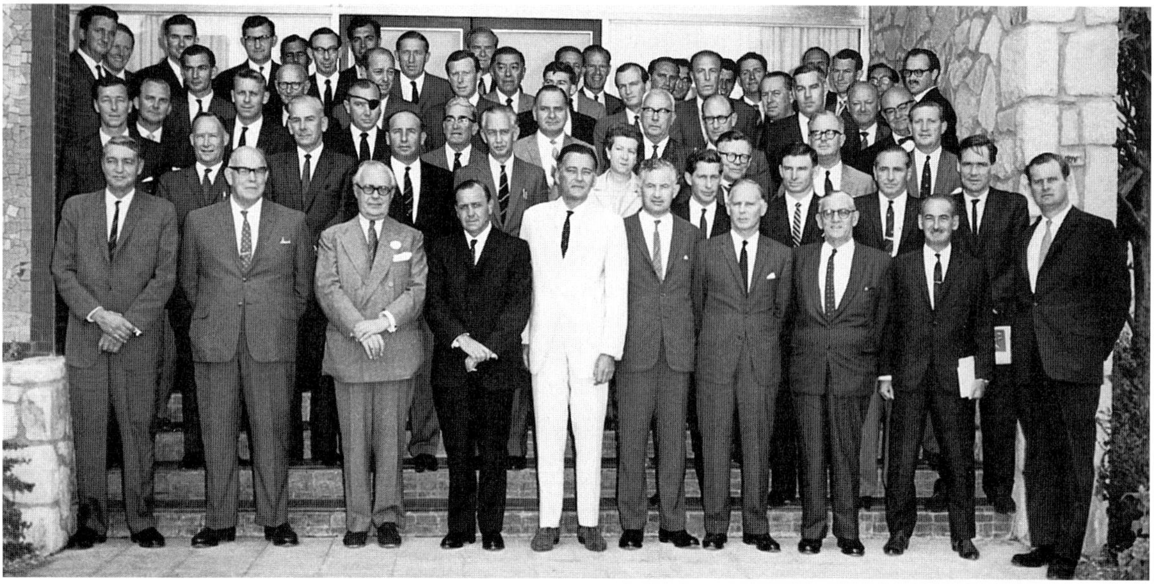

Delegates to the meeting in Canberra in 1963. Ian Potts is standing in the middle of the front row wearing the white suit. On his right is Hugh Pearson, President that year, and beside him are Leslie Pyrah (the principal guest), Henry Mortensen and Noel Bonnin. On Potts' left are Llew Wheeler (President elect), Alban Gee, Paul Hopkins, Lionel Jacobs and John Blackman. There are 61 urologists in this photograph, an indication of both the growing membership of the Society and the increased readiness of members to travel to meetings. Jim Gray (directly behind Henry Mortensen), with Norman Greenslade on his left, Humphrey Gowland (right at the back, directly behind Leslie Pyrah) and Bill Utley (directly behind Lionel Jacobs) had all come over from New Zealand. Perhaps the most remarkable member of the group, however, is the first woman to join the Society. Lorna Sisely is standing behind Ian Potts' left shoulder.

on the Executive. It was recognised that the interstate members would not attend many meetings of the Executive, but they would receive the minutes and have a vote when they did attend. Of the next ten Annual Scientific Meetings, two were in New Zealand, three were in Melbourne, two were in Canberra (run by the NSW members), two were in Sydney and only one was in Queensland.

The 1958 meeting in Christchurch did cause some concern. Edgar Reay tried to arrange the date to fit in with transport from the North Island and Australia:

> *It seems the best date we can arrange is Tuesday February 18th. The Sydney plane arrives on Monday and the boat arrives in Wellington on Tuesday, but it is really silly anyone coming by boat as the plane trip is so easy. Anyone coming by ship will have to come down by the ferry on Tuesday night, arriving here Wednesday morning.*[4]

Bill Utley was the local secretary and he produced a questionnaire to try and find out how many members were planning to attend. By October 1957 he had only eight acceptances and wrote to Llew Wheeler: 'If we cannot get a quorum, do we continue with the meeting or not?'[5] In the end, fifteen members attended.

The 13th meeting, in Queensland in 1960, would have been a landmark if Mick Hogg had lived. He planned to invite women to the annual dinner. After his death, Alex Inglis stepped in as President and a separate dinner for the women was back on the program. The change finally came at the Canberra meeting in 1963. The formal men only dinner was replaced at the last minute. Perhaps it was the proximity of the Queen, who was visiting Canberra at the time, that tipped the balance, or perhaps it was the presence of Lorna Sisely, the first woman to join the Society.

The Melbourne meetings of 1959 and 1962 were the occasion for significant innovations. The first trade exhibition was in Melbourne in 1959 and the idea of paying the travel expenses of guests was raised. Warwick Macky said the Society should pay. Woodward proposed commercial sponsors, and a major change was underway. Meanwhile, in an old school building across the road from the Children's Hospital, Douglas Stephens was experimenting with poster sessions.

In 1962 Jim Peters was President, and he appointed Mike Salvaris to run the trade exhibition. Together they decided it was time the Society had some money. That year, Frank Hinman Jr, from the United States, was the principal guest. The Society paid his first class air fares and Peters and Salvaris persuaded General Motors Holden to provide a car and driver to meet him at the airport. At first, space in the trade exhibit was slow in selling. They were charging £100 per stand. After about a month, Salvaris sent out a reminder saying that space was selling fast and putting the price up to £200. 'We filled the place in about three days.' Jim Peters recalled paying for the 'day in the country' (at a place on the Mornington Peninsula owned by his wife's family). They made a profit on the meeting of £1,700. 'That was the first occasion that the Society had any money.'[6]

Not all subsequent meetings showed a profit and not all were attended by guests whose fares had been paid through the Society, but the penny pinching days of the fifties had gone. The Society could not only afford a tape recorder but also the services of a professional projectionist and there was no longer a shortage of guests for the meetings. Many urologists—from England, from the United States, from SE Asia—were finding an excuse to be in Australasia at the time of the annual meeting, whether they were receiving financial assistance with their fares or not. They did not only come to give papers. They came to learn and they came to have a good time.

Amongst the best remembered visitors from that era are the members of the Urological Travelling Club, from England. Several of them attended the Melbourne meeting in 1965 and returned for the Surfers Paradise meeting in 1972. Dick Mogg from Cardiff was a particular hit with the locals.

The costs of the social side of the meetings continued to climb as the States tried to outdo each other in the provision of entertainment. Even by 1957, the cost of the President's At Home had become too high to expect one person to pay, and it was partly subsidised from registration fees. From 1958 onwards, the Society, or rather the members of the Executive, tried to ensure that the full cost was met by registration fees. They did not always succeed. Interstate presidents and their local committees showed a persistent inclination to cover some of the costs themselves, both on the Sunday outings and for the President's At Home. They were the hosts and they were determined to be hospitable. This warmth contributed enormously to the success of the meetings.

There is a story about the 1966 meeting in Auckland which illustrates at least something of the atmosphere during the social functions:

> *When delegates to Auckland stayed in the White Heron Lodge about a quarter of spouses attended. Bill Utley was fortunate that his wife Pat came. They left the drinkers Murnaghan, Gray and others after the dinner and retired early. Bill had to get up to the toilet a little later. In the dark he thought he opened the bathroom door but when he looked up he was in the hotel corridor and the door had snibbed shut. Pat was a heavy sleeper so there he was quite starkers. Ever resourceful he crept down the corridor and out onto the balcony. He was making his way back to his bedroom window when the drinkers flung back the curtains to clear the air only to reveal Bill in all his glory.*[7]

At around this time, sport also began to feature strongly in the social side of meetings. John Maddern recalled that 'golf was the key side show of the American meetings' and in about 1963 he and Steve Ferguson started playing in an exclusive four at the Australasian meetings. '[We] used to leave the meeting with noise and clatter.' 'The golf day became quite a feature of the meetings ... One of the highlights of the dinner was to present the golf trophy ...'[8]

Scientific Meetings 1968–1977 —Women and Children too

In this era, the Executive was increasingly busy with matters other than the Annual Meeting and the local committee took over a correspondingly larger proportion of the work. From the mid-1960s, Joe Murnaghan was generally involved on the scientific program committee and had a cumulative impact on the amount of academic urology featured at meetings.

In the search for variety in both guests and entertainment, the meetings were held in a wider range of cities. Between 1968 and

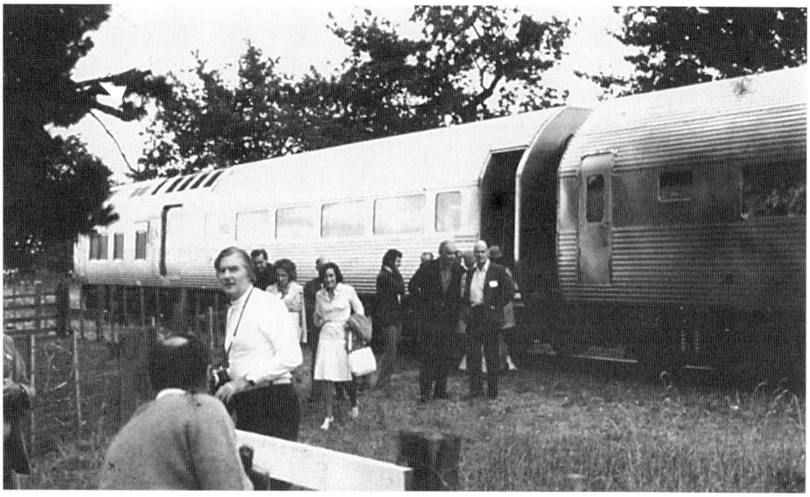

Humphrey Gowland's train, Wellington, 1973. Harry Learoyd, Gwyn Pearson, Elizabeth Macky, Humphry Gowland, Warwick Macky. (*Source:* Dennis Arnold)

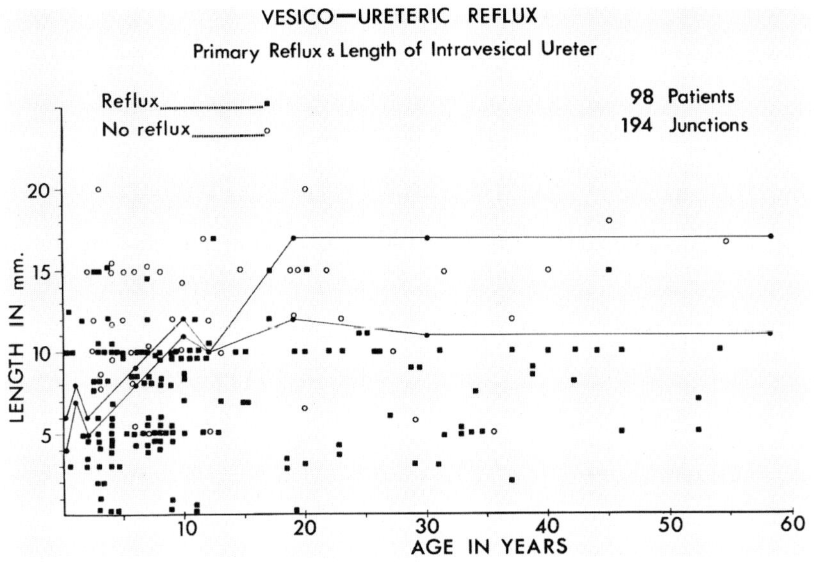

A typical Murnagram. In his efforts to bring academic urology to the meetings, Joe Murnaghan frequently showed slides of scattergrams. These were generally regarded as ranging from obscure to incomprehensible, so Warwick Macky christened them 'Murnagrams' and the name stuck. (*Source:* Joe Murnaghan)

1977, there were three meetings in Sydney, two in Melbourne, one in Surfers Paradise, one in Wellington and, for the first time, meetings in Adelaide, Perth and overseas in Hong Kong. Planning for the Hong Kong meeting in particular took years. The idea of an overseas venue was first officially raised in 1972, when Singapore was suggested, because the RACS was planning a meeting there in 1973.

Tourist brochures first began to accompany information on the meetings in 1971, for the Sydney meeting that year. The meetings were becoming almost too popular, and the costs at that meeting nearly got out of hand, partly because of inflation, but also partly because of 'an unprecedented number of visitors'. A special charge for the Ladies Program was introduced at the last moment, to help cover costs.

During this period, it became increasingly common for urologists to attend the meetings accompanied by their wives, and even partners and second wives, although this reflection of the rising divorce rate was frowned on by the more conservative members. The other major innovation during the 1970s was allowing children to attend some of the social functions. As usual, it was the Queenslanders who tried to lead the way in this further break with formality. Jeff Watson was President in 1972 and in his September 1971 newsletter about the forthcoming meeting in Surfers Paradise wrote:

> *The Sunday outing shall be by launch from the Nerang river at the end of Cavill Avenue, Surfers Paradise to Charles Roe's camp on Stradbroke Island. This time the Executive are experimenting by allowing a limited number of children to come. We have considered accepting applications for the children of members from southern states only. The ladies will have an all day outing on Monday. Tuesday afternoon shall be for golf and tennis. Wednesday afternoon shall be a half day outing when husbands may accompany their wives.*[9]

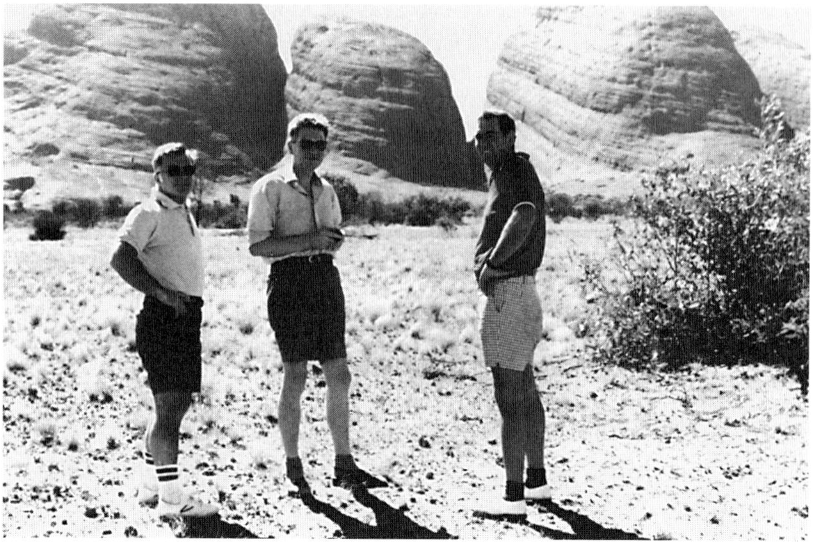

Before the Adelaide meeting in 1978, there was a trip to central Australia. The photograph shows *(left to right)* two of the international guests, Ralph Straffon from the United States and Richard Turner-Warwick from England with the President, Peter Harbison. (*Source:* Gwen Pearson)

At the Executive meeting on 11 February 1972, it was decided to revert to no children on the Sunday outing. The Society was a very conservative organisation and any change of this kind took years to become accepted.

By 1972 the meetings had become major events requiring considerable advance organisation. Jeff Watson, for instance, began looking for guests as early as 1969 and when he was in London for a meeting of the BAUS, he approached Dick Mogg, from Cardiff. Mogg indicated that 'the boys of the Urological Travelling Club would be extremely pleased to come.' Watson did not have so much luck with Professor Oetama, who was unable to attend, but Howard Hanley, John Williams, Philip Clark, Selby Tulloch and Dick Mogg made up a strong British Urological Travelling Club contingent. They were joined by Professor Nordin from Leeds, whose visit was funded by the Australian Kidney Foundation. Funding for guests was still a problem and the 1972 meeting benefited from the fact that the Nephrological Society Meeting was held the following week.

Despite the problems of funding and inflation, more and more visitors, especially from Asia, were attending the Scientific Meetings, and the fares of the principal guests were being sponsored by a range of organisations, including various drug companies.

Scientific Meetings 1978–1987—Registrars are invited

By the 1980s, the Scientific Meetings had become platforms for the display of the host city. Between 1978 and 1987 there were two meetings each in Adelaide and Melbourne and one each in Christchurch, Rotorua, Sydney, Canberra, Brisbane and Perth. The volume of business dealt with by the Executive had become consid-

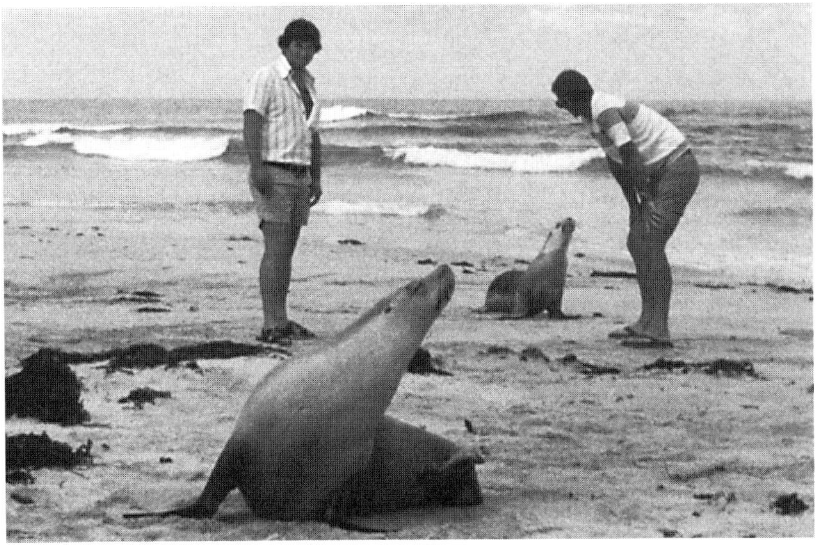

The 1978 Adelaide meeting incorporated a trip to Kangaroo Island, where Tony Tynan and Adrian Porter met a couple of sealions. (*Source:* Dennis Arnold)

erable, requiring more regular secretarial assistance. The meetings had also very much become the responsibility of the President and his organising committees, although ground rules were still laid down by the Executive.

By the time that Dennis Arnold became President, in 1981, the framework for rivalry between presidents over their meetings was well established. He arranged to hold the 1982 meeting in Canberra:

> *There was gentle competition among the presidents ... Humphrey Gowland put on a private train to take us up into the mountains ... I thought ... how can I outshine Humphrey? the High Court was the most impressive building [in Canberra] ... but how to influence a Government department? ... you could go from the bottom up or from the top down ... I went from the bottom up, started with the cleaners, got to the justices ... I had the President's Reception there at night.*[10]

The guests included J. Schüller who appeared on the program as the Storz Professor.

> *However, the Germans were unhappy to call Schüller a Professor as he was in fact a junior registrar in the Lithotripter Unit in Munich when we induced Karl Storz to provide the money to send him to our meeting and give us the first knowledge of ESWL.*[11]

During this period, presidents ceased to be chosen mainly on the basis of seniority. A positive contribution to the work of the Society became increasingly important and a number of presidents during the 1980s made their mark on the Society through involvement with the training program.

The running of the meetings was becoming increasingly complex and time-consuming as the number of registrants continued to rise. The Melbourne meeting in 1984, for instance, was organised by

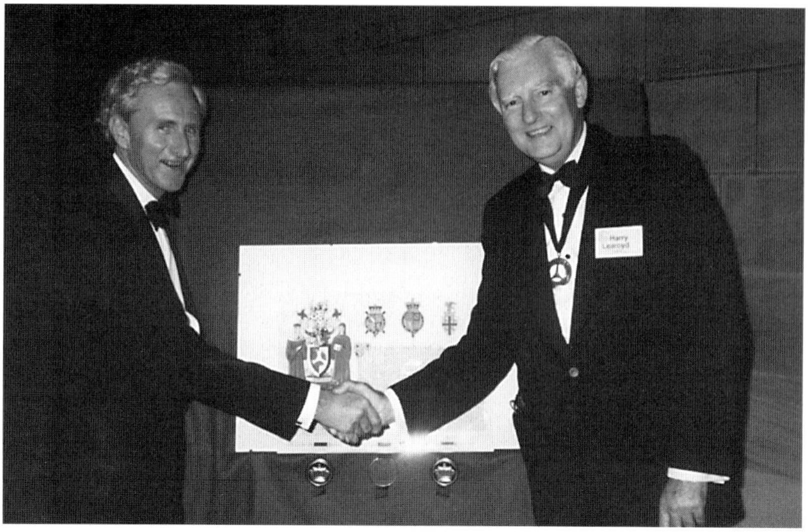

Harry Learoyd, President, accepting the Society's coat of arms from Don Urquhart-Hay, Sydney 1988

three committees, all made up of local people. One consisted of a professional conference consultant, plus the President (Dan Lenaghan) and Gerry Joyce. The second consisted of Ron Brown, Gerry Joyce and Dan Lenaghan and the third was the by now traditional ladies committee.

The principal guests in this era continued to be sponsored by the trade, plus some assistance from the RACS foundation, but the costs of the meetings escalated rapidly, as did the registration fees and the annual membership subscriptions. In 1969, the annual membership fee was $10.50, rising to $15 in 1970 and $25 in 1975. In 1983, the subscription was $50 Full, $40 Associate and in 1985 it rose to $80 Full, $65 Associate. Registration fees for the meetings rose even more rapidly and inflation was not the only explanation. The meetings were now generally held in five-star hotels, very much more expensive venues than the kind of hotels favoured in the 1970s, let alone the hospital halls of the 1950s and early 1960s.

This escalation in costs coincided with the acceptance of registrars as delegates to the meetings. In 1971 there were sixteen RACS-approved training posts and by 1988 this had risen to thirty. During the 1970s, despite the growing number of trainees, it was generally felt that registrars were not welcome at the meetings, although a few did apply for permission to attend, with varying success. The position changed dramatically in 1980. At the meeting in Christchurch, the Society decided to accept responsibility for training in urology throughout Australasia. Until then, there had been considerable co-operation with the College, but no coherent structured program.

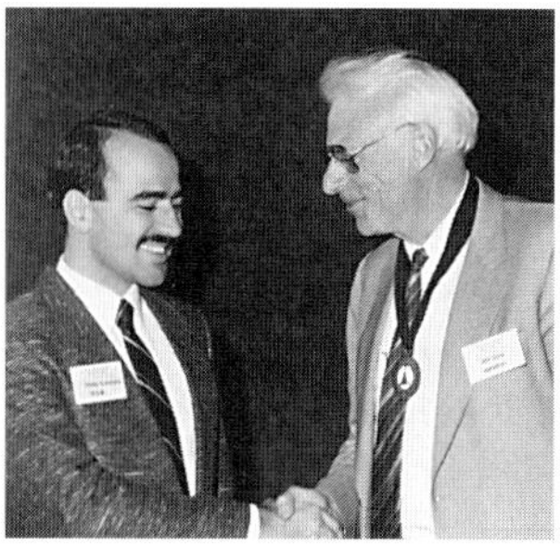

Jim Gray, President, congratulating Phillip Katelaris on winning the Keith Kirkland Prize at the Rotorua meeting, 1987. (*Source:* Jim Gray)

With the Society's increased involvement in training came a feeling that merely allowing registrars to attend the meetings was not enough. They should be strongly encouraged to attend. There followed a prolonged debate as to whether they should have to pay the full fees. The outcome of the argument varied from meeting to meeting. At the 1986 meeting in Perth, for instance, both registrars and New Zealanders were offered a 20 per cent discount, paying $280 instead of the full registration fee of $350.

Another indication of the Society's increased focus on training was the institution of the Keith Kirkland Prize. This was first awarded at the 1983 meeting in Brisbane, to the trainee who presented the best research paper (Stan Wisniewski). It was an instant hit and by 1984 had already become a highlight of the meeting. Besides the obvious rivalry between the registrars, it became a focus for the rivalry between urology units, as senior urologists took pride in the progress of 'their' registrars. From 1986, there was also the Alban Gee Poster Prize, for the best poster presentation. Together with the various sports prizes, these added a number of competitive elements to the program.

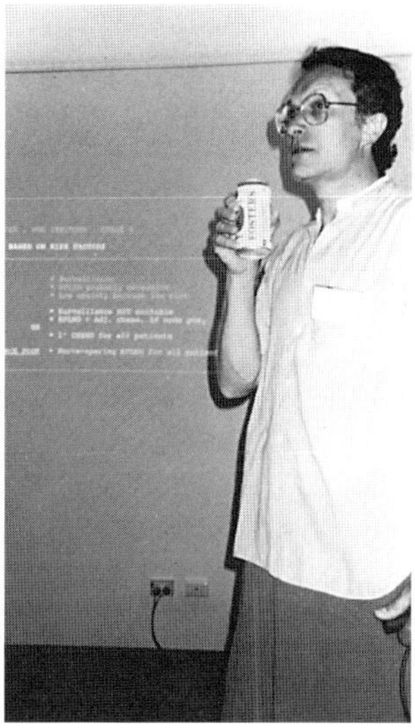

Reg Hall from Newcastle-on-Tyne was one of the principal guests at the 1990 Darwin meeting. Some of the scientific sessions took place in Kakadu National Park and Reg Hall is shown here presenting a paper Kakadu style. (*Source:* David Golovsky)

Scientific Meetings 1988–1997—and even Urological Nurses

By the late 1980s, the meetings were run by substantial local committees and over the years, the tasks had become fairly well defined. For the 1991 meeting on the Gold Coast, for instance, Graham Holmes was the President and overall meeting convenor, with considerable help from his wife, Pip. Philip McDougall and his wife 'Fred' ran the social program. Geof Hirst was in charge of the scientific program and Robin Spork dealt with trade sponsorship. The committee set out to raise a significant amount of money from the meeting in order to set up a fund for continuing medical education (CME).[12]

Despite this spreading of the workload, there was a growing recognition of the enormous amount of work now involved in running the Annual Scientific Meeting and acting as president. This was because the role of the president during the whole year of his term

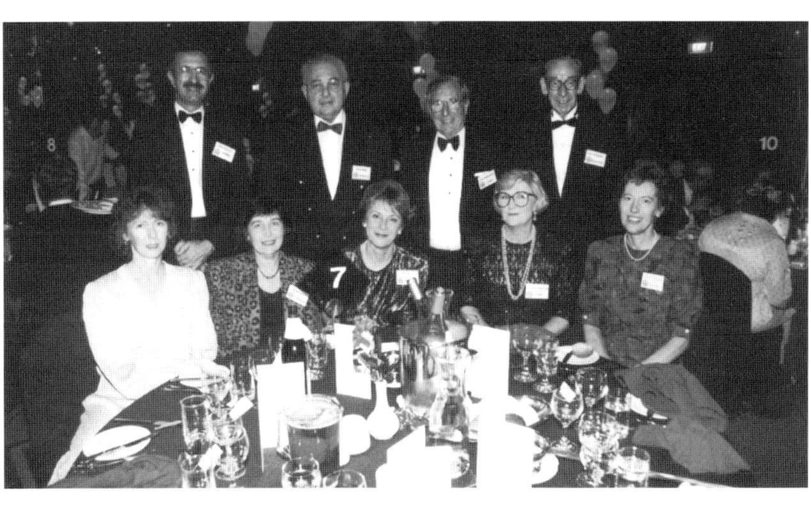

The Dinner Dance at the 1993 Hobart meeting was held in the ballroom of the Sheraton Hotel. The guests at this table are John Boulas, Ros Parisi, Joe Murnaghan and Dan Lenaghan plus Colleen Boulas, Marie Parisi, the Society's secretary, Gail Hill, Dulcie Murnaghan and Christine Lenaghan. (*Source:* Warren Johnson)

TABLE: ANNUAL MEETINGS OF THE UROLOGICAL SOCIETY OF AUSTRALASIA, 1937-1997

January 1937, Sydney, inaugural meeting, President Reg Bridge

I: *March 1938,* Sydney, President Jack Power

II: *March 1939,* Sydney, President John Tait

III: *March 1940,* Sydney, President Bobby Silverton (10 present)

IV: *April 1941,* Sydney, President Stanley Roe (Category of Associate Member introduced at special meeting, October 1941)

1942, no meeting, President Henry Mortensen

1943, no meeting, President Stanley Roe

V: *October 1944,* Lewisham, Royal North Shore and Sydney Hospitals, President Henry Mortensen (12 present; first scientific program in conjunction with Annual Meeting; Urological Correspondence Club founded)

VI: *October 1945,* Royal Melbourne, St Vincent's and Alfred Hospitals, President Henry Mortensen/Malcolm Earlam.[13] (13 present; first Annual Meeting with a social program)

VII: *1946,* Brisbane, President Malcolm Earlam/Jack Power

VIII: *April 1947,* Sydney, President Jack Power/Keith Kirkland. (37 present; *Proceedings* published for the first time)

IX: *February 1948,* Ballarat and Melbourne, President Keith Kirkland. (Last meeting of unincorporated Society)

1: *March 1948,* Sydney, President Henry Mortensen. (Procedural meeting only, first meeting of incorporated Society)

2: *June 1949,* Stawell Hall, Sydney, President Henry Mortensen/ Richard Harris. (34 present; guest E. Riches, England, first Honorary Member)

3: *July 1950,* Shell House, Brisbane, President Richard Harris/Pip Lukin. (26 present; guests A. J. Scholl and V. J. O'Conor, U.S., second and third Honorary Members)

4: *April 1951* Stawell Hall, Sydney, President Pip Lukin/Archie Telfer.[13] (28 present)

5: *February 1952,* Royal Melbourne Hospital, President Harold Moore

6: *April 1953,* Surfers Paradise Hotel, President Jack Power

7: *April 1954,* Stawell Hall, Sydney, President Colin Edwards. (Guest Roger Barnes, U.S., fourth Honorary Member)

8: *March 1955,* Royal Melbourne Hospital, President John Bowie Somerset

9: *April 1956,* Surfers Paradise Hotel, President Peter Row

10: *April 1957,* Blue Mountains and Stawell Hall, Sydney, President Malcolm Earlam. (Women's dinner, separate from men only formal Annual Dinner)

11: *February 1958,* Christchurch Hospital, President Edgar Reay. (15 present)

12: *March 1959,* St Vincent's and Royal Children's Hospitals, Melbourne, President Leonard Murphy. (31 present; guest Einar Ljunggren, Sweden; first trade exhibition)

13: *May 1960,* Broadbeach, Queensland, Presidents Mick Hogg[14] andAlex Inglis. (24 present; employed a professional projectionist for the first time)

14: *April 1961,* Stawell Hall, Sydney, President Alban Gee. (37 present)

15: *March 1962,* Prince Henry's Hospital, Melbourne, President Jim Peters. (Guest Frank Hinman Jr, US; first class air fares paid by Society; £1,700 profit)

16: *March 1963,* the Rex Hotel at Canberra, President Hugh Pearson. (First meeting where women joined the men for the Annual Dinner)

17: *April 1964,* Newport Motel, Sydney, President Llew Wheeler. (54 present)

18: *March 1965,* Southern Cross Hotel, Melbourne, President Doug Duffy. (67 present; four guests, members of the Urological Travelling Club, England)

19: *February 1966,* Medical Centre, Auckland Hospital, President Warwick Macky. (36 present; guest David Innes Williams, London)

20: *March 1967,* the Rex Hotel, Canberra, President Dick Craven. (36 present; guest Gustav Giertz, Stockholm)

21: *March 1968,* Chevron Hotel, Sydney, President Lionel Jacobs. (52 present; guest Dr Harry Spence, Dallas)

22: *March 1969,* St Vincent's Hospital/Southern Cross Hotel, Melbourne, President James Mortensen. (Principal guest Joseph J. Kaufman, LA; inaugural Harry Harris Oration)

23: *March 1970,* Hotel Australia, Adelaide, President John Maddern. (Principal guest Richard Turner-Warwick, first paper by a woman, Margaret Turner-Warwick)

24: *March 1971,* Wentworth Hotel, Sydney, President Jack Blackman. (Guests Willett F. Whitmore, New York, and G. B. Ong, Hong Kong)

25: *May 1972,* Iluka Motor Inn, Surfers Paradise, President Jeff Watson. (Guests, members of British Urological Travelling Club)

26: *March 1973,* James Cook Hotel, Wellington, President Humphrey Gowland. (Principal guest W. Gregoir, Brussels; wives could fly to New Zealand for less than their husbands)

27: *March 1974,* Old Melbourne Motor Inn, President Ken Burnside. (Several guests)

28: *April 1975,* Boulevarde Hotel, Sydney, President Bruce Pearson. (Principal guest Hans Marberger, Innsbruch)

29: *March 1976,* Queen Mary Hospital, Hong Kong, President Ian Potts. (Several guests from Japan)

30: *March 1977,* Perth, President Stan Watson. (English guests plus Madersbacher, Innsbruch; most Australasian papers from Perth)

31: *March 1978,* Australian Mineral Foundation & Gateway Inn, Adelaide, President Peter Harbison. (Principal guest Ralph Straffon, Cleveland)

32: *March 1979,* Melbourne Hilton, President Ian Nunn. (Principal guest Joseph C. Smith, Oxford)

33: *February 1980,* ChristchurchTown Hall, President Bill Utley. (Society accepts responsibility for supervising training in urology)

34: *March 1981,* Sydney Hilton, President Joe Murnaghan. (Guests included Victor Politano, Miami)

35: *March 1982,* Academy of Science, Canberra, President Dennis Arnold. (German guests provide early information on ESWL)

36: *April 1983,* Crest International Hotel, Brisbane, President Ros Parisi. (Guests included Johnston S. Passlow, alias Campbell McComas; inaugural Keith Kirkland Prize)

37: *April 1984,* Regent Hotel, Melbourne, President Dan Lenaghan. (143 participants, 89 accompanying persons)

38: *March 1985,* Adelaide Hilton International, President John Jose. (Guests included Michael Marberger, Vienna)

39: *April 1986,* Perth, President Ernie England. (Alban Gee Poster Prize inaugurated; features of the meeting included a view of Halley's Comet)

40: *March 1987,* Sheraton Hotel, Rotorua, President Jim Gray. (Guests included Patrick Walsh from Johns Hopkins, and Joseph Segura from Mayo Clinic)

41: *March 1988,* Regent Hotel, Sydney, President Harry Learoyd. (171 registrants, 107 associates; presentation of Coat of Arms to the Society)

42: *March 1989,* Hyatt on Collins, Melbourne, President Ron Brown. (Bought a computer for the Society office; urological nurses attended sessions)

43: *May 1990,* Beaufort Hotel, Darwin & Kakadu National Park, President Peter Maher. (From 1994, president no longer to convene meetings)

44: *April 1991,* Sheraton Mirage, Gold Coast, President Graham Holmes. (Guests included David Barrett from the Mayo Clinic; profit of $91 558 to start CME Fund)

45: *April 1992,* Convention Centre, Adelaide, President Villis Marshall. (Guests included Emil Tanagho and John Blandy; 201 registrants and 27 registrars)

46: *February 1993,* Sheraton Hotel, Hobart, President Warren Johnson. (Visitors included the presidents of BAUS, the AUA, the Japanese Urological Association and the Singapore Urological Association and the vice-president of the SIU)

47: *June 1994,* Cable Beach Club, Broome, President Stuart Taylor, convenor, Tony Low. (Guests included Paul Abrams, Helmut Madersbacher and George Webster)

48: *March 1995,* Sheraton Hotel, Auckland, President Ted Arnold, convenor Russell McIlroy. (Principal guests included Rolf Ackermann and David Neal)

49: *March 1996,* Hyatt Hotel, Canberra, President John Rogers, convenor Bob Wines. (Urological Nurses Association formed; guests included Christopher Woodhouse and Andrew von Eschenbach)

50: *May 1997,* Port Douglas, President Tony Low, convenor Robin Spork. (Guests included Paul Schellhammer, Laurent Bocon-Gibaud and Richard Haudmann)

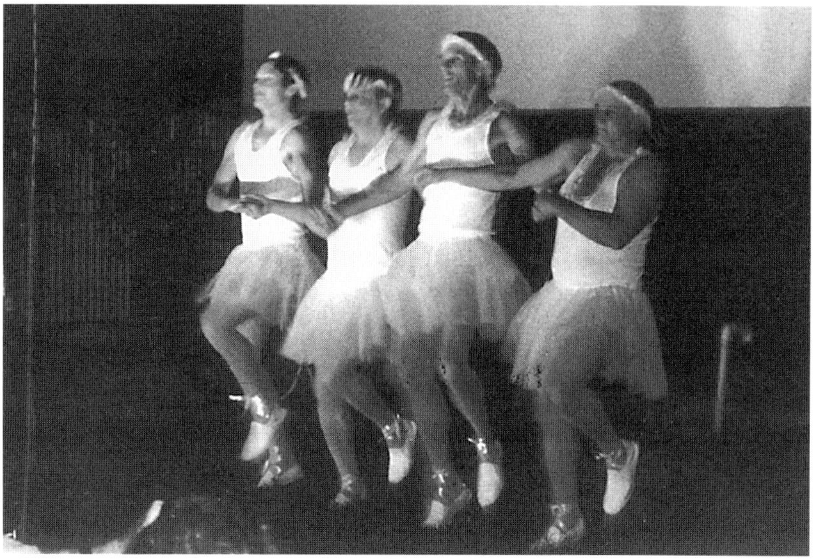

At the meeting in Broome in 1994, some 'swans' interrupted the showing of a film. Left to right: Tony Low, Alastair Tulloch, Andrew Low and Stan Wisniewski.

of office had increased enormously. The problem was first formally raised at John Jose's meeting in Adelaide in 1985 but a solution was not finally agreed until the 1990 meeting in Darwin. The first meeting run by a convener other than the president was in Broome in 1994, when Tony Low held the new position of ASM Convener.

The Broome meeting was also memorable for the after-effects of the golf. As has been noted, a number of urologists take their golf very seriously and various contests have come to have considerable significance as a part of the social rituals surrounding the meetings. In Broome, however, they were booby-trapped by the locals. Playing in high temperatures from spinifex fairways onto oiled sand greens, the urologists worked up a thirst. The only liquid refreshment provided was an esky full of beer at every other hole. At the Broome Golf Club that evening the golfers, more than one of them considerably the worse for wear, faced a large spit roast and piles of food, including a baking dish full of peas. Perhaps inevitably, it got knocked over and David Golovsky recalled the whole place turning green with wall to wall squashed peas.[15]

During the 1980s, urological nurses began to attend sessions at the meetings. A number of urologists were ambivalent about their presence. As Warren Johnson wrote in the report on his meeting in 1993:

> *Nurse registration again proved popular but there remains some controversy as to whether they are truly welcome and I think this should be discussed by the Executive with a view to the establishment of a policy and the level of charge.*

The nurses continued to attend meetings and in 1996 they formed the Urological Nurses Association.

CHAPTER 5

The Role of the Urological Society

~

Introduction

The Urological Society of Australasia is a highly successful professional organisation. That is to say, it has achieved for its members a high degree of professional autonomy and with this, the associated high status and income. The Society has not, of course, operated in a vacuum and this chapter outlines the activities of the Society in relation to other organisations, particularly the Australian Federal Government, the AMA and the RACS.

In its relationships with the College, the Society has acted as an Australasian organisation and in matters of training, accreditation, examination, continuing medical education and membership, New Zealand is fully a part of the picture. In its relationships with most other bodies, the Society acts as an Australian organisation, partly because of the balance of membership, but mainly because most of the outside organisations are themselves Australian and not Australasian.

The Society's success in achieving professional autonomy has been greater in some areas than in others and it has possibly been greater in Australia than in New Zealand. Economic autonomy—the degree of freedom that urologists have to determine their own rates of pay—was severely restricted in New Zealand even before the Society was formed. Political autonomy—the acceptance of the Society as representing the legitimate experts on urological matters and as the legitimate policy making body for matters affecting what the Articles of Association of the Society describe as 'the science of urology'—has generally been limited in both countries to matters of professional expertise. It is in the area of clinical autonomy that the Society has had greatest success.[1]

Through the Society, Australasian Urologists set urological standards and are largely self-regulating. They also choose, train and examine their successors, and provide for the continuing medical education of established specialists. The Society sets its own qualifications for membership and these have been widely accepted as defining the specialty of urology in Australasia. Through its control of membership and, from the 1980s, of training, the Society also has control of the qualifications for entry to the specialty. In addition, through its role in the accreditation of training posts and the selection of trainees it has the ability to directly influence the number of new entrants to the specialty. This is perceived, particularly from outside the medical profession, as a controversial area, not least because of the potential impact on the economic autonomy, bargaining power and incomes of urologists.[2]

Membership and Gatekeeping

The half century after 1948 was a time of rapid growth in the population of Australasia and a time of even more rapid growth in the membership of the Urological Society. While the population of Australasia grew from 9.5 million in 1947 to 20.7 million in 1991, the membership of the Urological Society grew from 42 to 251 in the same period. This represents a change from a population of about 226 000 per member of the Society in 1948 to about 82 500 per member in 1991.

While much of the rapid growth in the population of Australasia, especially in the late 1940s and 1950s, was the result of immigration from places other than the British Isles, the Society remained Anglo-Celtic in outlook. The Articles of Association specified that members had to be 'graduates of British Universities or Colleges'. From 1950 this was modified to 'be required to hold a surgical degree obtained by a two part examination of a British University or College'.

During the 1950s there was much debate about including graduates of non-British institutions, but it was decided that they should remain ineligible for membership in the normal manner. They might, however, be invited by the Executive to become members or associate members. This only appears to have happened twice. In 1953, B. Endelman, a Polish graduate and Fellow of the International Society of Urology, was invited to become an Associate Member and in 1966 Andrew Bogdan, a Hungarian graduate, was invited to become a Full Member.

Although the Articles of Association of the Society were racist, they were not sexist. Throughout the correspondence and minutes of the Society in the 1950s and 1960s the language was routinely sexist, but the Articles of Association referred to 'persons', 'graduates'and 'surgeons'. Consequently, when Lorna Sisely applied for Associate Membership in 1960, no special provision, or even official comment, was required before she was admitted. It was to be a long time before the next woman was admitted. Hilary Boucaut became a Full Member in 1989 and Helen O'Connell became a Provisional Member in 1993.

The membership rules as they stood in 1951 are reproduced in figure 5.1. They embody the ideas of the main figures in the Society at that time, particularly Henry Mortensen and Keith Kirkland, who seem to have been quite clear about what they wanted and to have held steadfastly to their view in the face of considerable opposition from other members of the Society.

5. Membership of the Society shall be limited to Persons (a) who are or have been engaged in the practice of urology, or (b) who take a special interest in urology' and the various classes of membership shall be further limited as follows:

(A) Full Member: to surgeons who in Australia or New Zealand Practise exclusively or having retired and having at the time of retirement practised exclusively the speciality of urology and are graduates of British Universities or Colleges <u>PROVIDED</u> that except in cases judged by the Executive to be special, an applicant for full membership shall as from the first day of January One thousand nine hundred and fifty be required to hold a surgical degree obtained by a two part examination of a British University or College.

Amended by Special resolution of 16/4/51.

(B) Fellow: to persons who are full members of the Society and have rendered distinguished service to the Society and the practice of urology.

(C) Associate Member: to graduates of British Universities or Colleges who

(i) being precluded by special circumstances from practising urology exclusively, practise general surgery or medicine in addition to urology or

(ii) being medical practitioners are engaged in Australia or New Zealand in the study of urology with a view to practising exclusively in that specialty.

(D) Honorary Member: to distinguished urologists who practise or have practised urology elsewhere than in Australia or New Zealand.

(E) Honorary Associate Member: to medical practitioners or scientists who do not practise urology but are actively interested in some phase or aspect of urology.

(F) Honorary Visiting Member: to visiting surgeons who are actively interested in some phase or aspect of urology.

The membership regulations of the Urological Society, 1951, from the Articles of Association

Keith Kirkland was, from the beginning of the Society, strongly of the view that membership should be restricted to full-time urological surgeons. It has already been noted in Chapter 3 that he maintained this view, even when it threatened the viability of the Society. Kirkland was also a key figure in upholding the same principles for the urological section of the New South Wales branch of the BMA.

The section met sporadically for a number of years during the war, while the Urological Society was floundering. After the war with improved scientific meetings, interest in the Urological Society increased and interest in the NSW section of urology of the BMA waned. There was no quorum for the annual meeting in either 1949 or 1950 and so the proposal to widen membership was revived.

An extraordinary meeting of the section was called for 5 November

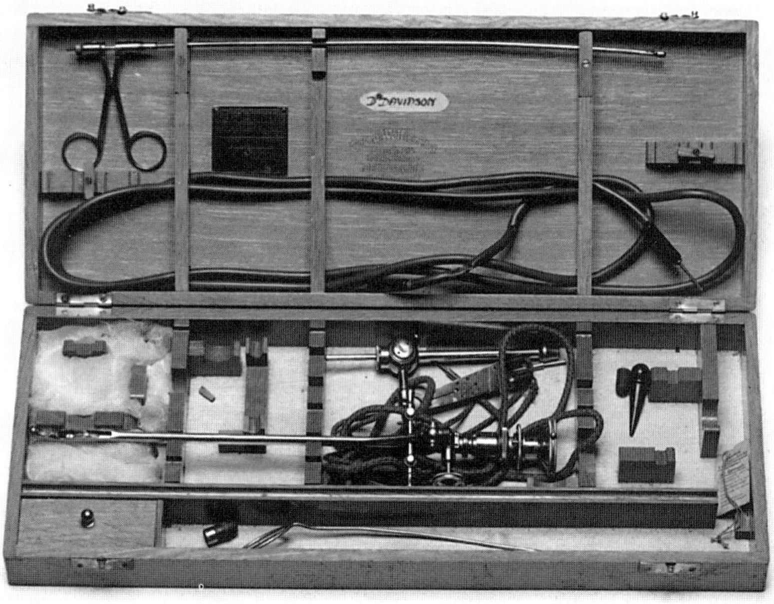

Ron Davidson's Wolf Operating Cystoscope. A style of instrument developed in 1910, this model was used by Ron Davidson in Ballarat from 1929. (*Source:* Urological collection, RACS)

1951 to discuss a motion to open membership to all NSW members of the BMA. Keith Kirkland was unable to attend, but made his views plain in a letter to the Secretary:

> *I feel very strongly that it would be a retrograde step to let down the barriers and allow membership to members of the profession, untrained in urology and doing other work.*[3]

The motion to widen membership was defeated, with the feared impact on attendances, and the section did not meet again until 26 July 1954. Fortunately, the Urological Society did not suffer the same fate, but the arguments over membership rules were only just beginning.

The Society's rules originally specifically excluded surgeons who were not 'graduates of British Universities or Colleges'. When drawn up, this was effectively an anti-American clause, but post-war migration from Europe forced the Executive to reconsider the position and in 1951 the rules were amended from the form in figure 5.1, giving the Executive the discretion to invite suitably qualified graduates from other colleges and universities to become members or associate members.[4]

The rules for full membership were both strict and clear and there seems to have been little debate over them in the Executive. The restrictions on full membership had a number of effects. Urologists still practising some general surgery were encouraged to become full-time urologists. This was in line with the objective of the Society to 'further the science of Urology'. Acceptance for membership of the Society increasingly acted as a form of accreditation. From an early date, the Society was prepared to lobby hospitals on behalf of members who complained when anyone who was not a member was appointed to a position as Urologist. The number of full members was strictly limited to those who were prepared to practise full-time

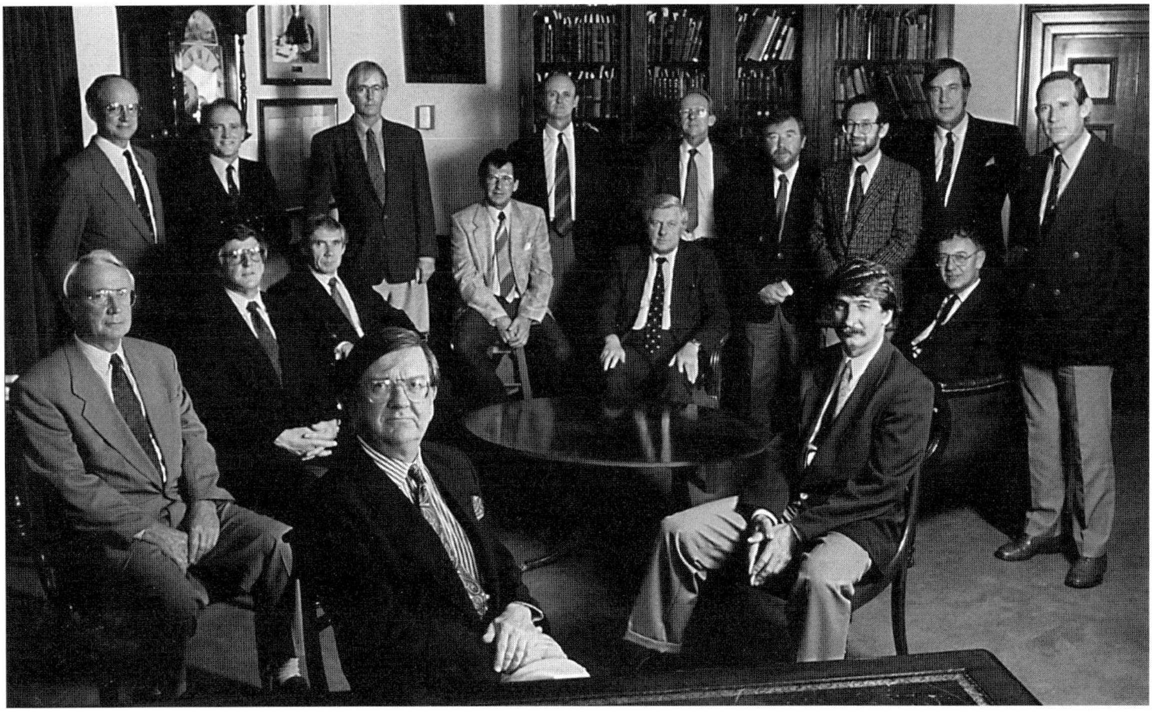

Members of the Executive of the Society at 145 Macquarie Street, Sydney, 1992. *Standing left to right:* Ted Arnold, Terry Morgan, Philip McDougall, Laurie Cleeve, Richard Millard, Peter Langdon, Alan Crosthwaite, Peter Maher, Tony Low. *Seated:* Russell McIlroy, Chris Farrell, John Hanrahan (President RACS), Warren Johnson, Geof Hirst, Villis Marshall, Andre Lalak and Stuart Taylor

urology and this helped to keep the number of urologists down. Most consequently enjoyed large practices and high incomes.

The Executive consistently acted to maintain this position and prevent any dilution of membership with surgeons who did not meet their criteria. Each candidate had to be proposed by two full members. All membership applications were circulated around the full Executive and each was carefully considered.

However, during the 1950s and 1960s, there was clearly too much work for the existing urologists, particularly outside Sydney, and this strict gatekeeping role was not inconsistent with encouraging promising young surgeons to take up urology as a specialty, provided they were prepared to meet the Society's requirements for admission to membership.

The rules for admission of associate members were more contentious. During the 1950s, when urologists were in short supply, there was something of a drift to allow considerable latitude in defining the 'special circumstances' that prevented a candidate from practising urology exclusively. Established urologists, particularly in Sydney and Melbourne, where the shortage of urologists was least acute, objected.

At the 1960 AGM in Brisbane, John Somerset proposed that associate membership be limited to those intending to progress to full-time urology and full membership. This may have been partly in response to the admission of Lorna Sisely. Not surprisingly, there were protests from Adelaide and Tasmania as the proposal would have disqualified all the associate members from the smaller centres.

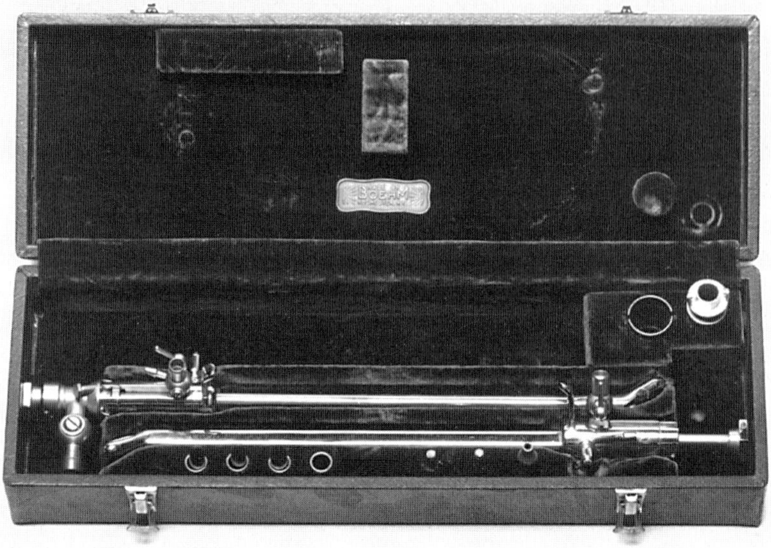

Gersham Thompson Direct Vision Prostatic Punch, Boehm, 1935. (*Source:* Urological collection, RACS)

Henry Mortensen and Keith Kirkland backed Somerset in principle, but the proposal was modified to one of instructing the Executive to strictly interpret the existing rules.[5]

Since then, the qualifications, especially for associate membership, have been debated and amended on numerous occasions, at times becoming almost a fixture of the agenda at the AGMs. This debate, in various forms, is not yet over, but has shifted to a discussion of the merits of permitting other specialists with a particular interest in an aspect of urology to have a formal association of some kind with the Society.

The problem of part-time urologists in country areas has not gone, but it has waned in significance and the membership rules have been amended accordingly.

John Somerset's idea of restricting associate membership to those intending to become full-time urologists has been raised many times but was never adopted in its most exclusive form. However, a category of membership for urologists aiming to become full members was adopted from1996 with the listing of Provisional Members, while specialists in other areas became Associated Members (previously Classified Associates), and a number of the old style associate members became full members.

Training and Accreditation

Until the 1970s, most members, whether full or associate, had obtained their senior surgical qualification from one of the British colleges of surgeons and this was reflected in the wording of the early membership rules. The Australasian College also awarded fellowships but the FRACS was not fully accepted as a substitute for a British fellowship

TABLE 5.1 EXAMINERS IN UROLOGY, ROYAL AUSTRALASIAN COLLEGE OF SURGEONS

AUSTRALIA:
1949 Henry Mortensen, John Laidley
1952 John Somerset
1954-60 John Somerset, Keith Kirkland
1960 John Somerset, Peter Row
1962 John Somerset, Keith Kirkland
1964-70 Alban Gee, Doug Duffy
1972 Alban Gee, Doug Duffy, Bruce Pearson
1974-80 Bruce Pearson, Peter Harbison, Joe Murnaghan, John Maddern
1982 Bruce Pearson, Joe Murnaghan, Peter Harbison, John Maddern, Ron Brown
1984-86 Ron Brown, Warren Johnson, Peter Maher, Villis Marshall, Ernie England, Tony Tynan
1988-90 Ron Brown, Warren Johnson, Peter Maher, Villis Marshall, Ernie England, Tony Tynan, Steve Stening
1990-92 Peter Maher, Villis Marshall, Tony Tynan, Steve Stening, Tony Low, John Rogers, Don Moss
1992-95 Peter Maher, Steve Stening, Tony Low, John Rogers, Don Moss, Laurie Cleeve, Graham Sinclair

NEW ZEALAND:
1947 Frank Macky, Edgar Reay, Bruce Rennie
1949-58 Frank Macky, Edgar Reay, Bruce Rennie, Patrick Treahy
1960-62 S. L. Wilson, Humphrey Gowland
1964-66 Humphrey Gowland, Warwick Macky
1968-72 Warwick Macky, Alexander Ferguson
1974-76 Alexander Ferguson, Bill Utley
1978-82 Bill Utley, Don Urquhart-Hay
1984-86 Don Urquhart-Hay, Colin McRae
1988-93 Colin McRae, Russell McIlroy
1993-95 Russell McIlroy, Ted Arnold

until the 1970s. This acceptance of the Australasian qualification emerged from a lengthy process of negotiation and argument between the College and the Society. Members of the Society normally date the major shift from overseas to Australasian training from the 1980s, but in fact the process began at least a decade earlier. The most important change in the qualifications for full membership of the Society came in 1975 when the reference to graduates of British Universities or Colleges was deleted and replaced by 'the Diploma of Fellowship of the Royal Australasian College of Surgeons in Urology or an equivalent degree or Diploma with similar training requirements'.[6] This formally recognised the widespread acceptance of the FRACS and the associated increase in the training opportunities for urologists in Australasia.

The RACS offered its first full examinations in 1946. Separate

Courts of Examiners were set up in Australia and New Zealand and they examined in a number of specialties, plus general surgery. Before 1946, the College had operated a combination of accepting senior surgical qualifications from elsewhere, an apprenticeship system and an interview.[7]

Henry Mortensen and John Laidley were the Australian examiners and the first two urologists to obtain their FRACS under this system were Leonard Murphy and Harold Cummine. The FRACS in urology was particularly helpful in providing a way to accredit the Gordon Craig Fellows without having to sit for the FRCS. Arthur Carrodus and Alban Gee were the next two FRACS in urology in 1948. The other urologists to pass under this system were Jim Peters in December 1948, Vernon Howarth in May 1950 and Warwick Macky in December 1950.

Interestingly, Frank Macky, Warwick's father, did not have a FRCS and so was ineligible for full membership of the Society, but he was admitted as a FRACS in 1931 and appointed a member of the New Zealand Court of Examiners from its inception in September 1947 until 1960. The other urologists were Rennie, Reay and, from 1949, Treahy, making the number of urologists on the New Zealand Court double that in Australia, where there were only two.

In December 1952, Searby and other generalists persuaded the College to cease holding the specialist examinations. John Laidley formally broke the news to the Executive of the Urological Society at the April 1953 meeting held in conjunction with the Society's AGM in Surfers Paradise. Both the Executive and the members of the Society at the AGM debated the matter at length.

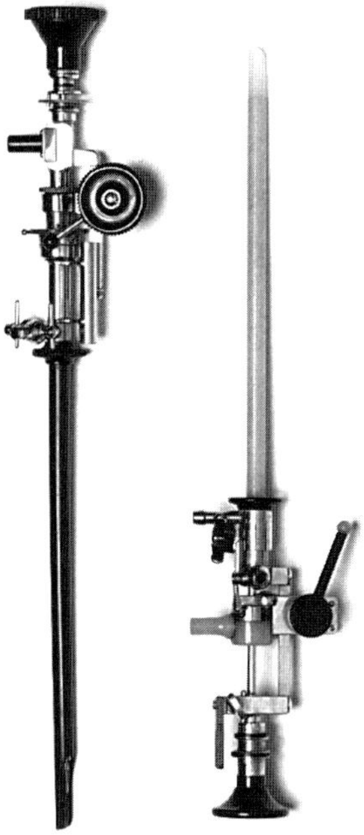

Left: Resectoscope, Stern-McCarthy pattern, made by Charles F. Thackray, Leeds. *Right:* Lorna Sisely's Stern-McCarthy resectoscope, c. 1949. (*Source:* Urological collection, RACS)

John Laidley, who in 1950 had been Chairman of the NSW section of the College, proposed a written protest from the Society. Henry Mortensen argued that:

> *it was essential for any graduate specialising in urology to obtain a general surgical degree by a two part examination and that his outlook should not be too narrow in regard to his specialty.*[8]

Mortensen was joined by Ian Potts and Doug Duffy in opposing the motion. Others sympathised with their view but still supported the protest to the College, which was duly written. That left the problem of the training of young urologists and members of the Society began to consider how and in what way the Society could 'undertake the responsibility of ensuring that the graduate's training in urology is of an adequate standard'.

Urologists were not the only specialists to protest and the College agreed to hold a further round of exams in 1954 as a stop gap measure. Meanwhile, Colin Edwards approached the other specialist bodies, hoping to discuss the matter with them before further discussions with the College. The BMA was also actively involved during 1954 in trying to obtain agreement on the definition of a specialist. This had the effect of stimulating further consideration of training

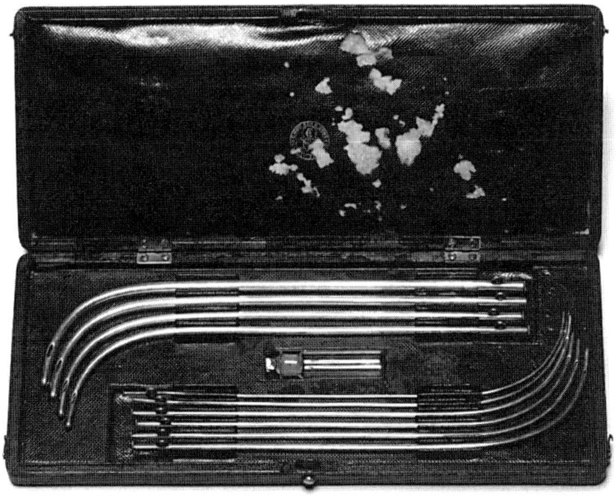

A set of graduated metal catheters, S. Maw Son & Sons, England, c. 1930. The vial in the centre was for oil. (*Source:* Urological collection, RACS)

and accreditation by the various specialist bodies, including the Society. Essentially, the Society's definition of a specialist in urology was someone who held a senior surgical qualification in general surgery or urology and would be acceptable as a full member of the Urological Society of Australasia.

The debate continued through much of 1954 with letters going to and fro between the Society and the BMA. Keith Kirkland noted that in America specialists were approved and issued with certificates. He considered 'that it might be necessary for the Society to act as an approved body in this regard at a future date'. The other approach was to try and obtain senior surgical qualifications from another body and John Laidley approached the Dean of the Faculty of Medicine at Sydney University with a view to reinstating the Master of Surgery in Urology. A combined approach to the Dean with the Neurosurgeons and Orthopaedic and ENT surgeons was proposed. This was in October 1954, but in December, Bowie Somerset indicated that the College was likely to change its mind and reinstate the Part 2 exam in the specialties. Meanwhile, the Post-Graduate Committee in Medicine was organising a conference on the training of specialists.

In February 1955, the generalists at the College submitted to all this pressure and notified the Society that the FRACS in urology was back. However, from then until 1962 the FRACS in urology met Henry Mortensen's objection to the earlier exam. Candidates had to have either the FRACS in general surgery or a FRCS before they could sit for the Part 2 FRACS in any of the specialties.[9]

The situation was stable from 1955 until 1961. In July 1961, the College held a conference with representatives of the specialist societies, with the objective of obtaining greater specialist participation in the scientific meetings of the College and a formal degree of affiliation. In April 1962, the Executive of the Society discussed affiliation to both the College and the newly formed Australian Medical

Association (AMA). No decision was made until the Society had found out what the other specialist societies were doing. This attitude recurred a number of times during discussions of relations with the College. The Society was keen to maintain its independence, but at the same time aware of a number of shared problems and the value of united action with the other specialties. When Alex Alder asked the Executive to suggest speakers for the Urological Section of the College ASM in May 1963, the reply was:

> *The Executive were of the opinion that its prime duty was to arrange for the meeting of the Society but that it may be in a position to help Mr. Alder at a later date.*

From 1962, the College changed the rules so that the Part 1 of the fellowship was the only prerequisite for sitting for the Part 2, whether general or specialist. On the whole, the specialists were not happy. A Conference of the Australian Post-Graduate Federation in Medicine in 1963 resulted in moves for the Society to consider formulating 'the basic requirements and qualifications for anyone wishing to enter into Specialist Urological Practice'.

At a special meeting of the Executive on 9 August 1963 a sub-committee was formed to consider the whole problem of training and accreditation. The members were Llew Wheeler, Bruce Pearson, Hugh Pearson and Joe Murnaghan. In the light of the recent changes made by the College, adequate training in general surgery before specialistation in urology was one of the main concerns. While this debate on training continued, the increasing recognition of the specialties was reflected in the proposal that the State Medical Boards set up Registers of Specialists.

The context of this debate on training was that most urologists still trained overseas. The Gordon Craig Fellows at Royal Prince Alfred Hospital were the largest group of Australasian-trained urologists, but at various times a number of other hospitals offered urology fellowships, including Sydney Hospital, Prince Henry Hospital in Sydney,

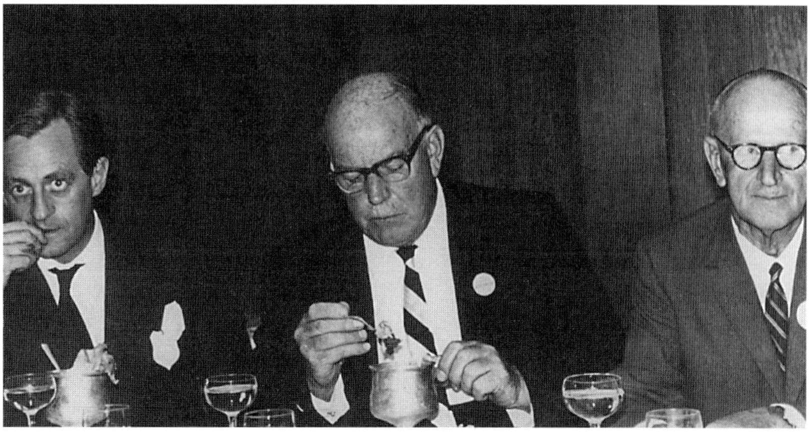

David Kennedy, Henry Mortensen and Colin Edwards at a lunch for those who had trained at St Peter's, ASM, Melbourne, March 1965. (*Source:* Harold Story)

St Vincent's in Melbourne and the Alfred Hospital, Melbourne. However, most Australasian urologists still trained in Britain and returned with a FRCS. It was therefore considered quite natural that the first grants for training urologists ever offered by the Society should be for training at St Peter's in London.

The Society's Travelling Fellowship in Urology

In September 1967, Joe Murnaghan raised the possibility of sponsoring a trainee in the three-year program at the Institute of Urology in London. The idea had arisen in correspondence between Murnaghan and Howard Hanley.

> *On the whole [wrote Hanley], I am quite sure that we can give one of your men as good a training as he will get anywhere in the world. After his three years we can send him home to you via one of the big American centres.*[10]

It was arranged that the Society would select a Senior Urological Registrar for the three- year appointment at St Peter's, St Paul's and St Phillip's. The position was advertised in Australia and New Zealand and the Society provided $500 for fares. It was not always easy to find suitable candidates, but over the years a number of Australasians went through the program.

Donald Macdonald, reporting back to the Society in February 1972, felt the training was generally very good, except that the London hospitals offered hardly any experience in resection. Returning to Australasia via the United States, therefore, generally involved a concerted effort to fill this gap in the London training.[11]

The Society's Travelling Fellowship added a number of Society-sponsored Registrars to the long list of Australasian urologists who had spent a year at St Peter's under their own arrangements. For a number of years, this tradition was recognised in a special lunch at the ASM, open only to members of the Society who had spent time at St Peter's.

Table 5.2 Urological Society of Australasia Travelling Fellows in Urology, in Association with the Institute of Urology, University of London:

1968 Geof Burfield	1986 Kim Moretti
1969 Don Macdonald	1987 Martin White
1973 Graham Sinclair	1988 Grant Russell
1975 Chris Switajewski	1989 David Winkle
1979 Anthony James	1990 Brian Landers
1980 Chris Farrell	1991 David Nicol
1983 Peter Langdon	1992 Neil Smith
1984 Daryl Stephens	1993 Roger Wa.tson
1985 Ken Vaux	

THE SOCIETY'S STANDARDS OF ACCREDITATION

During the period 1955-62, most of the specialist bodies seem to have been hapy with the FRACS and the way that the specialist Part 2 operated effectively as a Part 3—candidates had to have either a FRCS or the FRACS Part 2 in general surgery. There was a widely held view that specialists ought to have a good grounding in general surgery first and there was therefore considerable discontent among the specialist bodies when the College dropped this requirement.

In December 1965, for instance, the Secretary of the Australian Orthopaedic Association wrote to the Secretary of the Urological Society, asking for support in their approach to the College, requesting a reconsideration of the changes to 'the Fellowship regulations with regard to examination in the specialties'. 'It is our opinion that candidates wishing to do orthopaedics should first qualify in general surgery.'[12]

The Urological Society's sub-committee on training and accrediation broadly agreed. The sub-committee's recommendations of 1966 included the proposals that: Current trainees should obtain a general surgical fellowship from one of the Royal Colleges, plus at least two years full-time training in urology in a 'teaching hospital with at least two recognised urologists on the staff'.

For established urologists, Members of the Society with at least ten years' experience in full-time urological practice were recognised as fully qualified. The sub-committee made no specific objection to the recent change in the College regulations, but simply stated that it approved of the FRACS in urology. Significantly:

> *It is recommended that the Society communicate with the relevant bodies who are concerned with hospital appointments and inform them of what is regarded as sufficient qualifications. The Society request that such bodies appoint only such persons who have fulfilled such qualifications.*[13]

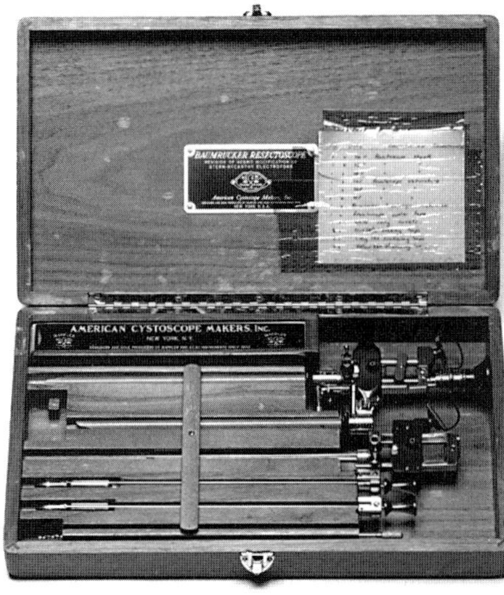

Baumrucker Resectoscope, ACMI. A revision of the Nesbit modification of the Stern-McCarthy Electrotome, 1950s. (*Source:* Urological collection, RACS)

THE SPECIALIST ASSAULT ON THE COLLEGE, 1969

The Society did not act as if the College was the only viable source of accreditation. The Society had its own standards of accreditation. If the College offered a suitable examination, so much the better. Otherwise: 'In the future it may be advisable to hold examinations and issue diplomata.'[14]

Other specialist groups, however, were more aggressive in their approach. The Ophthalmologists set up their own College, while the Neurosurgeons, Orthopaedic Surgeons and Plastic Surgeons all considered their own requirements for training and attempted to put pressure on the College.

By the late 1960s, Victoria, Queensland, South Australia and Western Australia had introduced a system of registering specialists, but there was no uniform national registration. In 1970, the Federal Government passed the National Health Act, which provided for higher fees for specialists than for other medical practitioners and at the same time set in motion procedures for the uniform national recognition of specialists. The National Specialist Qualification Advisory Committee was not set up until 1972, but the future importance of specialist training and accreditation was already very clear by 1969.

In July 1969, the Neurosurgeons set up a seminar on 'Specialist Surgical Training and Accreditation.' They invited representatives of the specialties and E. S. R. Hughes, the Censor-in-Chief of the RACS.[15] Doug Duffy was the representative of the Urological Society at the seminar and indicated that urologists had to train overseas, but the FRACS in urology could be the end point of their training. Other specialties trained in Australasia but thought the FRACS in their area was only the beginning, much in the same way as the Urological Society recommended a FRCS plus two years specialist experience.

There was unanimous discontent over the current Part 1 exam and a general agreement, even from E. S. R. Hughes, that general surgery was now itself a specialty. Throughout the seminar, there were numerous comparisons with the situation in the United Kingdom, where changes in the College Fellowships were also underway.

This was an important meeting because it established the principle of the College accepting advice from the specialist societies. As a result, each specialty was to set up an advisory committee on standards of training and accreditation and the RACS was to set up a joint advisory committee on surgical training, which would approach the specialist advisory committees for their recommendations.

In December 1969, a second seminar was held with a larger number of RACS examiners in attendance and there was further discussion of changes to both the Part 1 and Part 2 exams. Ian Nunn was the urologist present.[16]

In March 1970, the College formally approached the Society

requesting two nominees for the Specialist Surgical Training Committee. Basic surgical training for two years was to replace the concept of a year of general surgery. Advanced training was to begin in the fourth graduate year and run for a period set by the specialty concerned.

Each Specialist Surgical Training Committee was to consist of two RACS nominees and two specialist nominees. One of the RACS nominees would be chairman and at least one had to be a practising member of the specialty concerned. The Joint RACS Committee would then consist of the Chairmen of the Specialist Committees, plus Council nominees.

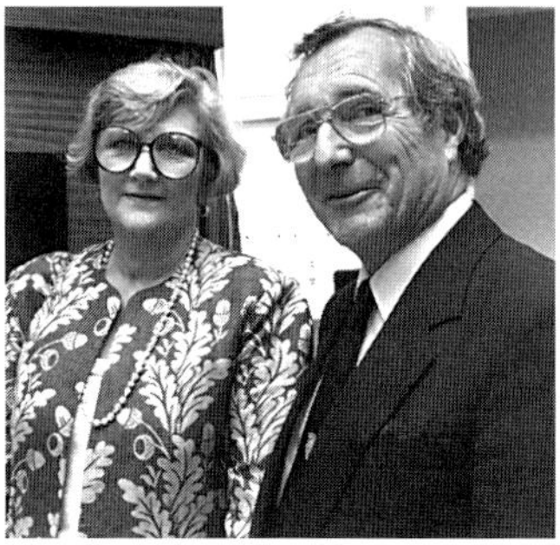

Joe and Dulcie Murnaghan at the opening of the G. F. Murnaghan Urology Unit, the Prince Henry Hospital, December 1992. (*Source:* Joe Murnaghan)

As a result, in March 1970 at its 23rd AGM, the Urological Society set up its Standing Committee on Standards of Training and Accreditation. It consisted of the Australian RACS examiners in urology, plus any Society members on the RACS Council, plus two others, including the President. At that date, Doug Duffy and Alban Gee were the Australian examiners; Douglas Stephens and Warwick Macky were both on the RACS Council and the other members were Jack Blackman (President) and Joe Murnaghan. Douglas Stephens later represented the Paediatric Surgeons and Jeff Watson from Queensland, replaced him on the Society's committee.[17]

There followed considerable debate as to whether advanced training (following the three years leading to taking Part 1) should be three or four years. Generally, the Society's sub-committee wanted four years and the RACS Joint Committee wanted three years. The eventual 1971 recommendation was three years, two in urology and six months each in general surgery and another specialty.

In March 1971, Joe Murnaghan presented the committee with the results of his survey of beds and urologists by hospital. It was to be another decade before this approach was taken to its logical conclusion, but the balance began to shift from an assumption of overseas training of urologists to an increasing proportion of training in Australasian hospitals. The 1971 RACS report on *Committees, Coordinators, Supervisors and Approved Posts in Surgical Training* listed twenty-one approved posts for Advanced Training in Urology in Australasia.

These moves changed the face of urological training in Australasia. The direct involvement of the Society meant that the FRACS in Urology was accepted as the norm for future urological surgeons. In theory the College could appoint a non-urologist to the Specialist Surgical Training Committee, but it did not do so. The members of the Committee in 1971 were Duffy (College-nominated Chairman), Blackman, Macky, Murnaghan and Watson, i.e. all members of the Society's own Committee on Standards of Training and Accreditation. Henceforward the Society played a leading role, under the auspices of the RACS, in the training and accreditation of Australasian urologists.

These changes represented a triumph for the College in bringing at least some of the specialties back into the College fold, but they also represented a triumph for the specialist societies in increasing their individual control over the standards of training and accreditation for entry to their own specialty.

Further changes during the 1970s generally consolidated this position for the urologists. In 1971, the College asked the Society to nominate regional advisors for each State and New Zealand and there was considerable overlap in personnel with the Training Committes of both the Society and the College. In 1976, the Specialist Surgical Training Committees became Surgical Boards and all five members of the Board of Urology were nominated by the Society. They were appointed for limited periods and in 1978 half of the original 1970 members had to resign, the other half coming due for resignation in 1980. In 1979, the Surgical Board of Urology consisted of Murnaghan (Chairman), Utley, Nunn, Bruce Pearson and Harbison.[18]

1979: Joe Murnaghan's Proposal and the Durham Smith Paper

In October 1979, Joe Murnaghan proposed a reorganisation of the Executive's Training and Accreditation Sub-committee. He proposed a more democratic Training, Accreditation and Education Committee of the Society, rather than the Executive, that would be built from the teaching hospitals up. Each hospital with a recognised training position in Urology (23 in 1979) would send a urologist to represent it on a State or New Zealand committee. The Chairmen of the State sub-committees would be nominated by their State sections and together would form the Training, Accreditation and Education Committee of the Society. The goal was then to persuade the College to increase the size of the Board of Urology from five to seven members to match, and to accept the Society's nominations.

This change was proposed at the same time as Durham Smith, from the perspective of the RACS, put forward his document on closer relations between the College and the specialties. Both documents were considered by the 1980 AGM of the Society in Christchurch. Unfortunately, Durham Smith could not attend, because the Christchurch meeting clashed with a College ASM in Sydney. Greater co-operation between the specialist societies and the College over their respective scientific meetings was one of the issues addressed in the Durham Smith discussion document. The problem had changed in detail but in essence remained the same as in the 1940s. The College could not survive without the specialties, but those, like the Urologists, who had their own scientific societies, had little commitment to the College or its scientific meetings.[19]

Over the next decade, as a Member of Council, as Chairman of the Court of Examiners and as President of the College, Durham Smith attempted to bring the College and the specialties closer together. His actions were undoubtedly informed by his own perhaps unusually wide experience of specialist groups. He took his FRACS in general surgery, did some specialist training in neurosurgery, became a general paediatric surgeon and a noted paediatric urologist. In this latter capacity he was a long time Associate Member of the Urological Society.

In 1979, Professor G. D. Tracy was President of the College and it was he who distributed the Durham Smith discussion document to the specialist societies. 'It is a document setting out ways in which co-operation might be achieved, and is offered as an initial draft upon which subsequent discussions may develop ... The College looks forward keenly to an extension of, and perhaps new direction to, our mutual goals', he wrote.[20] At the end of the 1970s, the context had therefore become a favourable one for fostering co-operation between the College and the specialist societies. In August 1980 the College agreed to accede to the Society's request to increase the Board of Urology to seven.

John Maddern was the new Chairman of the Board of Urology and in March 1981 he reported on progress to the Society's AGM in Sydney. The program was now to consist of two years basic training before taking the Part 1, then four years advanced training, including one year of general surgery and three years in an approved urological training post. Two of these three years had to be Australasian, but one could be overseas.

John Maddern was an examiner from 1974 to 1984 and identified a number of problems with the exam and with the experience of those presenting for it. He was concerned to expand the level of practical experience of trainees and to change the exam so that it rewarded those who were best equipped to become practical urologists. As Chairman of the Board of Urology he expressed his concerns to the College, concerns generally shared by the Orthopaedic surgeons. After Warwick Macky retired, Maddern was co-opted onto Council of the College as a representative of Urology under a scheme that gave representation to specialties without an elected Council member. Over time, the combination of pressure from the specialties and a changing attitude from a number of key people on the Council of the College saw progressive concessions to the specialities.

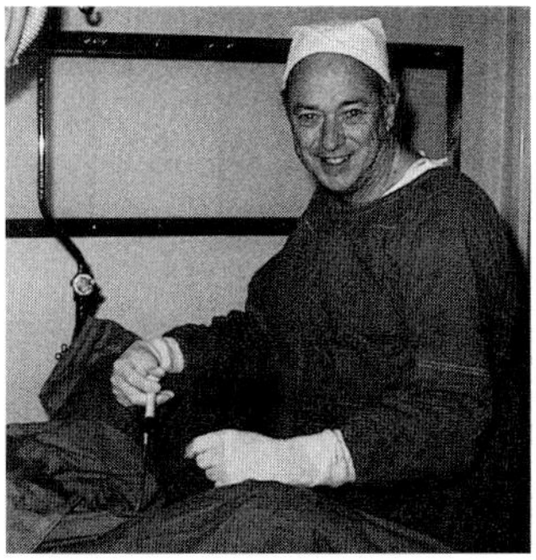

John Maddern. (*Source:* Don Moss)

By the time that John Maddern retired as Chairman of the Board of Urology in 1986, the College had agreed to changes in the exam, and the selection of examiners, to more closely meet the requirements of the Urological Society. There were twenty-four training posts and the trainees rotated through two or three posts, depending on the level of experience available in each. This had been achieved through considerable co-operation between the hospitals (who employed the Registrars) and the Society. Trainees were encouraged to attend Society meetings and to give papers, especially at the State and New Zealand section meetings. The balance had also shifted to a suspicion of the quality of overseas training posts and a confidence

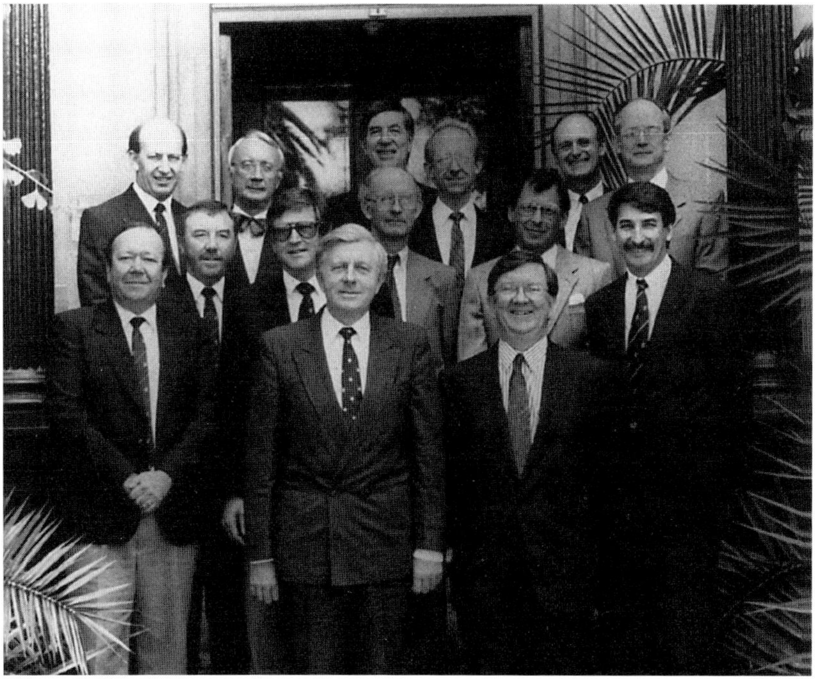

Members of the Urology Society Executive on the steps of the Royal Australasian College of Physicians building, 145 Macquarie Street, Sydney, 1992. *Back row:* Don Moss, Russell McIlroy, Peter Maher, Richard Millard, Laurence Cleeve, Ted Arnold; *Middle row:* Graham Holmes, Peter Langdon, Chris Farrell, Brian McGregor, Geof Hirst, Andre Lalak; *Front row:* Villis Marshall and Warren Johnson

in the Australasian positions. Young Australasian urologists were now substantially Australasian-trained and the State and New Zealand Sections of the Society had a new focus in their role of monitoring the selection and training of urological registrars.[21]

The 1970s, therefore, saw the beginning and the 1980s saw the full flowering of training programs and examinations designed and run by urologists to train and accredit urologists. The result was a very high degree of professional clinical autonomy. The Urological Society was not alone in achieving this. By the end of the 1980s many of the groups associated with the College had similar control over entrants to their own ranks. In 1994, Peter Baume published the result of the Government sponsored 'Inquiry into the Supply of, and Requirements for, Medical Specialist Services in Australia'. The report was called 'A Cutting Edge: Australia's Surgical Workforce 1994' but it was generally referred to as the Baume Report. The broad thrust of the report was an implication of restrictive practices and both the College and the Urological Society were outraged.

In its response to the Baume Report, the RACS expressed 'its extreme disappointment in the poor quality, superficial nature and lack of objectivity of the Report'. There were accusations of inaccurate data and hearsay evidence, but the core of the College's objection was to the report's attitude towards surgeons. 'It ignores the long established and well recognised professional ethos of the College, wrongly attributing its policies and actions to financial motives.' The reaction of the Urological Society was similar.

The fact remained that, from whatever motives, surgeons in general and urologists in particular had come to have an extraordinary degree of control over the training, accreditation (and numbers) of their successors. The period after 1994 marked a new era in the relationship between the College and the surgical specialties, including urologists, as together they faced the common problem of public and Government perceptions of their role, particularly in training.

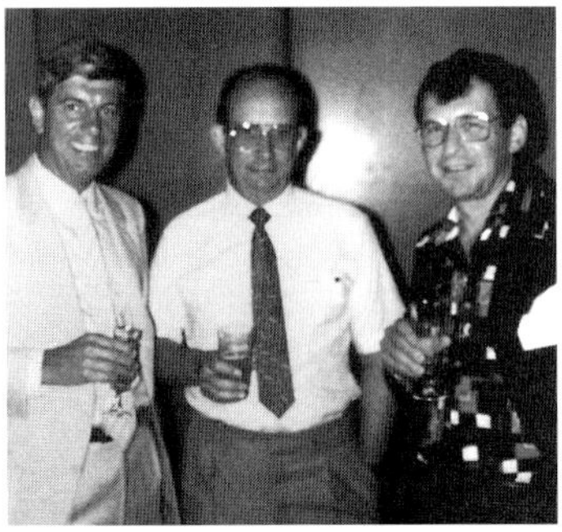

Frans Debruyne (Professor of Urology, Nijmegen, the Netherlands), David Evans (Urologist from Toronto and husband of Mary Gospodariwicz, radiation oncologist, Princess Margaret Hospital, Toronto) and Geof Hirst at the ICUC Meeting, Brisbane, 1987

The Chairman of the Society's Training, Accreditation & Education Committee in that era was Don Moss. He worked with the Australian Medical Workforce Advisory Committee to produce a report on 'The Urology Workforce in Australia, Supply, Requirements and Projections 1995-2006', which addressed most of the concerns expressed in the Baume Report. Don Moss was also involved in rewriting the training program, including changes designed to give trainees a wider experience of a range of training posts. During Don Moss' time as chairman, the number of training posts increased, but there remained problems in New Zealand.

> *There are accreditated posts that are not filled ... haven't had satisfactory applicants from New Zealand ... there are clearly too few urologists in Auckland ... In Australia we're close ... except for the provincial areas and Brisbane ... There weren't satisfactory posts in country Victoria ... were four posts in 1988 ... 10 posts plus [one in] Tasmania in 1998. Queensland is still short of a post but there are now some concerns that we're training too many.*[22]

There was the hope that more training posts outside the capital cities would encourage young urologists to set up in practice in the country but as Don Moss noted, although the Society had a dominating role in training, it had no say in the distribution of trained urologists. 'We have no role in where they work.'

In 1997 Don Moss' work was recognised by the College when he was awarded the Sir Louis Barnett Medal for his outstanding contribution to education, training and advancement in surgery.

Representing the Specialty

The first meeting of the Executive of the incorporated Urological Society of Australasia was on 4 March 1948. At the fourth meeting, on 14 October 1948, the Executive considered a letter from the Department of Trade and Customs containing a list of American urological instruments. The Society was asked to determine how essential they were, given the current restrictions on importing from outside the Sterling block.

This early acceptance of the Society as the authority on urology in Australasia was widespread. Without any planning or direct initiative from the Society, it became involved in an increasing range of matters as the acknowledged representative of Australasian urologists. Thus, in February 1950, the Department of Trade and Customs consulted the Executive on the case of Wallsend Hospital, which wanted to import a Hugh Young urological table. The Society informed the Department that it was the best table available, but not 'truly essential'. Most urological clinics in Sydney used local tables and found them adequate.[23]

A more lasting area of Government consultation was over the Pharmaceutical Benefits Scheme and the various elements of what the Society called the 'National Health Scheme', introduced by the Menzies Government in the early 1950s. A number of previous Government health schemes had failed to get off the ground because of opposition from the BMA, but the 1953 Pharmaceutical Benefits Act was introduced by Earle Page, a member of the BMA and a FRACS.[24]

Initially, the Executive of the Society as a whole dealt with correspondence over pharmaceutical benefits and was consulted regularly about deletions from and additions to the list. There was some direct lobbying from drug companies, to which the standard Society response was generally frosty, for instance in 1965:

> *The Secretary was instructed to write [to the drug company] explaining the accustomed procedure of the Society in these matters. i.e. should Canberra solicit our opinion concerning any drug, this was willingly given, but on the other hand, the Society, except in unusual circumstances, did not proffer opinion to the drug sub-committee in Canberra.*[25]

In later years, the Society was more likely to directly request that a drug of a particular type be listed, or, more commonly, that a drug of a specified type be restored to the Pharmaceutical Benefits List. In the 1960s, the Executive as a whole was still dealing with the increasing volume of correspondence over drugs. It was not until March 1970 that the Executive formed a sub-committee on Pharmaceutical Benefits.

From as early as 1955, however, the Executive began to delegate consideration of the National Health Service Schedules/ Commonwealth Medical Benefits Scheme to one individual. In the 1950s, this was Desmond Trainor and he was the Society's first expert on what later became known as fees and anomalies. By the 1960s, this role had largely been taken over by Lionel Jacobs and he was involved in collecting further information on this increasingly complex area, and reporting back to the Executive.

In the late 1960s, there was a marked change of emphasis from the Executive over the question of fees. The position until about 1968 was that each urologist charged the fee that they thought fit. This position was summarised on 6 May 1966, in response to a query from the Otolaryngological Society of Australia. The Secretary of the Urological Society was instructed to reply to the effect that: 'The Society has no schedule of fees laid down and that by and large there is no uniformity of fees and no standard first consultation fee.'[26]

Within two years, the Executive had set up a sub-committee on fees and anomalies. This sub-committee provided information to the

AMA, which was conducting a survey of most common fees to aid in negotiations with the Commonwealth Government. Over the next few years, this process was increasingly formalised and in 1973 Harry Learoyd, at that time the Society's expert on fees, conducted a relative value study for urological procedures. This relative value study was subsequently used in setting the level of both Commonwealth rebates and the (higher) AMA schedule of common fees for urological procedures. Urologists were under no obligation to follow either schedule, but during the 1970s both increasingly had a normative effect.

Between 1970 and 1975 there were increasing pressures on the Society to become involved in medico-political matters. Generally in the 1950s and 1960s, medico-political matters were dealt with through the BMA (AMA from 1962). In 1957, the BMA wrote to the Society (and other similar bodies) asking that medico-political matters be left in their hands and there was broad agreement that, provided there was no loss of autonomy, this made sense.

On the whole, the BMA had served the interests of the medical profession well, so much so that an article in the *Lancet* in 1963 described the Australian medical system as 'private practice publically supported'.[27] But in the late 1960s there was a change in the position of specialists that made it increasingly difficult for the AMA to represent all sections of its wide constituency equally.

State registers of specialists were considered as early as October 1963, and the Society was duly consulted over the definition of a urologist, but the major impetus for change came with the granting of higher rebates for specialists from 1970. The AMA supported the specialists in their claim for higher rebates and this led to a break away movement of some general practitioners, who formed the General Practitioners' Society in Australia in 1968. At the AGM in Wellington in March 1973, members of the Society discussed a circular from the General Practitioners' Society, which was compiling a register of specialists. The Society resolved that: 'a letter be sent to the A.M.A. notifying receipt of the circular and advising that Members of the Urological Society had no wish to co-operate in this matter.'[28]

Conflicting pressures within the AMA were associated with both rising levels of dissatisfaction and an increasing level of political awareness. In December 1970, the Executive of the Urological Society discussed how to become involved in medico-political matters without becoming liable for income tax and in July 1971 the Australian Association of Surgeons was formed. The Urological Society was happy to back the AAS and the August 1971 newsletter informed members that the AAS:

> *has been formed as a politically active organization to maintain and improve the conditions of service of surgeons. The Executive Council considers that the Association should be supported, but feels that the proposed Council should be representative of all States and all Surgical Specialties, and that State Committees of the Association should be elected by Members, and not*

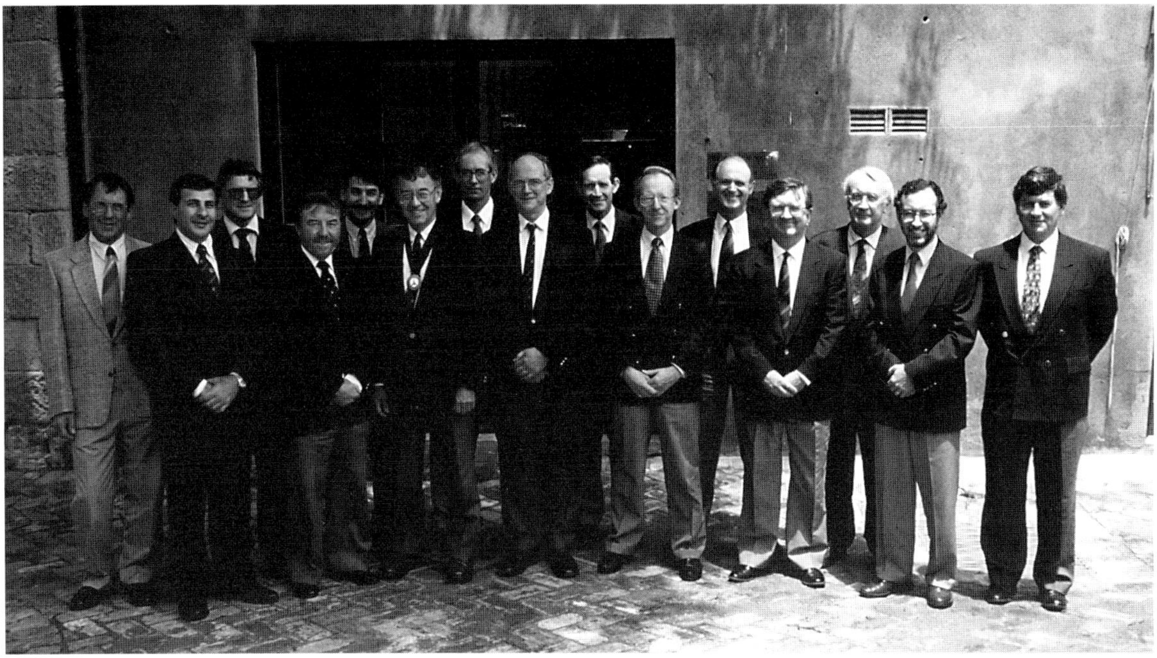

Members of the Executive outside 'the Stables', 1993. Geof Hirst, Mike Monsour, Chris Farrell, Peter Langdon, Andre Lalak, Stuart Taylor, Philip McDougall, Ted Arnold, Tony Low, Richard Millard, Laurence Cleeve, Warren Johnson, Russell McIlroy, Alan Crosthwaite, Adrian Porter

appointed by the Council. It is recommended that Australian Members of the Urological Society join the Australian Association of Surgeons and attend the inaugural Meeting in Melbourne on 29/9/71. If unable to attend, Members who have joined should send their proxy vote forms to the Society's representative, Mr. H.M. Learoyd, 143 Macquarie Street, Sydney, 2000.[29]

During 1972 and 1973, medico-political matters, fees and relations with the AMA began to take an increasing amount of the Executive's time and this process accelerated following the election of the Whitlam Government in December 1972. AMA opposition to Medibank during 1973 was expressed through a major press campaign and medico-political matters were very much in the spotlight. Members of the Urological Society were necessarily forming their own views.

In December 1973 and again in April 1974, Medibank was defeated in the Senate. In the resulting election, Labor was returned to office and the Medibank legislation became law in August. In the August 1974 newsletter of the Urological Society, Members were informed that:

The Executive has been concerned regarding the adjustment of fees, social aspects of Medical Practice and conditions of service. Legal opinion has been sought regarding the status of the Society in relation to these matters and it appears that as it stands at present, the Memorandum and Articles of Association do not allow the Society to become actively involved in these issues.[30]

The Executive called an Extraordinary General Meeting for 8 November to discuss three options:

1: resurrect the NSW section of urology of the AMA
2: form a separate body
3: amend the Memorandum and Articles of Association

The meeting favoured option 2 and the Australian Association of Urological Surgeons was formed, with the inaugural meeting set for April 1975, in conjuntion with the Sydney ASM.[31]

At the 28th AGM in Sydney, the main issue was not the AAUS but changes to the membership rules of the Urological Society. However, all three options for a body that could act in medico-political matters as discussed at the Extraordinary General Meeting in November were considered again and option 2 was accepted.

From 1975, the AAUS was generally called the Australia and New Zealand Association of Urological Surgeons, so that medico-political activity in New Zealand was also possible. However, changes to the constitution to set up ANZAUS took time to finalise. There was no perceived urgency, because Whitlam was dismissed in November 1975 and a Liberal Government elected. Although the Fraser Government campaigned on the platform that Medibank would be retained, it was soon clear that there would be substantial modifications along the lines suggested by the AMA.

In June 1976, the Executive of the Urological Society was still concerned with modifications to the constitution of ANZAUS, but was happy to 'wait and see' with regard to the organisation's future usefulness:

> *The matter was left in abeyance because of changing political situation but it was decided to finalise the constitution in case the Association had the need for a role in future political activity.*[32]

In September 1976, despite widespread strikes (not by doctors) in protest, there were substantial modifications to Medibank, including a phased return of fee for service. Over the next two years there were further modifications and by September 1978 there was little left of Medibank, although Medibank Private continued to provide health insurance.

In this period, the Urological Society showed little interest in overtly political activity. It was far too busy dealing with the continually growing volume of business arising from its role as the acknowledged representative of Australasian urology.

Some idea of the range of topics covered is provided by the list of correspondence dealt with at just one Executive meeting. On 29 October 1976, the Secretary tabled twenty-two items of correspondence. Subjects covered included the annual meetings (four letters); personal letters from members (three); queries about research funds (three); general society business (two); the National Library of Australia, the Victorian Post-graduate Foundation, a medico-legal query, the Austalian Kidney Foundation, the Health Commission of New South Wales, the Standards Association (one each), and what had joined the annual meetings as the bread and butter work of the Society: four letters from the AMA and AAS about various matters, including item numbers, and two from the Pharmaceutical Benefits Advisory Committee.

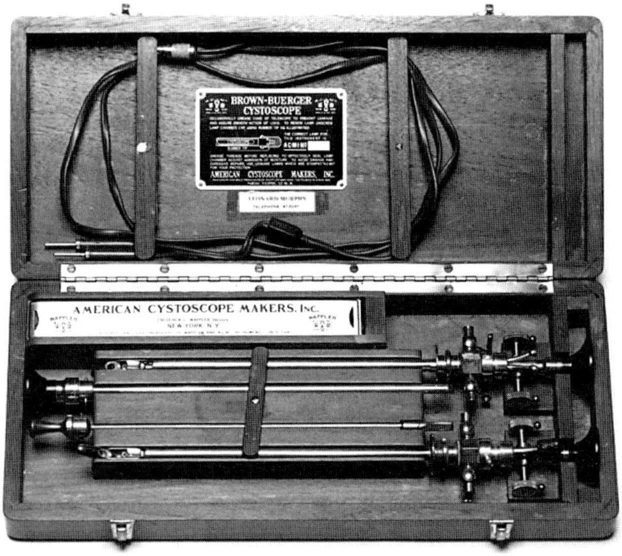

Brown-Buerger Cystoscope, ACMI, c. 1949, donated by Leonard Murphy. (*Source:* Urological collection, RACS)

The Pharmaceutical Benefits Advisory Committee

By 1976, the PBAC was holding regular meetings with representatives of the RACS and the specialist groups, including the Urological Society. There was also regular consultation between meetings. Harry Learoyd was the usual point of contact and in 1978 he complained 'It is obvious that the [Pharmaceutical Benefits Advisory] Committee has no member on it with any knowledge of Urology.'[33]

Generally, negotiations with the PBAC were protracted and purely technical. In particular, arguments about adding new drugs to the list, or keeping drugs the PBAC wanted to remove, involved the Society in preparing detailed submissions backed by long lists of academic references.

A slightly different issue was the Society's battle to have irrigating fluids used during TUR listed, and therefore eligible for benefits in private hospitals. There was no charge to the patient in public hospitals. In 1981, the Society lobbied Senator Peter Baume, at that time Minister for Aboriginal Affairs. Baume argued that irrigating fluids were a cost and not a benefit and therefore should be charged for equally in both private and public hospitals, if at all, but he did approach the Minister for Health on the Society's behalf.

The Fraser Government was concerned to keep costs down at a time of high inflation and there was a series of budget cuts. This put pressure on the PBAC to keep changes to the listings at least cost neutral. The impact of budgetary restraint reached a peak in 1982 when the meetings between the PBAC and the RACS/Society representatives were suspended in an attempt to save costs. They were not reintroduced until 1985, by which stage there had been a Labor Government for two years.

The Fees and Anomalies Sub-Committee

The other regular area of consultation and negotiation with representatives of the Federal Government was over the Medical Benefits Schedule. Interestingly, this was not seen as an overtly political matter until after the election of the Hawke Government in 1983. Until then, negotiations over the Medical Benefits Schedule were conducted through the Fees and Anomalies Sub-committee of the Executive, rather than through ANZAUS.

The 1973 relative values study conducted by Harry Learoyd was the basis of the 1974 Medical Benefits Schedule as it affected urological procedures. In 1978, there was a major review of the schedule and the relative value of item numbers. The Fees and Anomalies Sub-committee was involved in a series of consultations over these changes, through both the AMA and the AAS.

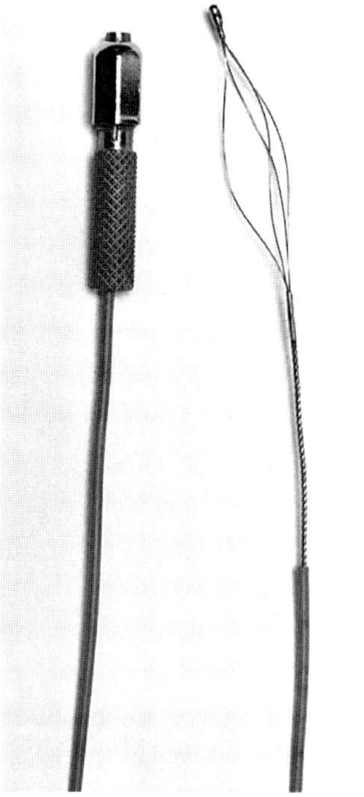

Dormia stone basket, invented in the 1930s. (*Source:* Urological collection, RACS)

In the 1980s, the consultation and decision making process became increasingly complex, with input from both the Medical Benefits Advisory Committee and the Medical Benefits Schedule Revision Committee. The Society, of course, like all the other interested parties, wished to be able to put its view. The result was a very slow and cumbersome decision making process.

By 1983, amendments to the Medical Benefits Schedule were generally made by the Minister for Health on the recommendation of the Medical Benefits Schedule Revision Committee. This included representatives of the AMA and the Commonwealth Department of Health. The Minister generally took the advice of the MBSRC, but the Committee was very slow in reaching an agreed position, at least partly because of the AMA's own lengthy consultation process. The net result was so slow that in October 1983 the Department of Health approached the AMA to see if they could come to an agreement without going through the MBSRC, because it was so slow.[34]

This was the system in place when the Hawke Labor Government was elected and the medical profession faced the re-introduction of Medibank. Stuart Taylor in his dual role as Chairman of ANZAUS and convenor of the Fees and Anomalies Sub-committee took ANZAUS into a new, more politically active era.

The Austrlia and New Zealand Association of Urological Surgeons

Although formed in 1974, the medico-political arm of the Society generally played a low- key role in the 1970s and mainly operated through the AAS. At first, there was no direct co-ordination. Bruce Pearson was the Chairman of ANZAUS 1974-77, but Harry Learoyd was the Society's representative on the AAS. In 1975 he was replaced by Stuart Taylor, who had been directly elected as one of the AAS's eight Councillors. He stood down in 1976 and was replaced by John Rogers as a co-opted member. This does not seem to have been a popular job at the time. John Rogers tried to stand down several times but was persuaded to remain until 1980. For the last two years of this term, he was also Chairman of ANZAUS and the dual role made such good sense that Tony Tynan continued the tradition 1980-83 before the return of Stuart Taylor to both roles in 1983.

The AAS seems to have been more radical than the AMA in the pursuit of the dismantling of Medibank and in 1979 disaffiliated from the AMA, although apparently without animosity. Generally, however, all the medico-political groups enjoyed a relatively quiet time between 1976 and 1983. The Fraser Government was broadly receptive to their views and confrontations were few. All that changed in 1983.

The period 1983-87 was a troubled time for the various medico-political organisations, including ANZAUS. Generally, both ANZAUS and the AAS were more radical in their opposition to Medicare than the AMA. The response of the AAS was particularly forthright. At a meeting on 18 June 1983, the Federal Council of the AAS passed a unanimous motion: 'That the Federal Council of the Australian Association of Surgeons rejects the Labor Government's Health Scheme—Medicare,'[35] and an alternative set of fundamental principles were proposed. In a letter to Ros Parisi, President of the Urological Society, Richard Colban, the Executive Director of the AAS, reported that:

> *It was further decided that the support of all medical, nursing, hospital and other health care related organisations, should be enlisted to inform the Australian people of the injustices and iniquities of Medicare with a maximum effort to prevent its introduction.*[36]

Nevertheless, Medicare was introduced and members of the medical profession had to learn to live with the details. In 1984, there was a Committee of Inquiry into Rights of Private Practice in Public Hospitals and in April, the ANZAUS prepared a submission, arguing for the continuation or restoration of the rights of patients in public hospitals to choose their doctor (not just from the hospital staff) and to choose to be private patients. The submission also argued against maximum fees, against any ceiling on the income of surgeons and against charging them for the use of public hospital facilities.

The Committee of Inquiry produced its report (generally known as the Penington Report after the chairman, Professor Penington) late in 1984 and the AMA called a meeting to discuss the recommendations. Stuart Taylor attended the meeting on behalf of the Urological Society and afterwards wrote:

> *Penington's stand is a very interesting and a very dangerous one. The stand is this, simply put, that he in his report has achieved absolutely everything possible from the Federal Government, and therefore it is critical that we accept his report, particularly the important linked recommendations, as a package, otherwise the Government will turn nasty and destroy us. By that he means, and illustrates, that they will put such restrictions on us that the practice of medicine will become most unpleasant.*[37]

In fact many members of the AMA did accept Penington's Report, but the AAS and ANZAUS did not. During 1984, both organisations appear to have come to the view that they no longer wished to bargain over rebates through the MBAC, because this was in danger of being regarded as bargaining over fees. In fact, over the previous decade many surgeons had come to charge the AMA common fee at most and quite frequently the lower schedule amount for rebates for medical services, or as Stuart Taylor put it:

During the last two and a half years my wide contact with my colleagues on these matters has made it clear to me that the majority of Urologists follow the Medical Benefits Schedule of fees, and accept the rebate now paid by Medicare ... What is happening in my opinion is that a precedent is being set as a result of all this that means that the level of fees is becoming a matter between Medicare and we Doctors.[38]

Stuart Taylor argued that surgeons should charge the fee they felt to be appropriate for the work and use their own discretion to vary the fee, depending on the ability of the patient to pay. Meanwhile, neither the AMA nor the Government were including the AAS in their deliberations over fees.

Events came to a head at the end of 1984 with the Doctors' strike in New South Wales. The concern was over loss of income and a 'backdoor' civil conscription of doctors. Stuart Taylor, through ANZAUS, strongly supported industrial action:

If the battle in N.S.W. is lost, then we can all look forward to a reduction of our incomes ... Very few of us if any would not suffer a severe reduction in income, and those less well established, in my opinion, would be ruined throughout this Country.[39]

There was a feeling by many that the AMA had lost touch with the views of members, but certainly the medical profession as a whole, like the AMA, was not united behind the strike. Like virtually all strikes, it was a most unhappy period for those affected, whether or not they took part in industrial action. Looking back over the period, Tony Low wrote:

The Australian Association of Surgeons ... I think reached its height of importance over the confrontation with Dr Blewitt and the infamous Section 39 Legislation, leading ultimately to the doctors' strike. I think at that stage

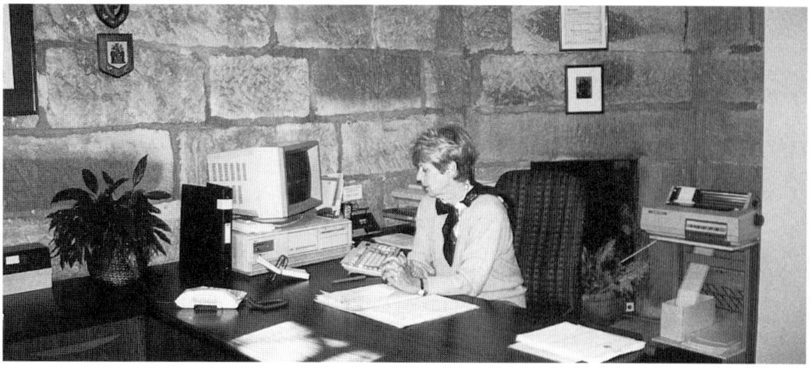

Gail Hill at work in 'the Stables', 1993

the AAS and the AOA [Australian Orthopaedic Association] carried the can for surgeons, and perhaps for doctors in general, though it was a pretty sad day in my opinion, that strike action became necessary. Unfortunately, the AAS did appear to become increasingly right wing after that time, perhaps not surprisingly, and I think has waned in importance in recent years, and I understand has a decreasing membership.[40]

By 1987, ANZAUS was once more involved in detailed negotiations over fees. Geof Hirst joined Stuart Taylor and the emphasis shifted from confrontation to co-operation. The AMA had been negotiating on behalf of the Society, but in this era Geof Hirst and Stuart Taylor began travelling to Canberra and meeting directly with members of a sub-committee of the Department of Health. In 1988, Geof Hirst took over as Chairman of ANZAUS and the new urological schedule of rebates was accepted by the Government in February 1989. The Government had made it clear that there was no more money for rebates, but the relative values could be rearranged and this was the most significant change in relative values since 1973.

During the negotiations, ANZAUS was provided with the number of procedures by item number and worked out how much money was spent. First Stuart Taylor and Geof Hirst and then Laurie Cleeve and Geof Hirst worked on the schedules. The rates for cystoscopy went down, but the rates for other procedures went up. As Geof Hirst noted, the principle was to keep rebates down where other specialists were involved but to raise them for procedures performed only by urologists. The result was generally of significant financial benefit to the members of ANZAUS. However, ANZAUS took care to emphasise that these were rebates, not fees. The level of fees was a matter for the individual surgeon. The new AMA's (considerably higher) schedule of common fees appeared shortly afterwards. In 1991, Laurie Cleeve succeeded Geof Hirst as Chairman of ANZAUS.[41]

In 1988, the Executive of ANZAUS ceased to be the same as the Executive of the Urological Society, a recognition of the ever increasing workload of the latter body. The focus of relations with Government was shifting to manpower issues, particularly after the Baume Report of 1994, and this involved the Society rather than ANZAUS. The mid-1980s was a time of important change for the Urological Society. The range and complexity of issues dealt with by the Executive had increased considerably since the 1970s and in addition the Society was involved in a number of issues that aroused strong feelings. Political matters and the doctors' strike have already been discussed, but there was also the issue of extracorporeal shock wave lithotripsy (ESWL) and discussion over the re-organisation of the Society, the separation of the role of the President from that of Convenor of the ASM and alterations to the manner in which the President and the site for the ASM were chosen.

Extracoporeal Shock Wave Lithotripsy

Discussion of this new technology first appeared in the Minutes of the Executive during 1984 and rose to a peak in 1985-56. The key characteristics of the technology were that it was:

a) very expensive and only economic to operate for a large population, involving co-operation between several urologists and/or hospitals

and

b) very popular with patients so that there was considerable pressure to purchase a machine before any other hospital/group of urologists in the same city cornered the market.

From an early date it was clear that the financial pressures involved led to strong feelings and at the Executive meeting on 3 May 1985:

> *It was decided that the responsibility of the Society would be to advise Government on the availability and the use of E.S.W.L. in Australia. It would negotiate with regard to the fee for usage and would not be involved in the setup or entrepeneurial activity which only produced division among Society members. The Society would urgently set up strict guidelines to facilitate the introduction of the machines without chaos in the country.*

Even this limited role led to conflict. The AMA was recommending three machines for Australia, but groups of urologists and private hospitals were already well on the way to importing machines for Sydney and Melbourne without regard to the Australia-wide picture. The main players were a group associated with the Epworth Private Hospital in Melbourne, a group of urologists in Sydney and an international private hospital group with a hospital in Sydney.

Access to the machines for urologists and their patients was generally agreed amicably, but besides the number of machines and their location, both of which were controversial, there was the issue of fees/rebates and the question of whether a qualified urologist needed to oversee treatment.

These last two matters were negotiated broadly by the AMA and conflict between the AMA and the Society ensued. Geof Hirst was Chairman of the Society's ESWL sub-committee and involved in submissions to the MBSRC via ANZAUS and the AMA. On 22 November 1985, he reported to the Executive that the AMA was not prepared to support the principle of urological referral only to the ESWL.

By the end of 1985, the issue had turned into a general argument over the level of Society representation to the MBSRC and, significantly, was more and more frequently dealt with by the Executive as a whole, rather than mainly through ANZAUS. This direct involvement of the Society further added to an already increasing workload.

Representing the Specialty in Other Areas

Something of the range of business dealt with by the Society in the mid-1980s can be gathered from the 1984 Annual Report of the Executive. During the year, the Executive dealt with the organisation of the ASM and membership applications, which had been the basic work of the Society from its foundation, but it also dealt with training, accreditation and education, including the co-ordination of training positions in Australasia; relationships with the RACS; restructuring of the FRACS examinations in urology; proposed changes to the structure of the Society; the Medical Benefits Schedule Revision Committee; the International Congress on Urological Cancer held in Sydney in September 1983 and Paediatric Urology.

The sub-committees of the Society included one for Training, Accreditation and Education, Convenor John Maddern, and one for Fees and Anomalies, Convenor Stuart Taylor; there was also responsibility for the Society's video library (David Golovsky). In addition, the Society had representatives on a range of outside bodies, including the Australian Standards Association (Bill Straffon, plus Dennis Arnold with special responsibility for the Standard for urethral catheters); the Pharmaceutical Benefits Advisory Committee (Bob Wines); the Australian Kidney Foundation (Gwynne Brockis); Clinical Oncology Society of Australia (Geof Hirst); and the AAS (Stuart Taylor). This enormous volume of work led to consideration of the structure of the Society.

Reorganisation of the Urological Society of Australasia

The single biggest workload in the Society every year had always been that of the Convenor of the Annual Scientific Meeting. In the years when the President had a limited involvement in the rest of the Society's business, particularly when he was not from Sydney, this had worked very well. The principal role of the President was as Convenor of the ASM. By the 1980s, this had changed. The principal role of the President was as representative of the Society and Australasian Urology, nationally and internationally. The additional workload of running the ASM no longer made good sense. However, the proposal to separate the two roles opened up the ever controversial question of the rotation of both the presidency and the ASM around the States and New Zealand.

John Jose raised the matter at his ASM in Adelaide in 1984, but given the potential for interstate rivalries, it is not surprising that the first meeting at which the President was not also the Convenor was a decade later. The matter was debated at every meeting between 1984 and 1990 until agreement was reached on the new system. Tony Low was the Convenor of the 1994 Broome meeting, but the President, Stuart Taylor, was from Newcastle in New South Wales.

Office and Administration

During the 1930s and 1940s, the small amount of secretarial work involved in running the Society was performed by the secretaries of members of the Executive, particularly Keith Kirkland's secretary, Marie Corbey. As the members of the Executive all had their rooms in Macquarie Street, this caused few problems. Every year, the secretaries concerned were paid a small honorarium and storage for the

Society's records does not seem to have been an issue. However, during the 1960s and 1970s, members began to move their rooms away from Macquarie Street and the Society's records were handed on from Secretary to Secretary in a series of carrier bags.

Lewisham Hospital provided one point of stability and during the 1970s and 1980s the Society's 'treasures' were stored there in two display cabinets, until the hospital closed in 1988. The other point of stability was the Royal Australasian College of Physicians building at 145 Macquarie Street. The Society had been holding meetings there since the 1940s and came to an arrangement over office space. A number of specialist societies used the RACP facilities and they shared both rooms and secretaries. Ruth Lilian worked for the Society on this basis and so did Audrey Gordon. Gail Hill was appointed in 1987, after Audrey Gordon's death. She had half a room, a desk, a chair and a filing cabinet. The space was shared with the secretary who worked for the Cardiac Society and the Nephrologists were next door.

In about 1990, the Society began to consider buying its own premises. The New South Wales branch of the RACS was buying a building on Albion Street and for a while it seemed that the Society would acquire the old stables at the back of the premises on a strata title arrangement. However, that fell through, causing considerable bad feeling between the Society and the College, and in 1993, the Society's office moved to Albion Street as a tenant of the RACS. This left the Society still looking for premises to buy and arguments over what had, or had not, been done were a feature of the AGMs in this period. In 1996, while Tony Low was President, the Society finally bought premises in Edgecliff, which were leased out for three years until the move could be arranged.[42]

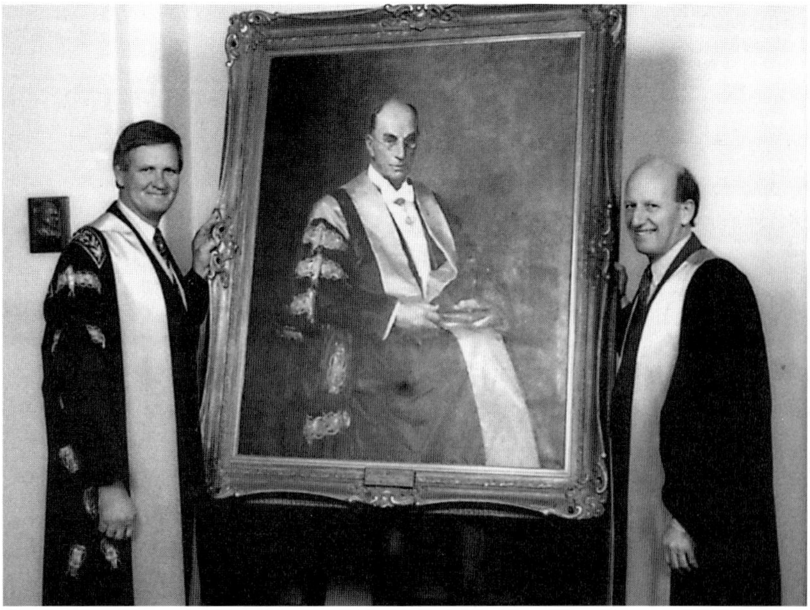

Colin McRae (President RACS 1997-98) and Don Moss (President USA 1998) in front of a portrait of Sir Louis Barnett (President RACS 1937-39). In 1997 Don Moss' work was recognised by the RACS when he was awarded the Sir Louis Barnett Medal for his outstanding contribution to education, training and advancement in surgery.

International Links

Urology in Australasia has never been isolated from urology in the rest of the world. Most of the pioneer Australasian urologists did at least some of their training in Britain or the United States and their international travel and international contacts did not end with their appointments as consultants. Keith Kirkland and Henry Mortensen in particular travelled extensively, and many other early urologists made several trips overseas. Both were corresponding members of the exclusive American Association of Genito-urinary Surgeons, which strictly limited its overseas membership. Many more members of the Urological Society attended meetings of the American Urological Association and, once it was formed in 1945, they attended meetings of the British Association of Urological Surgeons. Many were Commonwealth members of BAUS and the relationship between the two societies was particularly cordial.

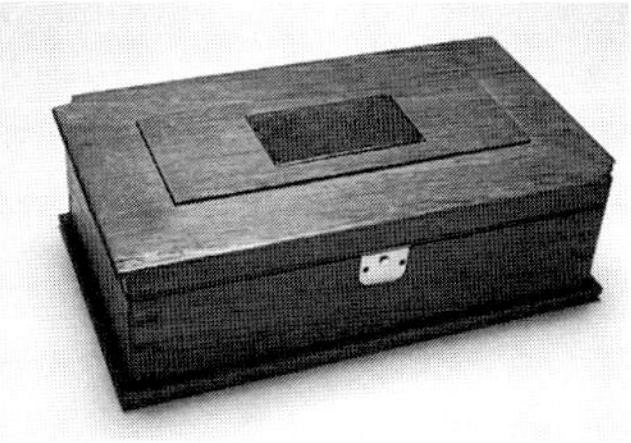

Gavel and case presented to the Society by the British Association of Urological Surgeons, 1949, made from an anatomy table in the Royal College of Surgeons of England that was damaged by bombing in 1941

In 1949, BAUS presented the USA with a gavel and case made from an anatomy table that had been damaged by bombing in 1941. In 1994, the USA presented BAUS with a gong, in honour of their fiftieth meeting. Links with the United States were also strong, but lacked the sense of belonging to the same club that characterised relations with BAUS.

From the beginning, Australasian urologists were also members of the Societe Internationale d'Urologie. In 1937, when the USA was formed, the Australasian section of the SIU was limited to ten members, eight from Australia and two from New Zealand. All the positions were filled and in 1940 the Society wrote to the SIU asking that the quota be increased. Australasian members of the SIU held their section meetings at the Society's ASMs and many found time to attend the international meetings. In some years, numbers were sufficient to justify group travel arrangements through the Society. The SIU meetings were held every three years, usually in Europe, and the principal language was French. This became increasingly inconvenient over time as fewer doctors learned French as a matter of course and by the 1970s the SIU meetings were burdened by the very heavy costs of simultaneous translation.

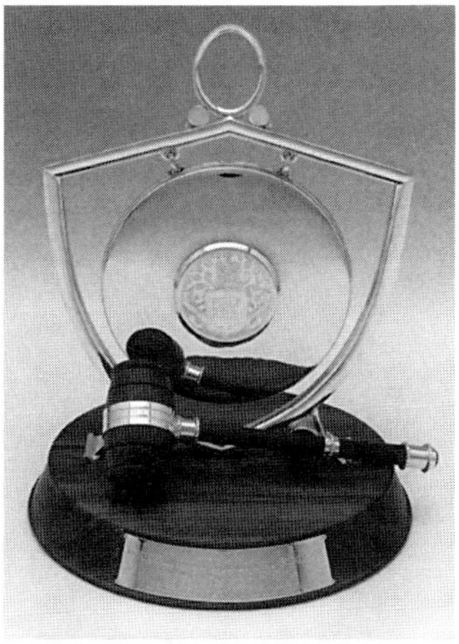

Gong presented by the Society to the British Association of Urological Surgeons at its fiftieth AGM, Birmingham, June 1994

During the 1960s, Australasian urologists began to develop increas-

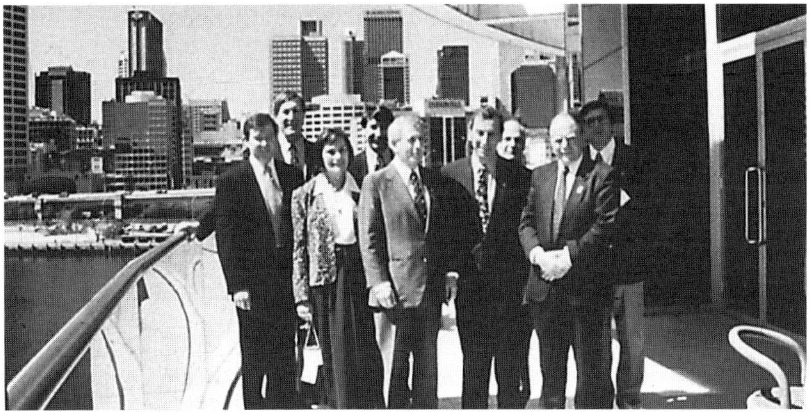

The organising committee for the 1994 SIU Meeting, Sydney: Bill Lynch, Peter Maher, Gwen Pearson, Andre Lalak, Ted Korbel, David Golovsky, John Rogers, Michael Rochford and Chris Farrell ing links with urologists to the north, particularly in India, Singapore and Malaysia. As air travel became faster and less expensive, Australasians travelled overseas more frequently and overseas urologists started to travel to Australasia in greater numbers. As a result, it became possible to hold viable international meetings in Australasia. As early as 1953, the British Medical Association began arranging a joint meeting for members of all its branches around the Commonwealth. It was held in Auckland in February 1961. International meetings in the southern hemisphere were becoming an attractive prospect for Europeans and North Americans. The number increased during the 1970s and by the 1980s, international meetings were quite common. Just three examples give some indication of the variety involved:

In August 1979, Gwynne Brockis from Perth convened the first International Urinary Stone Conference in the southern hemisphere. Delegates from thirty countries flew to Perth and the proceedings were published in the United States.

In September 1987, Graham Holmes and Geof Hirst convened an International Congress of Urological Cancer in Brisbane. The conference featured a large international faculty, particularly from Europe and the United States, and an interactive style.

In September 1994, Sydney was the venue for the largest international urological conference held in Australasia until that date. Bruce Pearson had long been a keen member of the SIU and he was one of those who lobbied to have the principal language changed from French to English. At the meeting in Seville in 1991 he was successful and the Executive of the SIU voted that the next meeting, in 1994, be held in Sydney. Bruce Pearson died in 1992, but the Australasian members of the SIU voted that the Chair of the Australasian President at the 1994 meeting would remain vacant in his honour. David Golovsky and Michael Rochford ran the meeting in his absence.

The SIU meeting in Sydney was a huge affair by Australasian standards, with 2700 delegates, and it ran at a very significant profit. The resulting funds put the SIU on a better financial footing than ever before and also provided $2 million as the basis of the Australasian Urological Trust, to support urological research in Australia and New Zealand. The first recipient of a scholarship from the Trust, the Bruce Pearson Fellowship, was Mohamed Khadra from Sydney.

The location of the 1994 SIU in Sydney indicated that international urologists recognised the standing of Australasian urology and as such, it marked a significant point in the history of the specialty in Australia and New Zealand.

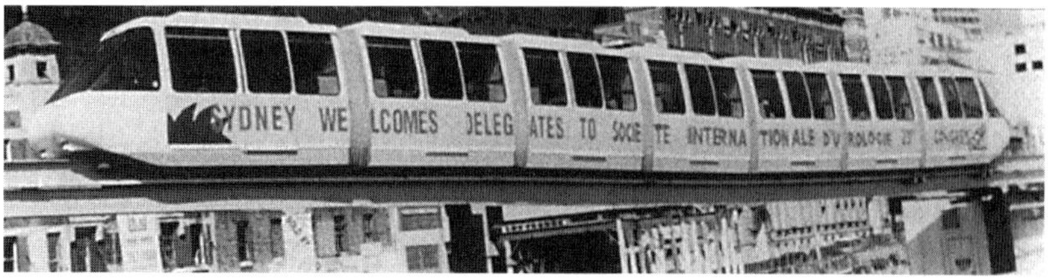

The Sydney monorail welcomed guests to the Société Internationale d'Urologie Meeting in September 1994.

PART 3

~

The Regional Sections of the Urological Society, 1948–1996

~

~

The regional chapters place considerable emphasis on the role of the heads of units in the major public hospitals, particularly in the early years of the development of the specialty.

Several—perhaps most—of the pioneering urologists were more or less competent managers. Their departments had good patches and bad patches, but generally ran amicably enough. Some fostered enthusiasm and team spirit. Some have even been described as inspirational. Others ran stifling departments where any deviation from their way of doing things was severely frowned upon. In the worst instances, a clash of personalities produced two senior urologists who refused to talk to each other and left the registrar carrying messages between them. A strong personality that furthered the Society's goal of 'advancing the science of urology' by standing up to the general surgeons, could also be a tyrant in his own department.

However, this is perhaps to overdraw the picture. Surgery is not a career that attracts unassuming 'yes' men (or women) and the history of the Urological Society is full of strong and colourful characters. The younger generation of urologists were generally very good at standing up for themselves. Nevertheless, the varying leadership styles of the early heads of units had a major impact on the careers of younger urologists.

Public hospital appointments were seen as vital, especially before the 1980s, to the development of the private practices where urologists made their money. Competition for posts was fierce, but largely based on seniority and prior association with the hospital—as medical students, residents and registrars.

During the 1950s and 1960s, younger urologists had little room for manœuvre if they wanted to practise in a city. As one senior urologist put it: 'you got established by steering your little ship between favouritism and nepotism.' Generally, they looked for a public hospital appointment in the city where they had done their initial clinical training, and at the same hospital. This gave the heads of those units considerable power, not because they made the appointments (generally they did not, although they might have some influence over the decision) but because those who were appointed were reluctant to leave, whatever the conditions. Heads of units themselves could not be sacked, although there were one or two instances where they were forced to resign. Young urologists did resign major public hospital posts, and in Sydney and Melbourne they were still able to build private practices, perhaps with appointments at suburban hospitals. But it was seen as a risky thing to do, especially in the smaller cities and especially in the early years. A move to a country centre might be the only real alternative.

The senior urologists used their power and influence in a variety of ways. Some were very helpful to their younger colleagues, inviting them to join them in private practice, for instance. Others used their position to pass on some of their (unpaid) public hospital workload and concentrate on building their private practices. Favouritism was common, nepotism was not unknown and in one or two extreme cases senior urologists used their position to attempt to frustrate the careers of those they did not like.

The regional chapters are organised around the major public hospitals because that is where the power lay. Until the 1980s, for instance, the presidents of the Urological Society were virtually all heads or senior members of urology units at the major metropolitan teaching hospitals. In the 1950s and 1960s as these units grew in size and number they were the building blocks of the Urological Society where groups of urologists were most likely to meet and interact.

Most of these units were initially strictly hierarchical. Prince Henry's in Melbourne, for instance, had a Urologist, plus a First Assistant and a Clinical Assistant and in 1962, when it became a teaching hospital for the newly established Monash University, the post of Second Assistant was added.

By the 1990s, this picture had changed substantially. The structure of most units had become more egalitarian and promotion to the position of head of the unit had ceased to be quite so rigidly based on seniority, as opposed to merit. In addition, the development of urology at suburban and private hospitals, especially in Sydney and Melbourne, and the development of urology in towns and cities outside Auckland, Christchurch, Wellington and the Australian State capitals provided a far wider range of opportunities for young urologists. They were no longer constrained to attempting to obtain appointments at one particular hospital and the power of the heads of the major units was consequently reduced.

Changes in training also had a major impact. Throughout Australasia, the number of accredited training posts increased particularly rapidly during the 1980s. Partly this increase was a response to perceived manpower needs, but 'it was also in response to good training opportunities created in hospitals by urologists wanting accreditation.'

The development first of State selection of trainees and then of rotating registrars through posts led to important changes in the relationship between senior urologists, particularly heads of units, and their younger colleagues. As one urologist put it: 'In the old days, the head of the unit put you in; you did all your training in one unit.' With the end of this system, the opportunities for nepotism and favouritism were much reduced.

However, perhaps the biggest dilution of the influence of the major units came from the increasing number of urologists who were finding that they could build up successful private practices without the need for any public hospital appointment at all. This was true even in Queensland and New Zealand which had traditionally had a form of socialised medicine.

These major shifts in the career opportunities for urologists took place at the same time as a period of rapid changes in the specialty–percutaneous surgery, developments in chemo-therapy for testicular tumours, extracorporeal shock wave lithotripsy, sophisticated urodynamics, laparoscopic surgery and alternative therapies for BPH. Urology as a specialty has evolved very rapidly since the 1930s and the pace of change has certainly not slowed in more recent years.

CHAPTER 6

Urology in New South Wales and Canberra

~

Background

Urology as a profession has generally provided remarkable job security. It is not at all unusual for urologists, once their initial training is complete, to spend all their working lives associated with one hospital or group of hospitals. This is in stark contrast to professionals in many other areas—scientists and engineers, for instance—who in the late twentieth century have learned to live with short-term contracts, redundancy and retraining.

The number of urologists has grown enormously since 1948, but so has the available work. Population growth has contributed to this expansion, but the number of urologists has grown far faster than the total population. At various times, there have been concerns that there might be too many urologists, particularly in Sydney, but there have been no significant problems of shortage of work. Fewer general surgeons doing urology, an ageing population and an increase in the number, sophistication and effectiveness of urological procedures have all contributed to this expansion.

As a result, the common pattern for young Australian urologists has been to obtain one or more public hospital appointments and a growing private practice. (Until recently, the private practice was a less important element in the picture for New Zealand urologists.)

Both the public hospital appointments and the private practice tend to keep the urologist in one place. They are not easily transferable. There is no tradition, as with GPs for instance, of buying and selling urological practices simply in order to move. More commonly, a young urologist is invited to join a group when a senior urologist is thinking of retiring.

This combination of penalties for moving—having to start again building a private practice—and rewards for staying—a growing private

TABLE 6.1 POPULATION (IN THOUSANDS) PER UROLOGIST# NEW SOUTH WALES, 1950–1991

	NSW Total	Sydney	Newcastle	Wollongong	Rest of NSW
1950*	129.8	67.5			1 501.0
1958*	107.0	68.9			498.2
1961	83.3	60.3			232.5
1966	90.1	63.5	109.2	149.5	1 215.5
1971	80.7	63.8	87.9	99.5	177.5
1976	73.5	60.4	90.8	105.5	196.8
1981	73.2	60.5	97.3	111.3	187.1
1986	72.0	70.1	57.9	75.1	100.5
1991	74.4	72.2	71.3	59.0	102.0

#Calculated on full + associate members of the Urological Society
* Dates refer to members of the Urological Society; census years were 1947 & 1954 because these figures are far more sensitive to changes in the number of urologists than to changes in population.
Source: Censuses of New South Wales; membership records of the Urological Society

practice in an expanding field of work—have combined to produce enormous stability.

The exceptions are the academic urologists who, like their fellow academics in other fields, move around the English-speaking world in search of Associate Professorships and Professorships, and the trainees, who have always shown a remarkable propensity for globe trotting.

This pattern was clear from the beginnings of specialist urology, right through until the 1970s. World War II only reinforced the tendency to stability with hospitals taking pains to make room for 'their' surgeons returning from service with the armed forces.

Since the 1970s, however, the pattern has been markedly fractured in Australian (but not New Zealand) inner cities, and it has not been fractured as a result of decisions made by urologists. Many have had to rearrange their practices because their hospitals have been run down or moved or closed. The process of suburbanisation of hospitals, particularly major public hospitals, has followed many years behind the process of suburbanisation of population and it has generally been driven by politicians rather than the medical profession. It has resulted in a significant shake-up to the kaleidoscopic pattern of providing urological services and this shake-up has been particularly marked in Sydney.

The New South Wales Hospital System

Since 1948, the New South Wales hospital system has grown broadly in line with population growth. Between 1948 and 1991, the population of Sydney more than doubled, but growth in the rest of NSW was very much more modest. This increased dominance of Sydney was reflected in changes in the number of hospital beds. Within Sydney there was a significant time delay between population growth in the outer suburbs and a change in the distribution of hospitals.

TABLE 6.2 THE NEW SOUTH WALES HOSPITAL SYSTEM, 1949-1989

	1949	1960	1970	1979	1989	%change
Public hospitals						
Sydney	53	61	64	95	71	+34%
Rest NSW	190	206	199	194	174	-8%
Total	243	267	263	289	245	+1%
Beds						
Sydney	7 693	10 527	11 910	15 499	16 494	+114%
Rest NSW	10 144	12 356	13 638	13 778	12 989	+28%
Total	17 837	22 883	25 548	29 277	29 483	+65%
Private hospitals						
Sydney	139	139	92	77	74	-47%
Rest NSW	123	62	30	23	23	-81%
Total	262	201	122	100	97	-63%
Beds						
Sydney	2 579	3 270	3 413	4 088	4 884	+89%
Rest NSW	909	578	512	1 094	1 334	+47%
Total	3 488	3 848	3 925	5 182	6 218	+78%
Population	**1947**	**1961**	**1971**	**1981**	**1991**	
Sydney	1 484 434	2 289 747	2 807 828	3 204 696	3 538 448	+138%
Rest NSW	1 501 030	1 627 266	1 793 352	1 921 521	2 193 458	+46%
Total	2 985 464	3 917 013	4 601 180	5 126 217	5 731 906	+92%

Source: New South Wales Year Books; Censuses of New South Wales

During the 1980s, there was a fall in the number of public hospitals in Sydney, after a sharp rise in the 1970s, and this broadly reflects the process of adjustment in the distribution of hospital beds.

Private hospitals have consistently formed only a small part of the system—16 per cent of beds in 1949, falling to 13 per cent in 1970 and rising to 17 per cent in 1989. Until 1975, private and intermediate beds in public hospitals made an equally important contribution.

During the 1950s and 1960s the traditional NSW pattern was for most major public hospitals to have a number of beds set aside for paying patients, often in a separate building, although typically sharing diagnostic and operating facilities with the public beds. Generally, the number of private beds remained stable, but the number of intermediate beds, where patients paid part fees, rose steeply. This category, along with the institution of Honorary medical staff, disappeared in 1975 as a result of changes in Commonwealth funding.

The broad pattern in NSW, as in other Australian States, was for the State Government to be notionally responsible for the hospital system, but with an increasing reliance on Commonwealth funds. Until 1975, there were two major classes of public hospital, those in

TABLE 6.3 BEDS IN NEW SOUTH WALES PUBLIC HOSPITALS, 1949-1978

	Private	Intermediate	Public	Total
1949	1 131	2 564	14 142	17 837
1960	1 250	4 639	16 994	22 883
1969	1 219	6 617	17 712	25 548
1978	-	-	29 277	29 277

Source: New South Wales Year Books

country areas generally being under greater State control. After 1975, the schedules under which hospital administration and funding were regulated became more complex. In particular, greater differences were introduced between hospitals run by religious groups (mainly Catholic) and other major public hospitals.

Post-war changes in Commonwealth health provision have frequently been bitterly fought by the medical profession and the impact on the Urological Society is discussed at greater length in Chapter 5. However, changes in the late 1940s and early 1950s increased Commonwealth funding with a general principle of encouraging and rewarding individual health insurance. The 1970s saw much sound and fury on all sides and changes that maintained Commonwealth support for the State hospital system, but based on the idea of individual insurance as an added extra, not the norm. Politicians of both major parties engaged in a tug of war through the health system and there were a number of changes and counter changes in a short period of time.

The wash-out in NSW was that from 1975 the Honorary system went and so did private and intermediate beds in public hospitals. The private beds were more or less replaced by an increase in beds in private hospitals, but the intermediate beds were lost to the system.

Royal Prince Alfred Hospital

Dennis Arnold recalled that when he was training, in the early 1950s, the 'Royal Road' to success was either a year as RSO at St Peter's in London or a Gordon Craig Fellowship at Royal Prince Alfred in Sydney.[1]

When Dennis Arnold returned from London, the money for the Gordon Craig Fellowship had more or less run out. Over the years, the University of Sydney had been eating into the capital to pay for the fellows and Bruce Pearson, who was the fellow before Dennis Arnold, had to moonlight to pay his way. Similarly, Dennis Arnold was appointed as Registrar at Concord Hospital and this helped to cover costs while he was the Gordon Craig Fellow. It was 1957 and Malcolm Earlam was the senior man in the Urology Department at RPAH. The other members of the team, in descending order of seniority, were Angus Walker-Smith, Arthur Carrodus, Harry

TABLE 6.4 THE GORDON CRAIG FELLOWS

1926	John Laidley	1964	Glen Coorey
1927	Malcolm Earlam	1967	John Rogers
1931	Bobby Lee-Brown	1971	Malcolm Drummond
1934	Angus Walker-Smith	1974	John Boulas
1937	Arthur Carrodus	1977	Andrew Brooks
1945	Harry Cummine	1980	Peter Langdon
1947	Vernon Howarth	1983	David Eisinger
1949	Llew Wheeler	1986	James Wong
1954	Bruce Pearson	1990	Robert Thomas
1957	Dennis Arnold	1993	Mohamed Khadra
1960	Harry Learoyd		

Cummine, Llew Wheeler and Bruce Pearson. They had all been Gordon Craig Fellows.

The Gordon Craig Fellowship was set up in 1926 by Robert Gordon Craig, using money he had made from shares in Malaysian tin mining. He also set up the Gordon Craig Research Institute at the University of Sydney and persuaded Adolph Bolliger from Chicago to come to Australia and set up the research facilities. Bolliger's specialty was the biochemistry of skin and feathers, but over the ensuing years he supervised the Gordon Craig Fellows in research more closely linked to urology.

In the years before World War II, Arthur Carrodus worked on possum hormones. This was shortly before Huggins' work in Chicago on female hormones and the prostate. Harry Cummine was awarded a PhD for his work on anti-coagulants for post-operative blood clots.

Not all the Gordon Craig Fellows did so well, but they all had to spend time on pure research, besides working as registrar to what was initially a 16-bed urology ward in RPAH. Dennis Arnold argues that

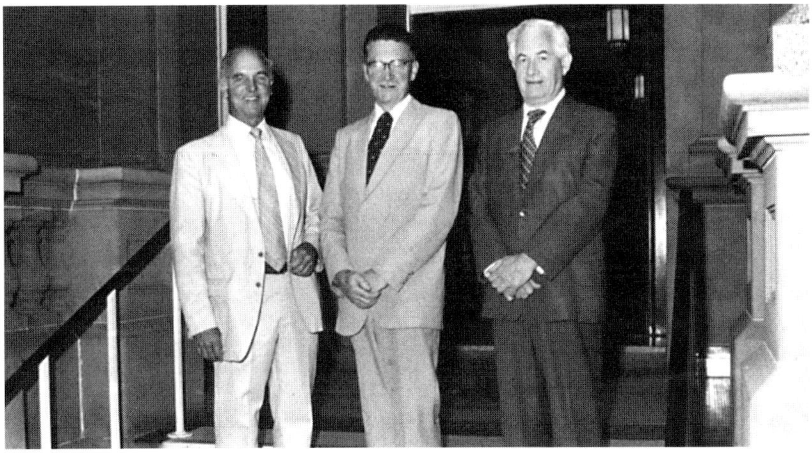

Bruce Pearson, Richard Turner-Warwick and Llew Wheeler outside Royal Prince Alfred Hospital, 1979. Richard Turner-Warwick was the inaugural Penfold-Collins Visiting Professor. (*Source:* John Rogers)

until Bruce Pearson's day, the fellows were somewhat 'sequestered' from the rest of the RPAH surgeons, but that in later years they were exposed to more general surgery. The first two fellows, Laidley and Earlam, were proud of the fact that they were entirely Australian-trained. Most later Gordon Craig Fellows had a broader background and some overseas training. Llew Wheeler, for instance, spent some time in England and so did Dennis Arnold.

As the only training post in urology for many years, the Gordon Craig Fellowship made an enormous contribution to Australasian urology, but it made an even bigger contribution to RPAH. Essentially, the urologists at RPAH were, and are, the Gordon Craig Fellows. Urologists elsewhere in Australasia chose and contributed to the training of their successors, but at RPAH they did so in a particularly systematic fashion.

When John Laidley died in 1955, Malcolm Earlam wanted to go into partnership with Vernon Howarth but, after a brief period, Howarth moved to Newcastle. He appears to have been only the second Gordon Craig Fellow to leave RPAH. The first was probably Lawson Tait, who gave up urology and went to England to become a novelist.[2]

Rule 80 of the Royal Prince Alfred Hospital regulations was supposed to ensure that Honorary Surgeons at Prince Alfred held no similar appointments elsewhere. However, there were a number of exceptions, most notably at the Royal Alexandra Hospital for Children where Laidley and Earlam had both held honorary appointments. Dennis Arnold continued the tradition, pursuing his interest in paediatric urology. Another way around the rule was to obtain appointments as a consultant surgeon and Bruce Pearson, among others, managed a number of consulting appointments when he was still in his thirties.

Royal Prince Alfred was a public hospital, but followed the general pattern for major New South Wales public hospitals in the 1950s and 1960s in also having private and intermediate beds. The intermediate beds were paid at half the private rate. In those days, the Urology Department had one undivided male ward with 25 beds and 6-8 female beds in the ward next door. The operating theatres were on the same level, but the private beds were in a separate building—Gloucester House. They shared the operating theatres and other facilities with the public beds.

Harry Learoyd, Bruce Pearson and Ernie England at a meeting in Melbourne, 1989. (*Source:* Harry Learoyd)

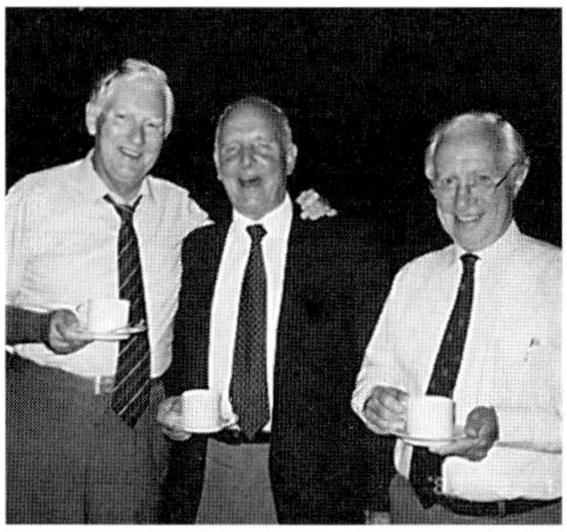

This was rather different from the Catholic Hospitals, which generally had completely separate public and private facilities. 'They dealt with the government better. Everyone thought the Labor Party didn't really understand the operation of the Honorary system.'[3] The system ended in the mid-1970s with the changes brought to health care by the Whitlam Government.

Another important element in the income of surgeons in Sydney was provided by the availability of beds in private hospitals. During the 1950s, 'John Laidley and Malcolm Earlam tied up the Scottish Hospital, Paddington—the private hospital.'[4]

Macquarie Street

In 1958, 75 per cent (21 out of 28) of the Sydney members of the Urological Society had their rooms in Macquarie Street. The exceptions were the four RPAH urologists, with their rooms near the hospital, plus three others, all associate members of the Society.

In 1989, only 15 per cent (7 out of 46) of the Sydney members of the Urological Society had their rooms in Macquarie Street. Of those seven, five were older members who had had rooms in Macquarie Street thirty years earlier. The new pattern was for urologists to have rooms near their principal public hospital, for example three at Newtown, near RPAH, three at Little Bay near Prince Henry, three at Beecroft near Westmead and three at St Leonards, opposite the Royal North Shore Hospital.

While most members of the Executive of the Urological Society had their rooms in Macquarie Street, the office of the Society was always there, unofficially. From 1984 there was a more formal arrangement and the Urological Society had a room in the Royal Australasian College of Physicians building at 145 Macquarie Street. In 1993 the office left Macquarie Street and moved to 177A Albion Street, Surry Hills.

In the early years of the Urological Society, the RPAH urologists had their rooms in Macquarie Street, particularly at 'Ardrossan', number 139. Soon after John Laidley's death, they moved to the Royal Prince Alfred Hospital Medical Centre, 100 Carillon Avenue, Newtown, and when Malcolm Earlam was President for the second time, the Executive of the Society broke with tradition and met in his rooms there.

However, Laidley, Earlam, Wheeler and Pearson were all at 139 Macquarie Street when Llew Wheeler became Secretary of the Society in 1955. He recalled that either Laidley or Earlam told him he was going to be Secretary. 'Everybody knew everybody' and the Executive met in the University Club, 'just across the lane at the back of 139 Macquarie Street'. When Dennis Arnold became Secretary in 1966, the Executive still met in the card room at the University Club in Phillip Street.

From 1979, the Penfolds-Collins Visiting Professor added another element to the mix at RPAH. Many eminent urologists spent some time in the department, including Richard Turner-Warwick and John Blandy from England, Lester Persky, Donald Skinner, Mark Soloway and Jean de Kernion from the USA and Rudolf Hohenfellner from Germany. 'Most of the visiting professors had their operations shown on closed circuit television and Members of the Society were invited to watch the procedures.'[5]

Over the years, the contribution of RPAH to the Urological Society has been enormous, providing six presidents, seven secretaries and three treasurers. In addition, three of the RPAH urologists have been made Fellows of the Urological Society—Angus Walker-Smith and Malcolm Earlam in 1967 and Bruce Pearson in 1987. John

Rogers remembers that it has always been a happy department and a microcosm of multi-culturalism. The Urological Society has never been exclusively Protestant in membership and over the years it also ceased to be exclusively Anglo-Celtic or white. RPAH played an important role in legitimating this change.

Sydney Hospital

Sydney Hospital is a most attractive collection of buildings, but it is squashed in beside State Parliament House on the east side of Macquarie Street. This location has been both its strength and its downfall. Over the years, Sydney surgeons have found it particularly convenient to have their rooms just across the road and down the hill, clustered around BMA house with its views of the Botanic Gardens. However, the hospital site ran out of room to expand, there was fierce competition with the politicians for what little parking space there was in the area and the patients began moving out from the city centre long before World War II. As a result, plans to relocate the hospital provided a constant undercurrent of uncertainty from at least the 1950s.

Despite this, for many years Ward Seven of Sydney Hospital was a serious rival to Royal Prince Alfred as the major centre for urology in Sydney and it was also the cradle of the Urological Society. This was where Keith Kirkland began his career and the base from which he pioneered urological services at a number of other hospitals. While Harry Harris was responsible for bringing international recognition of Australasian operating procedures and Gordon Craig was responsible for initiating Australasian training, it was Keith Kirkland who was mainly responsible for giving Australasian urologists a sense of their own identity as a proud and exclusive group of skilled specialists.[6]

Besides Reginald Bridge, who died in 1944, the other early urologists at Sydney Hospital were Archie Telfer, who died in 1953, and Alban Gee, who was at Sydney for three years before taking up an appointment at Royal North Shore in 1949. Alban Gee had trained in London and it was he who showed Keith Kirkland the Terrence Millin retropubic prostatectomy, although he later reverted to a version of the Harris prostatectomy.[7] Ian Potts wrote:

> *Archie Telfer was a terribly enthusiastic fellow, of a charming disposition, and universally liked. I think he was the first ever to use a watch chain to outline the urethra in the lateral film in the female incontinent. He was always up to some new type of thinking.*[8]

He died aged only forty-nine.

By 1954, Keith Kirkland, ex-Olympic swimmer, big, strong, self-confident, was not only the boss at Sydney Hospital, but had been there seventeen years longer than anyone else. Next in seniority was Hugh Pearson, who joined the department in 1949. In the early 1950s, John Blackman returned to Sydney after a period of training in London:

In 1954 the department consisted of Keith Kirkland, H. H. Pearson, and L. A. Jacobs, I. F. Potts and J. E. Blackman assistant urologists. At that time the Department of Urology at Sydney Hospital was the biggest in N.S.W. operating all Wednesday with two open theatres and two closed theatres working side by side. It was a wonderful atmosphere with challenging activity, lots of dialogue and discussions about urological problems. Every week there were many visitors to the department from Australia, New Zealand and indeed other parts of the world.[9]

Lionel Jacobs and Ian Potts also remembered Sydney Hospital in the 1950s as extremely busy with out patients on two days, cystoscopies on one-and-a-half days and a full day of operations.

Operating started at eight in the morning and last on the pecking list, of course, had the last listed operation. This was the traditional practice in those days, but any irritation involved waiting in the wings, was really dissipated by assisting one's seniors and seeing the volume of work done, which was self instructive.[10]

Ward Seven was the male urology ward with about 20-25 beds and there were also scattered female beds, mainly in Ward Fifteen. The tradition was for Saturday morning ward rounds starting at 8 a.m. with all the staff, including Miss Ogilvy the almoner, the sister, the senior

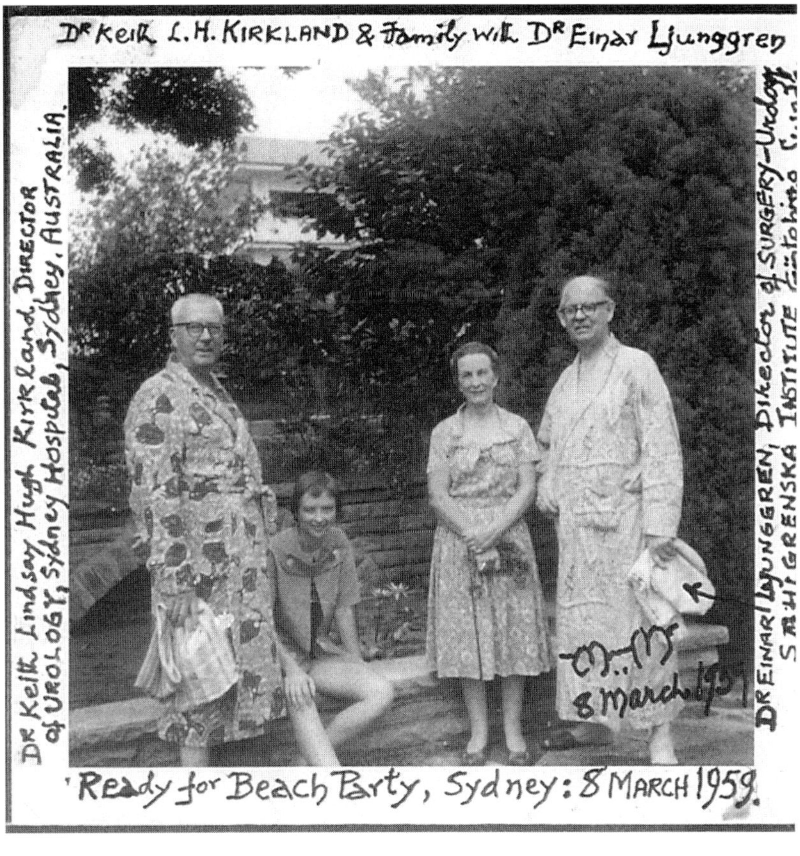

nurse and Kevin Dedman, the instrument man. Afterwards, they would go up to the Board Room and look at X-rays.

Sydney had its fair share of territorial battles with the general surgeons and Keith Kirkland's attitude is a good indicator of the line taken by the Urological Society: The only real urologist was a full-time urologist. 'The acute retentions came in on the surgeon of the week, on the general surgical ward. Some would even operate on them.' The Urology Department would not see a patient unless they took charge clinically and John Blackman tells the story of sitting with Keith Kirkland in the surgeons' room at the Maitland Theatre:

> *One of the sisters came in from the theatre to ask Keith Kirkland whether he would step into the Maitland theatre to help one of the general surgeons who was having trouble enucleating a prostate. Keith's reply was that if the surgeon was happy to transfer the care of the patient to the urology department he would be pleased to step in but on no other account.*[11]

While the unit at Sydney was at its busiest, the urologists instituted a training fellowship and Donald Duncombe, Geoff Gibson and Brian Storey went through the three-year program. 'Renal transplantation was a regular event and we had some children, ample females with incontinence, and a good cross-spread of diseases of both sexes.'[12]

The Australian Kidney Foundation

Sydney Hospital was involved in kidney dialysis from an early date, with an artificial kidney from 1959 and the Kidney Unit from 1962.

> *Keith Kirkland was an inveterate overseas traveller and went to most of the American and International meetings. He returned from one in the Scandinavian countries and was highly impressed with the Kolf artificial kidney machine. He was instrumental in raising funds (the rest of the Unit were flogged along to beg and beseech funds from all wealthy patients) to organise the first Dialysis Machine in Australia at Sydney Hospital. One of our bright young medicos, Malcolm White, took over the management of this machine and finally developed the first renal disease ward within the hospital.'*[13]

The Sydney Institute of Urology, which became the Australian Kidney Foundation, was formed in 1964. The Sydney Hospital urologists involved were Keith Kirkland, Hugh Pearson, Ian Potts, Harry Learoyd and John Blackman, but probably the single most important moving force was Hugh Pearson. Other urologists involved at various times were Lionel Jacobs, Dick Craven, Joe Murnaghan and Geof Watson, plus Jim Mortensen from Melbourne. Businessman Lionel Coppleson provided administrative and fundraising expertise and the Institute of Urology was involved in raising funds to help set up the renal transplant units at Sydney, Royal Prince Alfred and Prince Henry Hospitals.

In 1968 the name was changed to the Australian Kidney Foundation and, as a national body with representation from the Urological Society and the Nephrological Society, the office moved to Canberra. Hugh Pearson was the first Medical Director and later Medical Secretary. In 1971 he resigned and was succeeded by the Melbourne nephrologist, Priscilla Kincaid-Smith.[14]

The energy in this urological hothouse was diffused somewhat during the 1960s. In 1963, the pattern of teaching hospitals was rearranged and Sydney, Prince of Wales and Prince Henry Hospitals became the teaching hospitals for the University of New South Wales. At the same time, there were moves to relocate Sydney Hospital to the Prince of Wales site.

'Ward Seven people were sent out to the Urology Department at Prince of Wales.' There was a diathermy machine and an X-ray unit at Prince of Wales and John Blackman began to build up some experience with TUR. 'The older fellows preferred cutting ... so I got the TURs.' This was a general pattern in Sydney.

During the 1960s Lionel Jacobs went to Prince of Wales and then went on from there to Prince Henry. Hugh Pearson moved to Canberra in 1968 and in the next decade the department was gradually run down. Ian Potts was the boss at the time.

'The introduction of a Government unfavourable to our cause resulted in severe contraction of work at Sydney Hospital, so that the Urological Unit literally withered on the vine.' John Blackman moved to St Vincent's and Brian Storey went to the new hospital at Westmead.

However, Sydney Hospital played a pivotal role in the development of the Urological Society. Until 1955, when Llew Wheeler took up the position, the Secretary of the Urological Society had always been from Sydney Hospital. After that, apart from Jim Blackwood from St Vincent's, the position alternated between Sydney and Royal Prince Alfred until Peter Maher in 1978. In this era, the Society was run from Macquarie Street where most Sydney urologists had their rooms.

John Blackman and Hugh Pearson, who took over from Keith Kirkland as the boss at Sydney Hospital, were in partnership together with rooms at 135 Macquarie Street (BMA House). Between 1952 and 1971 (by which date Hugh Pearson had gone to Canberra) one or other of them was Secretary, Treasurer or President of the Society for eleven out of those twenty years. Alban Gee, Ian Potts and Harry Learoyd were other Sydney Hospital urologists who served the Society as both Secretary and President. Lionel Jacobs spent time as both Treasurer and President and was a pioneer in obtaining trade funding for the ASMs. In addition, Geoff Gibson was Secretary and Brian Storey was Treasurer. Keith Kirkland, of course, was Secretary for ten years and Treasurer for twelve, besides spending a year as President. In 1963 he was made a Fellow of the Urological Society.

Prince Henry (The Coast) Hospital

The first urologist at Prince Henry was Bobby Silverton. He was appointed in 1922 and also spent a considerable amount of his time across the far side of Sydney Harbour at Royal North Shore Hospital.

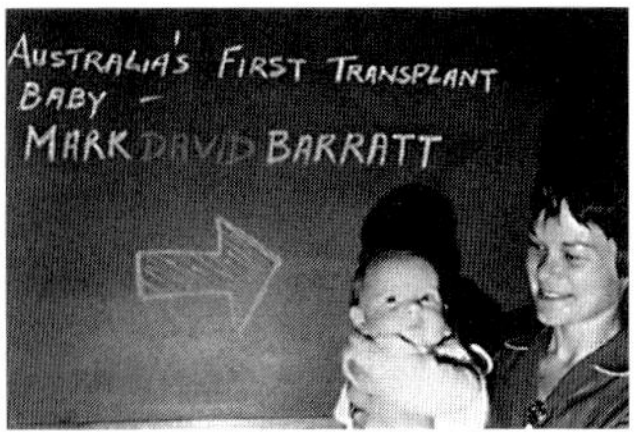

'The urological unit at Prince Henry Hospital undertook the first cadaver kidney transplant procedure in New South Wales and David Barrett was the first transplant baby from the third recipient on our program.' (*Source:* Joe Murnaghan)

In 1934 he was joined by Angus Walker-Smith, who also had an appointment at Royal Prince Alfred Hospital.

Throughout the 1950s, the position of Prince Henry within Sydney urology was peripheral. 'Prince Henry is at the coast ... you have to drive out past Long Bay Gaol ... it was the infectious diseases hospital.' 'The old fever hospital down at the coast ... a long way out of town ... past the golf courses ... you were running out of tarmac ... sand track eventually.'[15]

The location of the hospital, far to the south of where any of the urologists had their rooms or their private patients, and its history as an isolation hospital for everything from tuberculosis to leprosy ensured that both in site and status it was a long way from the centre of things.

In contrast to Royal Prince Alfred and Sydney Hospitals, Prince Henry was on a relatively spacious site with distinct groups of buildings. In the 1950s 'anyone operated on had to go out in the open down to the operating theatre.'[16]

In 1963, the new University of New South Wales began offering clinical courses and took over Prince Henry as a teaching hospital. The politicians were prepared to back the development with money, particularly as Sydney Hospital was resisting the proposed move to the Prince of Wales site.

In 1962, Joe Murnaghan arrived from Edinburgh as Associate Professor of Surgery.

He found that the standard of clinical urology in Sydney was extremely good, but there was very little research except that done by the Gordon Craig Fellows. The work of his team at Prince Henry essentially transformed that picture. From the late 1960s, Murnaghan was Professor of Surgery and the research budget at Prince Henry grew rapidly. 'Prince Henry built up quickly mainly on the efforts of Joe ... a political animal ... got money.'[17]

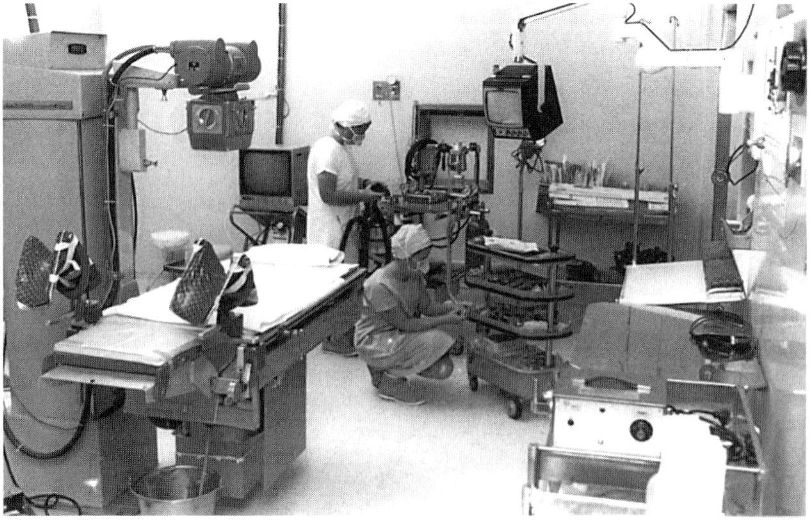

'This was the ultimate appearance of the major urological theatre in my unit (1965) and the operating table, though large and cumbent was probably the first all inclusive urological table in Australasia. It was quickly overworked but was very effective. Though the tabletop was urgently replaced within a few months because of rust developing from our use of 12.5% sodium iodide as the contrast agent.' (*Source:* Joe Murnaghan)

Murnaghan took over a cottage that had been an isolation ward for skin diseases and turned it into a diagnostic urology unit with X-ray tables and diagnostic tables.

> *A very modern urological diagnostic service was designed and equipped whereby a single patient could be almost totally evaluated with any cystourethroscopy, pyelography, cystography, cystometry and very special studies available in one visit to a urological theatre. The provision of this facility was unique in Australia and unusual in the rest of the world and it was evaluated from the cost benefit analysis by the Department of Health Administration in the University.*[18]

Work on renal dialysis, paediatric urology, urodynamics and spinal injuries all followed. The department began to train urologists in academic as well as clinical urology and performed the first kidney transplant in New South Wales. Over the years, Bob Farnsworth, Lionel Jacobs, Harold Thomas, Tony Tynan and Richard Millard joined the department and those who worked there believed that the centre of excellence in Sydney urology had moved from Royal Prince Alfred and Sydney to Prince Henry.

Margaret Rose, the vet who wrote the Government guidelines on using animals in experiments, ran the monkey colony. She did research on liver metabolism while the urologists did research on the neurogenic bladder in primates. Stuart Gowland worked there for a while on a Commonwealth Fellowship. When he needed to take X-rays, the monkeys were put in primate restraint chairs under blue drapes and he drove them over to the radiology department in a VW camper van. They were taken through the back door in between human patients. 'We had a terrible time with the animal welfare people ... they used to paint Margaret Rose's car ... we had to change the locks quite often.' Changes in thinking on the ethics of using primates, from Margaret Rose and Joe Murnaghan, among others, eventually led to the closure of the colony.[19]

Joe Murnaghan's main disappointment from his time at Prince Henry was that he was not able to persuade even one of the urologists to take up full-time research. Richard Millard came out from England to set up video urodynamics but even those like Bob Farnsworth and Richard Millard who continued to do basic research had busy clinical practices. Living on a lecturer's salary was not an attractive option for a surgeon who had the alternative of building a private practice in a growing field.

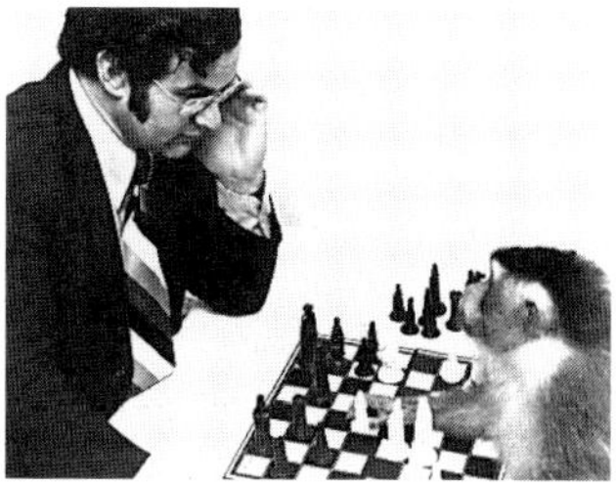

'Stuart (Sid) Gowland playing chess with one of his monkeys at a successful conclusion of a very fundamental and useful year of research in our laboratory in 1975.' (*Source:* Joe Murnaghan)

Despite this, the contribution of Prince Henry to academic urology in Australasia was enormous and this wider perspective on changes in the specialty was clearly reflected in the programs of the Annual Scientific Meetings. Joe Murnaghan was a pioneer of academic urology in Australasia. Some Sydney surgeons may have had their reservations about Murnaghan's clinical skills, but none dispute his contribution to academic urology. From the time of his arrival in Sydney, Murnaghan was heavily involved with the Urological

Society and served on the Executive from 1962 until 1983. He was President 1980-81 and in 1984 was made a Fellow of the Society.

Other urologists at Prince Henry have also played an important role in the Society, Bob Farnsworth, for instance, as Treasurer 1974-77 and Richard Millard for many years as the Society's representative on the Pharmaceutical Benefits Advisory Committee. Richard Millard was also involved in the Continence Foundation of Australia. This was an organisation that grew during a period of specialisation among nurses. The number of nurse continence advisers and urological nurses grew rapidly during the late 1980s and 1990s and led to a revolution in continence care. This was an unfashionable area but as Richard Millard put it: 'The urology input stopped it being just old women.'[20]

Royal North Shore Hospital

Two of the foundation members of the Urological Society had appointments at the RNS—Bobby Silverton, who founded the urology department there, and Colin Edwards, who was appointed in 1932. John Blackman remembers Colin Edwards in the 1950s as lightly built, balding with a moustache and 'a very nice fellow'.[21] He had a ride with him in the first Holden, after Chifley opened the factory. Doug Keller remembers Bobby Silverton as small, assertive and talkative. Silverton and Edwards do not seem to have been friends and they went their own ways at the hospital. However, there is evidence in the minutes of the Executive of the Urological Society that they backed each other in rivalries with urologists from other hospitals.[22]

In 1949, Bobby Silverton and Colin Edwards were joined by Alban Gee and all three played an important role in the early days of the Urological Society. Silverton was President in 1940 and Edwards was President in 1953-54, Treasurer in 1955-57 and was active on the Executive of the Society from its inception until the late 1950s. In 1967 he was made a Fellow of the Society.

Alban Gee was a Queenslander by birth, although educated in New South Wales. He graduated from Sydney University in 1935 and was FRCS (Ireland) in 1940. Gee did his residency at Lewisham under Richard Harris and then served in New Guinea and New Britain during World War II.

Alban Gee, whose involvement with the Society began when he was at Sydney Hospital, was Secretary in 1946-52 and President in 1960-61. Gee also had appointments at Lewisham and Hornsby Hospitals, among others and was in partnership with Richard Harris. He was an acknowledged master of the Harry Harris prostatectomy and was generally regarded with affection as well as respect: 'a thorough gentleman, good at his work, loved by the patients.'[23] Alban Gee was examiner in urology at the RACS from 1964 to 1975. In 1978 he was made a Fellow of the Urological Society of Australasia and in 1983 awarded the OBE for services to medicine. He died on 2 March 1986.

In later years, the urologists at Royal North Shore Hospital had little involvement with the Society. Neither Broadfoot nor Doug Keller, who were both at RNS from the early 1950s, ever held any office in the Society. Doug Keller was not even a full member until the 1970s because he continued to perform some general surgery.

From 1948, Royal North Shore was a teaching hospital attached to Sydney University and from the 1950s, with five urologists, the department was large and busy. Initially, the beds were shared with the general surgeons but new building in the 1970s included a 25-bed urology ward. In 1981, RNS had nearly 1000 beds but by the mid-1990s it was down to about half that size as the hospital was starved of funds. Meanwhile, the urologists at RNS were once more playing a leading role in the Urological Society. Frank Breslin, who moved to RNS when the Mater closed in 1982, was Treasurer in 1968-71 and Ken Vaux was Treasurer in 1994-6. The other urologists at RNS in 1996 were John Saalfeld and Harvey Alexander.

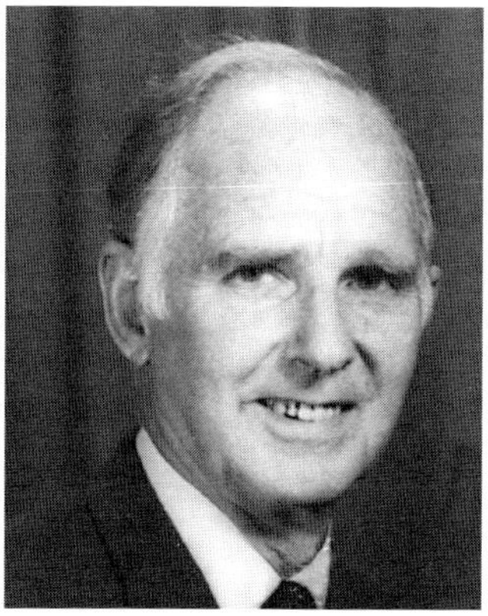

Alban Gee, in whose honour the Alban Gee Poster Prize is awarded each year at the Society's ASM. (*Source:* Muriel Gee)

St Vincent's Hospital

The first urologist at St Vincent's was William Perry, appointed in 1941, but he died the following year. Keith Kirkland took over and built up the department to a position of some prominence. John McNamara was appointed in 1948 and in 1955 the Department consisted of Keith Kirkland, John McNamara, Richard Craven and J. Blackwood. That was the year that Kirkland retired and McNamara took over as head of department. He was never particularly involved in the Urological Society but many of the other St Vincent's urologists were. Richard Craven was Treasurer in 1957-61, President in 1966-67 and an active member of the Executive throughout the 1950s and

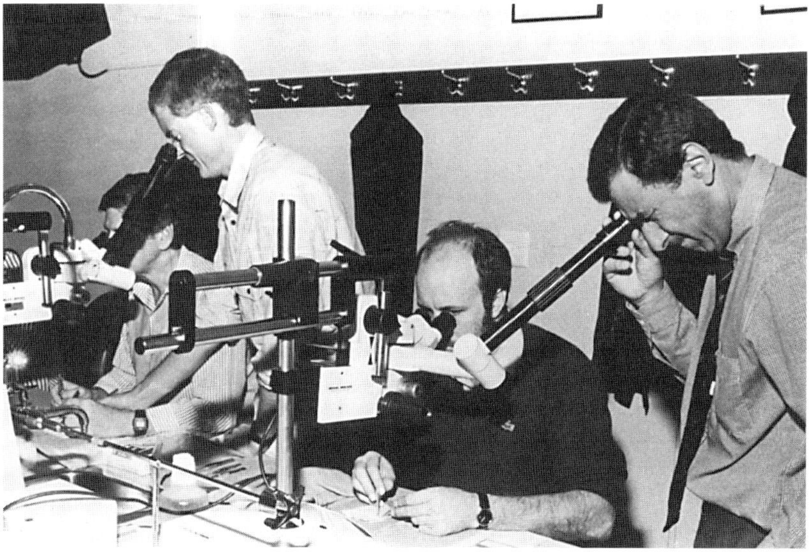

Microsurgical workshop 1991. *Standing* are David Golovsky and M. McCluskey. *Seated* closest to the camera is Les Yeaman and behind him Chris Farrell. (*Source:* David Golovsky)

1960s. He retired in 1971. James Blackwood, who was appointed in 1954, was Secretary in 1961-63. He retired in 1970. George Schnitzler, who was appointed in 1961 was Treasurer in 1971-74.

During the 1970s, the department was very busy, performing more than 1200 operations in 1974-75, for instance.[24] From the 1980s, however, like a number of other Catholic hospitals, St Vincent's was under threat of closure. As an inner city hospital, it served Kings Cross and had a reputation as the 'AIDS' hospital. St Vincent's Private next door had no such image problems and continued to thrive with surgeons such as David Wilson, David Golovsky and Philip Stricker. In the 1990s it was known as the Prostate Hilton, inheriting that position from another Catholic hospital—Lewisham.

Lewisham and the Mater Misericordiae Hospitals

After Harry Harris' death in 1936, Lewisham remained a centre of excellence in urology, particularly in prostatectomy. The dedicated nursing staff of the Little Company of Mary remained and so did Richard Harris. He was always somewhat in his older brother's shadow, but he was a fine surgeon and an active member of the Urological Society, serving on the Executive for many years. He was President in 1949-50. As a result, working in the rather unexpected location out at Lewisham remained attractive for leading urologists and Desmond Trainor, Richard Craven and Alban Gee were among those with appointments there. All were notable figures in the history of the Urological Society, working hard on various committees in the days when it was still a small and cosy society.

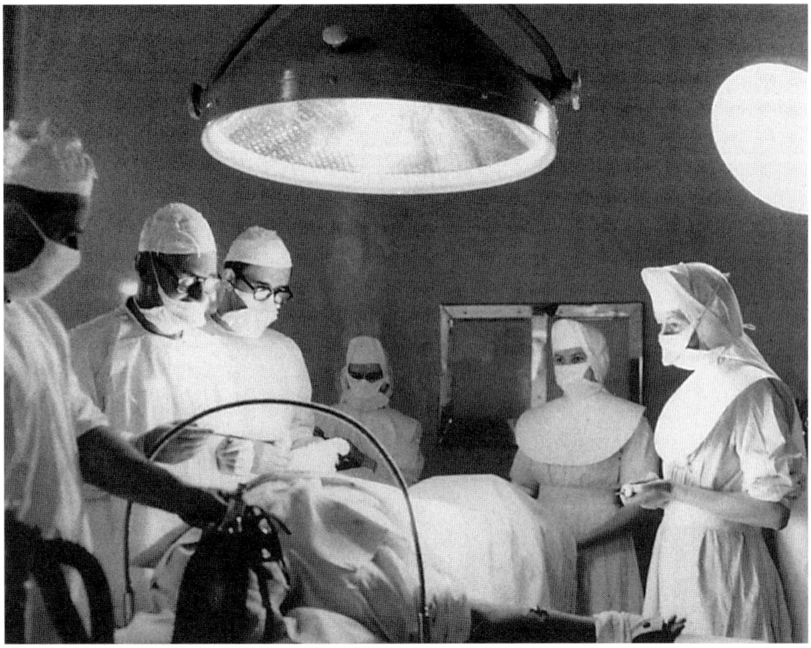

Operating theatre at Lewisham Hospital in about 1960. (*Source:* the archives of the Little Company of Mary)

Frank Breslin was appointed at Lewisham in 1963, after Richard Harris died. The Lewisham team were enormously proud of their tradition. The hospital was in a run down area and Frank Breslin said that it must have been irritating for the Royal Prince Alfred people to come out and see what Harry Harris was doing.[25] Llew Wheeler, who was at RPAH from the early 1950s, agreed.

> *The Royal Prince Alfred Hospital was the biggest hospital. There was jealousy between them and Harry Harris at Lewisham. Harris used to get closure [in his prostatectomy operation] ... the Prince Alfred people couldn't get round to doing this for some years afterwards.*[26]

The status of Lewisham as the pioneer hospital for urology in Australasia was recognised by the Urological Society which set up a small museum there for old surgical instruments and other of the Society's treasures. When Lewisham closed in 1987, as part of the program of running down metropolitan Catholic hospitals, there was no obvious home for either the display cabinets or their contents. By that date, the Society had an office in the Royal Australasian College of Physicians building on Macquarie Street, but it was shared with the secretarial staff of other societies and there was little room. One of the cabinets ended up in David Golovsky's care and the instruments were stored in boxes until the office of the Society moved to more spacious premises in the old stables behind the Royal Australasian College of Surgeons building in Surry Hills.

The disruption of the established pattern of Catholic hospitals also affected the Mater Misericordiae on the North Shore. The urology department was founded by Keith Kirkland. He trained Errold Maloney in urology and retired in 1956, leaving Maloney and Angus Walker-Smith to run the department. Angus Walker-Smith was made a Fellow of the Society in 1967. Maloney died suddenly in 1964 and Frank Breslin, and later Glen Coorey, ran the department until the Mater Public was closed in 1982 and the new (and very busy) Mater Private Hospital was built.

Concord and Prince of Wales Repatriation Hospitals

In 1969, Peter Maher was appointed to Concord Hospital as a registrar. Eric Parry, the only urologist before him, had been an associate member of the Urological Society since the early 1960s. In 1970, Maher was appointed Staff Specialist in urology and remained as head of department until early 1995, when he became Visiting Medical Officer.

The hospital was founded in 1942 as a part of the special provision for returned servicemen and was a free Commonwealth hospital with salaried staff. Even the Visiting Medical Officers (equivalent to Honorary staff elsewhere) were paid an hourly rate. Until the

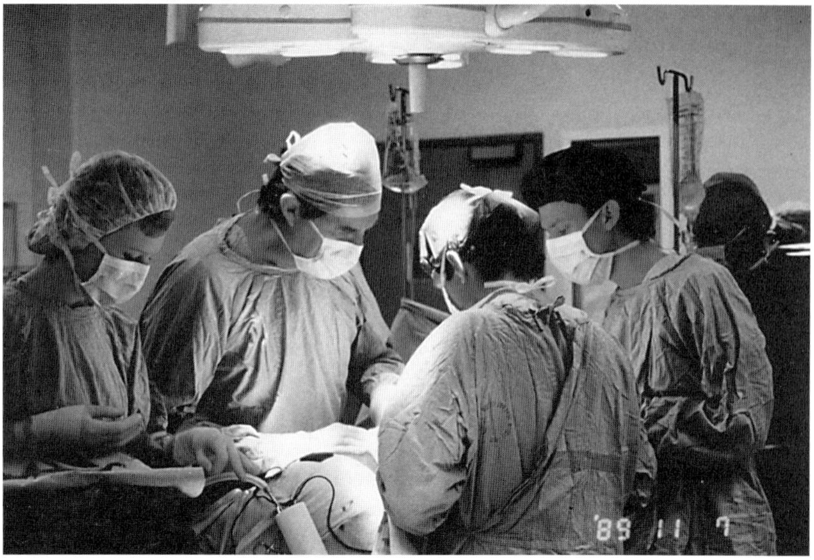

Peter Maher operating at Concord Hospital with Bill Lynch, registrar, assisting in the foreground, 1989. (*Source:* Peter Maher)

1970s, most of the Visiting Urologists at Concord were from Royal Prince Alfred Hospital, people like Arthur Carrodus, Llew Wheeler and Harry Cummine who would 'do their bit for the digger by coming across'. As the phrase suggests, Concord was more or less west of RPAH. Once Peter Maher was appointed and there on a regular basis, the Visiting Urologists began to spend less time at Concord.

Maher built up a department that dealt with virtually everything except paediatric urology. He was particularly interested in incontinence, impotence and lithotripsy but because of the clientele of 'old diggers' there was a 'very large exposure to prostatic disease ... Joe Murnaghan called us the prostate shop.'[27]

From the late 1960s, Concord was involved in the training scheme with a position for a urology registrar and a stream of notable urologists went through the program. David Golovsky was appointed in 1971 and Andre Lalak was also among those who gained experience in the prostate shop.

In the 1990s, the urologists at Concord were, besides Peter Maher, Enzo Lazarro, Andre Lalak, Andrew Mitterdorfer and David Eisinger. Andre Lalak was Treasurer of the Society in 1991-94. Peter Maher was Secretary in 1978-81, President in 1989-90 and in 1995 he was made a Fellow of the Society.

During and immediately after World War II, the Prince of Wales Auxiliary Hospital at Randwick was also a Commonwealth repatriation hospital but by 1960, it was a part of the State hospital system. The original links were with Sydney Hospital, but as one of the teaching hospitals for the University of New South Wales, it also developed close links with Prince Henry and in the 1980s the urological staffs at both hospitals were the same. The Prince of Wales site also included a children's hospital.

Westmead Hospital

There was a considerable time delay between the outward spread of Sydney's population and the outward spread of Sydney's hospitals, but Westmead represented the new generation. At the beginning of the 1980s, as Sydney Hospital ran down, Westmead built up. The first Matron was Jacky Harris, who had been the sister in charge of Ward Seven, the urology ward at Sydney. In theory, the urology beds were transferred to Westmead, but there were only two urologists at Westmead in 1996—Andrew Brooks and Malcolm Drummond, both Gordon Craig Fellows.

In 1995, the Royal Alexandra Hospital for Children closed and The New Children's Hospital opened, adjacent to Westmead, where there is more space and new facilities. In 1996, Grahame Smith was the urologist there. Generally, the older generation of surgeons preferred not to move west and left the jobs to the younger generation.

The major exception to this pattern is Michael Rochford who worked in the western suburbs from 1969. Nepean was the major hospital in the west before Westmead was built in 1977 and suffered from poor facilities. Despite this peripheral position, Michael Rochford played an active role in the Society and was Treasurer in 1983-88, besides playing a leading role in running the SIU meeting in Sydney in 1994.[28]

St George

Like Nepean, St George Hospital is in a suburban area. It began as a cottage hospital for the community at Botany Bay and was attached to the University of New South Wales. By the 1990s the area contained not only the old diggers but also a large Greek and Moslem community.

The first urologist at St George was Gordon Pfeiffer. He had spent a year as RSO at St Peter's and was one of those invited by Keith Kirkland to the first meeting of the Sydney Urological Association. However, he continued to do some general surgery and was therefore ineligible for full membership of the Urological Society.

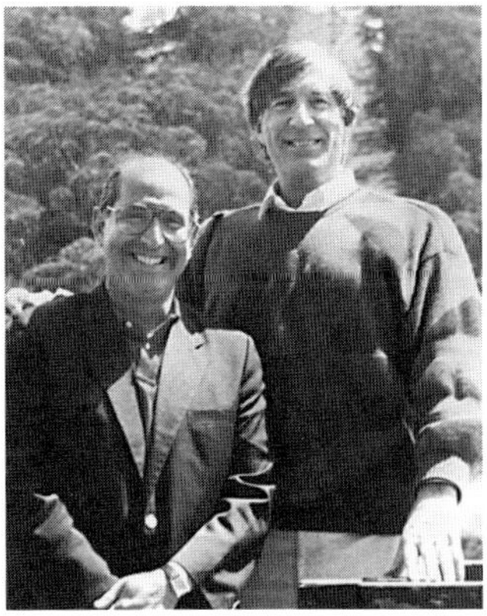

Peter Maher and Professor Michael Lieber from the Mayo Clinic, New South Wales State Section Meeting, Thredbo, 1989. (*Source:* Gwen Pearson)

The era of urological procedures performed by full-time urologists really began with Bill Lucas in the mid-1960s. Bill Lucas began his career at Sydney Hospital, after training in Britain and the United States. 'In those days Sydney was the best urology unit ... a happy hospital, good staff, tragic to cut it back ... patients would come from all over NSW and the Pacific Islands ... it had charm.'

St George was also by and large a happy hospital, although the politics involved with building the new hospital caused some tension. By the 1980s, St George was in a marginal State electorate and a considerable amount of money was invested in the building of both private and public hospitals on the same campus.

Tony Tynan, Chris Farrell and Bill Lynch all had appointments at

St George and between them made a significant impact on the Society. Tony Tynan was Chairman of ANZAUS in 1980-83. Chris Farrell was on the Executive from 1989, Secretary in 1990-93 and subsequently Chairman of the CME Committee. Bill Lucas' contribution to the Society was less official. He had considerable expertise in matters pertaining to the stock market and was a Fellow of the Securities Institute of Australia. His witty talks at the Society's ASMs might or might not assist Members interested in that area.[29]

Canberra

The first associate members of the Society practising in Canberra were Peter Hughes and A. G. Robson. By 1966, Hughes was a full member, but Robson retired and in 1965 Graeme Heap agreed to join Peter Hughes. They had met in Birmingham and co-operated to set up a haemodialysis service at the Canberra Community Hospital. In 1966, Hugh Pearson moved to Canberra so the area enjoyed the services of three full members of the Urological Society. One of them, Hugh Pearson, had given up his position at the pinnacle of Sydney urology as Head of the Department at Sydney Hospital, in order to move to Canberra, where he ran the Australian Kidney Foundation. In 1971 he retired from the AKF and concentrated on his private practice.

Hugh Pearson retired in 1978 and in 1982 Richard Nugent set up in private practice, keeping the Canberra team at three until the 1990s, when it increased to four urologists. In 1991, they applied for

TABLE 6.5 MEMBERS OF THE UROLOGICAL SOCIETY OF AUSTRALASIA IN NEW SOUTH WALES AND CANBERRA

	1950	1958	1963	1966	1971	1976	1981	1986	1991#
Canberra	-	-	*/2	1/1	3	3	3/1	3	3
Sydney	14/8	21/7	22/16	24/16	30/14	40/10	42/11	41/7	49
Newcastle	1	1/2	1/4	3	3/1	4	4	4/3	6
Wollongong	-	-	1	1	1/1	2	1/1	2/1	4
Lismore	/1	/1	/1	/1	/1	1/1	1/1	3	1
Wagga	-	-	-	- /2	/1	/1	1/1	1	1
Singleton	-	-	-	-	/1	/1	/1	-	-
Albury	-	-	-	-	-	/1	1	1/1	2
Tamworth	-	-	-	-	-	/1	1	1	1
Taree	-	-	-	-	-	/1	/1	1	1
Gosford	-	-	-	-	-	-	1/1	2	3
Nowra	-	-	-	-	-	-	-	/1	1
Orange	-	-	-	-	-	-	1/1	2	2
Tweed Heads	-	-	-	-	-	-	-	/1	1
Camden	-	-	-	-	-	-	-	-	1

* Left of /= full member; right of /=associate member; # 1991 figures are full+associate.
Source: Membership records, Urological Society of Australasia

a urology training post at the Woden Valley Hospital and the first year with an accredited trainee was 1995.[30]

Newcastle

The first NSW urologist outside Sydney was J. Broughton in Newcastle. He retired in the 1950s and Vernon Howarth, a Gordon Craig Fellow, set up in practice. By 1958 there were three urologists in Newcastle: Vernon Howarth, who remained until 1983, plus two associate members of the Urological Society : O. J. Ellis and D. D. Henry. They did not remain long, but in the early 1960s, two general surgeons, Kevin Johns and Keith Walker, began to specialise as urologists. Both were based at the Mater Misericordiae Hospital.

The other major hospital in the area was the Royal Newcastle. In the late 1960s it was a 450-bed hospital but then underwent a considerable building program. Among the new facilities were a dedicated urology diagnostic and endoscopic suite. Funding was made available to equip this with the latest operating tables, video and X-ray facilities and endoscopic instruments. Stuart Taylor, who had trained in Britain and then spent 1969 as a registrar with Joe Murnaghan at Prince Henry, moved to Newcastle in 1970.

Over the years, Stuart Taylor was joined by Sandy Grant, James Patterson, Martin White, Phillip Sprott and Stephen Clarke.

> *On 27th December 1989 Newcastle was struck by Australia's worst earthquake, which resulted in major structural damage throughout the region and 13 deaths. The York and North wings of Royal Newcastle Hospital were severely damaged and rendered structurally unsafe. This included the dedicated urology ward of 20 beds, Ward 5. After immediate evacuation onto the adjacent lawn, the unit was moved to Wallsend District Hospital, some 15km to the west.*[31]

After protracted negotiation with the Hunter Area Health Service, a dedicated urology ward was opened in the refurbished Royal Newcastle Hospital.

Stuart Taylor was a very active member of the Urological Society and played a particularly important role in medico-political matters. He was chairman of ANZAUS in 1983-88, President of the Urological Society in 1993-94 and subsequently the Society's representative on the RACS Council. Sandy Grant was also active in the Society and on the Executive in the 1990s.

Other New South Wales Towns

G. M. McFadden was the first urologist in Wollongong, the next largest town in New South Wales. He joined the Urological Society in the early 1960s. In 1969 he was joined by Michael Rosen, who did pioneering work in incontinence. In 1974, Rosen designed an artificial sphincter which was simple but effective and clear proof that innovative urologists were not only to be found in the capital cities.[32] During the 1980s, the number of urologists in Wollongong grew rather faster than the population and there were four by 1991.

N. E. Brand, an associate member of the Urological Society, practised in Lismore from 1951 to 1995. In 1976, he was joined by Stuart Siller from Sydney, and David Kerle joined them in 1988. David Siller, a nephew of Stuart, started in 1996.

Few other towns could sustain more than one urologist. Wagga Wagga had P. R. McNeill in the 1970s and there was a period of overlap before John Smith arrived in 1981. Orange had both Peter Bilenkij and Mark Morrissey in 1996, managing to overcome problems of professional isolation and finding locums in country towns.

Over the years, the Urological Society acknowledged the problems of practising full-time urology in regional centres and therefore supported associate members in country areas. However, the overall policy remained that it is in the best interests of patients that whenever possible only full-time, fully trained urologists perform urological procedures. Generally, the country urologists were fighting battles in the 1980s that the city surgeons had won in the 1950s, such as general surgeons wanting to perform urological procedures when there was a urologist on the hospital staff.

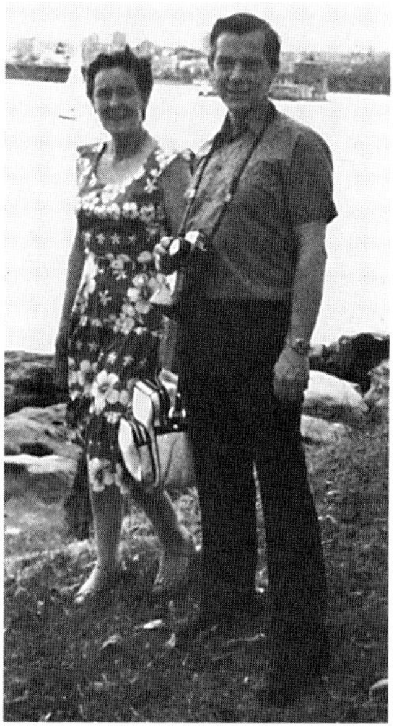

Anne and John Blandy in Sydney, c.1975

Providing adequate coverage for country areas remained a problem in the 1990s, but there were a number of moves to improve matters. City surgeons such as David Wilson, Geoff Gibson and Peter Maher visited country areas, such as Dubbo and Armidale. Meanwhile, the central coast, Wollongong and Canberra were well supplied with their own urologists and in other areas such as Orange and Lismore two or three urologists would get together. 'They bump off each other quite well. Some very good work is presented and done.' This was despite the problems of attracting young urologists to country areas when they had been trained to be interested in the big operations.[33]

The New South Wales Section of the Urological Society

From 1940, the section of urology of the NSW branch of the BMA operated effectively as the NSW section of the Urological Society. However, by the late 1950s, it had ceased to meet regularly. NSW members did, however, meet on an informal basis from time to time, particularly when distinguished visitors were in Sydney. For instance:

> *On Wednesday 10th August [1955] at 8.15 p.m. Sir Stanford Gade and Professor Windeyer will lecture to the Society (in conjunction with the Post-graduate Committee in Medicine) on 'New growths of the Penis and Testis' (not 'of the Penis and Scrotum' as previously stated.)*
>
> *There will be a dinner at the University Club (6.15p.m. for 6.45p.m.) before the lecture, and so far eighteen members have signified their intention of being at it. All NSW Members have been circularised about this dinner.*[34]

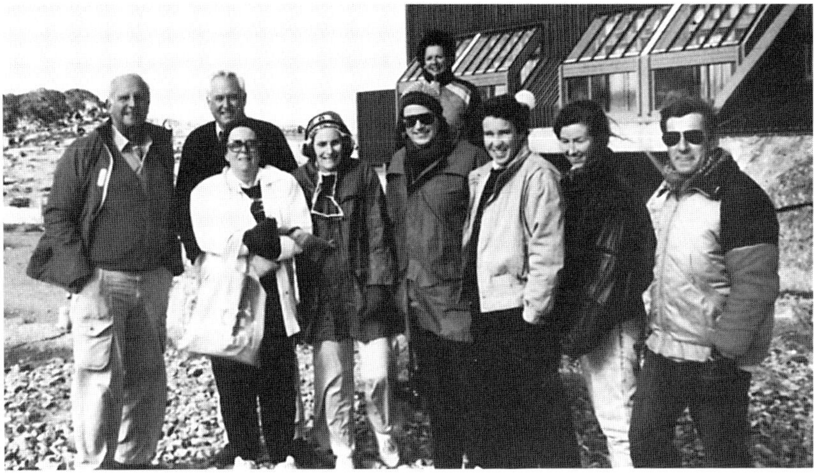

New South Wales State Section Meeting, Thredbo, 1989. Bruce and Gwen Pearson, David Wilson, Joanna Maher, unknown, Nina and John Saalfeld, Bill and Donna Lynch. (*Source:* Gwen Pearson)

This was the state of affairs when, in early 1958, urologists in Queensland proposed setting up a Northern Branch.

The Executive hurriedly formed a sub-committee consisting of Colin Edwards, Hugh Pearson and John Blackman and on 14 April they met to discuss the question of State Branches. The general opinion was that members of the Society were free to form branches, but all members of each branch must be members of the Society.

The first meeting of the Northern Section was on 27 May 1958, with Hogg as Chairman, and the first meeting of the Victorian Section was on 21 October, with Leonard Murphy as Chairman. This was also the year that, as a result of an initiative from Henry Mortensen, State representation on the Executive was agreed. The first meeting of the enlarged Executive with State and New Zealand representatives was on 13 November 1959.

Meanwhile, the section of urology of the NSW Branch of the BMA was still not meeting regularly and it was not until 13 March 1962 that a NSW Section of the Urological Society first met, with Keith Kirkland as Chairman and Joe Murnaghan as Secretary and Convenor. From then on, the section met more or less regularly, providing younger members with the opportunity to present papers, as well as a forum for informal discussions.

Over the years, Section Meetings grew and regularly included distinguished guests, whether from overseas or from elsewhere in Australasia. In 1989, for instance, the AGM of the NSW Section was held at Thredbo in October and guests at the Section Meeting included John Fitzpatrick from Dublin, and Richard Turner-Warwick and Tony Mundy from London.[35]

CHAPTER 7

Urology in New Zealand

~

Background

In 1951, New Zealand had a population of about two million and by 1991 this had risen to about three and a half million, but over this period, the distribution of the population changed considerably. The population of the North Island in general and the Auckland region in particular grew much more rapidly than the population of the South Island. In 1951, 32 per cent of the population lived on the South Island and by 1991 this had fallen to 25 per cent. By that date, the population of greater Auckland exceeded the entire population of the South Island.

By 1951 there was already a strong tradition of specialist urologists in the three centres of Christchurch, Wellington and Auckland. Over the next forty years, the number of urologists grew more rapidly than the population as specialist coverage was progressively extended outside the major cities. Although more than one in four New Zealanders live in Auckland, there are a large number of other important towns and the dominance of Auckland is by no means as great as that of the capital cities of the Australian States.

During the second half of the twentieth century the relative importance of Christchurch and Dunedin declined, but other towns continued to grow strongly, especially on the North Island. Besides Auckland, Hamilton, Palmerston North and Napier/Hastings all more than doubled in population between 1951 and 1991 and there was also significant growth in Wellington.

As a result, New Zealand's urologists are far more evenly spread across the country than is generally the case in Australia. In 1996, eight North Island and five South Island towns had specialist urologists.

New Zealand's urologists were also far more likely to work mainly within the public sector than was the case in Australia. The 1938 Social Security Act set up the Social Security Fund to help provide, among other things, hospital funding. From 1939 hospital benefits

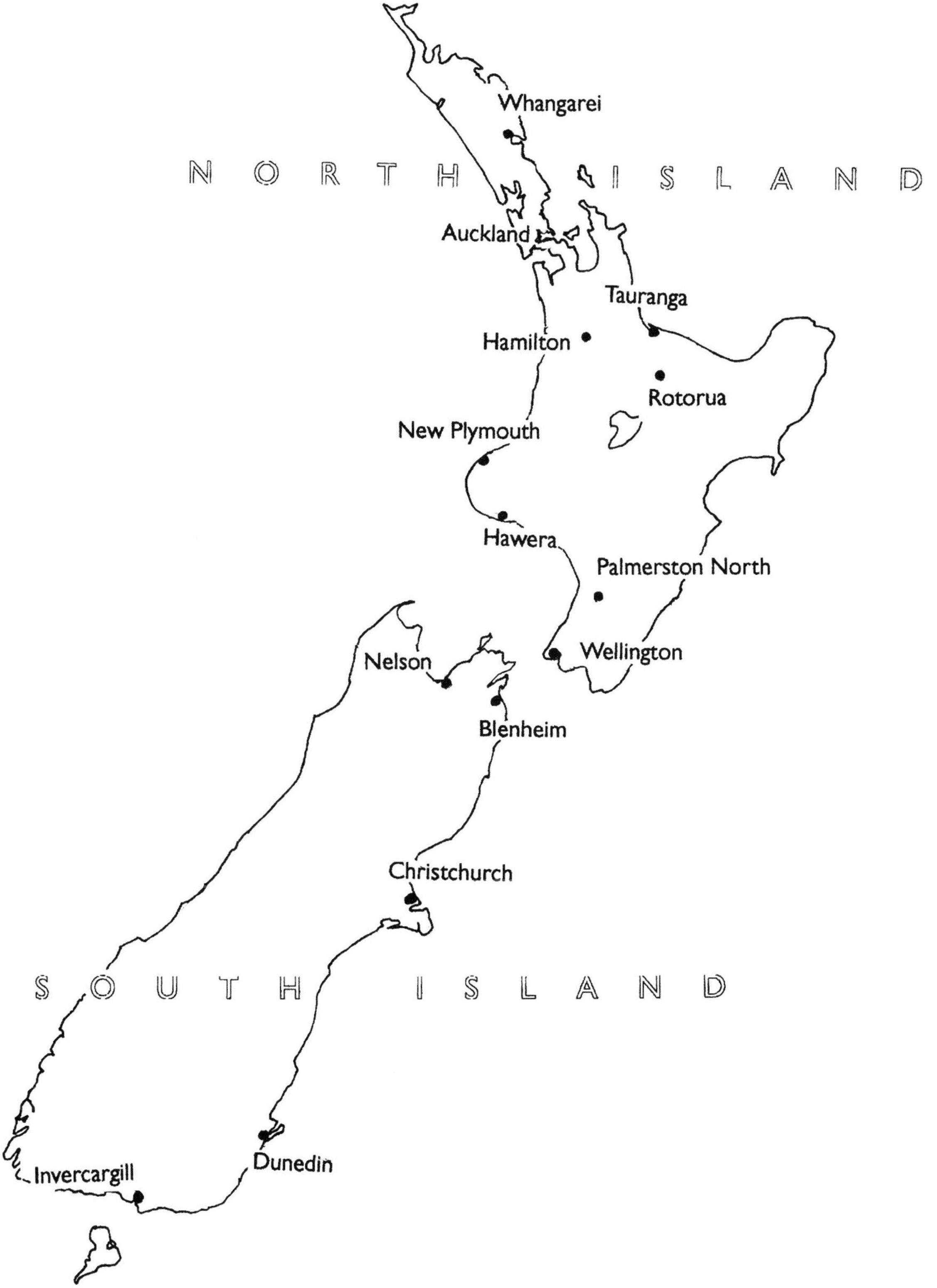

New Zealand cities and towns with one or more specialist Urologists, 1991

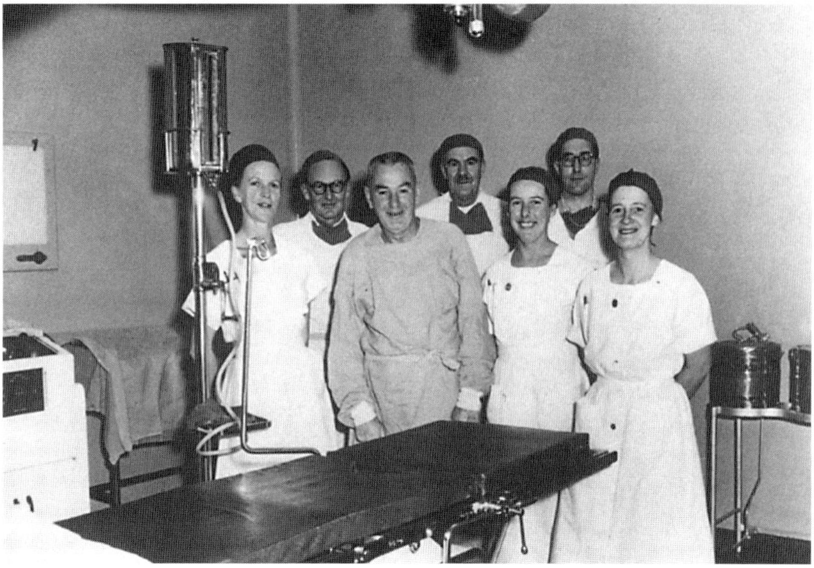

Christchurch Urology team, 1962. *Left to right:* Sister Jan Turnbull, Dr C.J. Morkane, Edgar Reay, Dr E. T. H. Taylor, Sister B. M. Reynolds, Dr B. Jones, Sister M. L. Wright. (*Source: The History of the Canterbury Area Health Board*)

were provided for in-patients and until the late 1950s, hospitals were funded from three main sources: the Social Security Fund, a Government subsidy from general taxation revenue and the Local Authority levy collected through the hospital boards.

The LA levy was more visible than other forms of taxation and was progressively reduced. From 1946 it was limited by law to 5d in the £1 and by 1957 it had been phased out completely. This had the double effect of reducing the power of the hospital boards and increasing Government involvement in the running of hospitals. The 1957 Hospitals Act formalised this position and from 1958 the Minister of Health was responsible for the provision of hospital beds, but still acting through the hospital boards.

Public hospital beds remained free, but the number of private hospital beds was already growing. By the mid-1980s, about one in four beds were in the private system, compared with about one in ten in the 1940s. This pattern of change was accelerated during New Zealand's period of Rogernomics when, under a Labour Government, the New Zealand Welfare State was subjected to a large dose of economic rationalism led by the Minister of Finance, Roger Douglas. In 1989 the hospital boards were abolished and replaced by 14 Area Health Boards. There were hospital closures and general complaints of lack of consultation with the medical staff.

In 1993 there was further major change with the formation of Crown Health Enterprises (CHEs), based around the major public hospitals, and the public system continued to struggle through a period of major turmoil. Four Regional Health Authorities (RHAs) were provided with funding and the CHEs and private health care providers were encouraged to compete with each other for RHA contracts. By 1994 there were more private than public hospitals in

TABLE 7.1 POPULATION CHANGE IN NEW ZEALAND, 1951-1991

	1951	*1961*	*1971*	*1981#*	*199 1*
Auckland	382 003	514 497	698 382	770 362	885 377
Wellington	217 270	263 440	324 032	320 979	324 792
Hamilton	80 313	109 955	136 022	133 571	148 168
Napier/Hastings	57 420	75 989	86 882★	107 481	109 875
Palmerston North	53 251	68 719	75 944★	91 821	
Total North Island	**1 313 865**	**1 684 785**	**2 051 363**	**2 322 989**	**2 550 370**
Christchurch	202 184	253 017	302 610	290 680	306 856
Dunedin	102 674	112 338	117 740	108 029	109 423
Total South Island	**625 603**	**730 199**	**811 268**	**852 748**	**878 994**
Total New Zealand	**1 939 472**	**2 414 984**	**2 862 631**	**3 175 737**	**3 429 364**

Source: New Zealand censuses. #The figures for city population are not strictly comparable because of changes in the statistical areas over time. The 1951-71 figures are for Statistical Divisions. The 1981 and 1991 figures are for the (smaller) urban areas. ★1966, not 1971, figures.

TABLE 7.2 NEW ZEALAND MEMBERS OF THE UROLOGICAL SOCIETY OF AUSTRALASIA

	1951	*1963*	*1971*	*1981*	*1991*
NORTH ISLAND					
Auckland	3	5	6	8	7
Wellington	2	4	3	3	5
Hamilton	-	2	1	1	2
Palmerston North	-	1	1	2	2
Rotorua	-	1	1	2	2
Tauranga	-	-	1	1	2
Whangarei	-	-	-	1	1
New Plymouth	-	1	-	1	1
Hawera	-	-	1	-	-
Total North Island	***5***	***14***	***14***	***19***	***22***
Popn/Urologist	**262 277**	**120 342**	**146 526**	**122 263**	**115 926**
SOUTH ISLAND					
Christchurch	2	3	2	5	6
Dunedin	-	1	1	1	3
Nelson	-	-	1	1	1
Invercargill	-	-	-	1	1
Blenheim	-	-	1	1	1
Total South Island	***2***	***4***	***5***	***9***	***12***
Popn/Urologist	**312 801**	**182 550**	**162 254**	**94 750**	**73 250**

Source: Membership records, Urological Society of Australasia; New Zealand censuses

TABLE 7.3 HOSPITAL BEDS IN NEW ZEALAND 1949-1989

	1949	1959	1969	1979	1989
Public	14 129	16 695	16 753	17 517	15 553
Private	1 814	2 662	3 629	5 139	6 194
Total	15 943	19 357	20 382	22 656	21 747
%Private	***11.4%***	***13.8%***	***17.8%***	***22.7%***	***28.5%***

Source: New Zealand Year Books

New Zealand, although the private hospitals tended to be smaller. The number of private beds had risen to 7652, or 31.7 per cent of the national total. Treatment in public hospitals remained free but many private hospitals were also partly subsidised by Government funds and the health insurance companies also came to play a greater role in the hospital system. Whereas at the end of World War II it was virtually impossible for a specialist surgeon to make a living without a public hospital appointment, by the 1990s the private sector had grown sufficiently to make this possible, if still uncommon.

The Pioneers of Urology in New Zealand

In 1948, when the Urological Society of Australasia was incorporated, three New Zealand hospitals already had well established urological departments.

Edgar Reay, a foundation member of the Urological Society, was head of the department at Christchurch Hospital and his assistant was Norman Greenslade.

In Auckland the senior urologist was Frank Macky. He was never a full member of the Urological Society, but both Howard Gaudin and Lesley Parton were, from at least 1950.

In Wellington, Patrick Treahy and Bruce Rennie were both full members of the Urological Society. Treahy had been at the Wellington urology unit since 1930 and Rennie joined him in 1937 when Campbell-Begg left for South Africa.

Together, these eight men were the pioneers of New Zealand urology, but only Reay was ever president of the Urological Society and as a group they did not play a major role in the early years of the Society. Regular flights across the Tasman date from 1949, but until at least the mid-1950s travel between New Zealand and Australia was difficult and expensive and those who played the greatest role in the affairs of the Urological Society were those who most regularly attended meetings. The Urological Society did not meet in New Zealand until the 1958 AGM in Christchurch.

Christchurch Hospital

In 1958 the urology team at Christchurch Hospital consisted of Edgar Reay, Norman Greenslade and Bill Utley. All trained in England,

Reay at St Peter's and Utley with Terrence Millin. Greenslade began as a general surgeon, but specialised in urology from 1945.[1] His major contribution to medicine, however, was probably in helping to put New Zealand on the international medical map.

Norman Greenslade was behind the 1953 proposal that eventually saw the BMA meet in Auckland in February 1961 and he was President of the New Zealand branch of the BMA in 1967.

This move to bring members of the BMA from all over the Commonwealth to New Zealand had repercussions for the Urological Society. From 1953 onwards, the idea of holding an Annual Scientific Meeting in New Zealand was raised repeatedly and a number of members were in favour of holding it in Auckland in 1961 to take advantage of the eminent visitors to the BMA meeting. The problem was the tradition of meetings personally run by the President. Edgar Reay, in Christchurch, was the senior member of the Society in New Zealand.

In the event, the first New Zealand meeting of the Urological Society was held in Christchurch in 1958 with Edgar Reay as President. (The 1961 meeting was held in Sydney, in April, too late for any of the visitors to the February meeting in Auckland.)[2]

When Edgar Reay retired in 1959, Norman Greenslade took over as head of the department. Among his initiatives was the idea of integrating urology and nephrology. In 1967, Peter Little was appointed as Renal Physician and from the 1970s the shared ward became known as the Nephrourology Ward.

The older generations of urologists frequently talk of the struggle to maintain their specialty in the face of opposition from the general surgeons and the *History of the Canterbury Area Health Board* provides an interesting example. From 1962, the urology ward, Ward XI, had its own operating theatre, but this was supposed to be for cystoscopies only. Surgery, it was proposed, should be performed later in the week in the main operating theatre suite, entailing two general anaesthetics for the patient, apart from other problems. The urologists went 'on strike'.

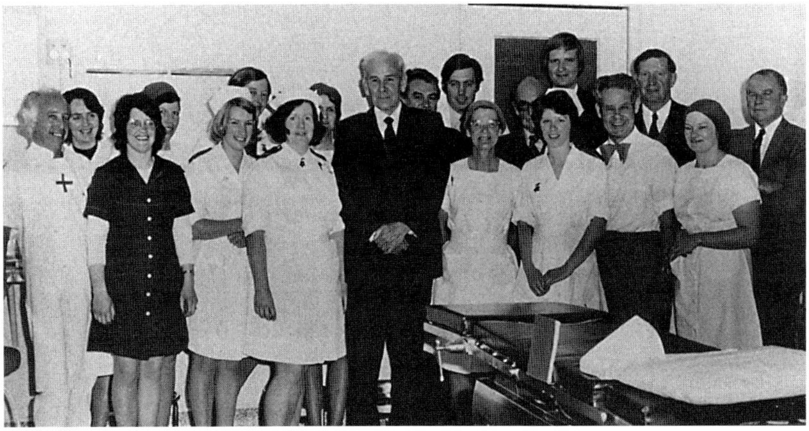

Department of Urology, Christchurch Hospital, Mr N. F. Greenslade's retirement, October 1975. *Back row:* E. Graham, M. Jones, J. Webley, N. Wright, V. G. McGirr, W. Sugrue, C. J. J. Morkane, C. V. McRae, W. L. F. Utley, S. C. Peddie, *Front row:* S. Coldron, S. Rennie, J. Abbott, M. Price, N. F. Greenslade, M. L. Wright, C. Walls, J. Davis, P. Leith. *(Source:* Ted Arnold)

The urologists subsequently agreed between themselves that if they were not allowed to operate in Ward XI theatre then no arranged urology surgery would be performed anywhere in Christchurch Hospital, although emergency surgery would be performed in the main theatre suite.[3]

After that, urologists were allowed to operate in Ward XI theatre on a 'trial' basis, an arrangement which continued for nearly thirty years. Despite, or maybe because of, these problems, the department developed a strong and stable operating team with Charles Morkane as anaesthetist from 1946 until his retirement in 1980. The first kidney transplant was in 1972, with Bill Utley, Bob Donahue, a visiting surgeon from New York, and Colin McRae. Over the thirty years that Ward XI and its theatre worked together, there were only three ward sisters and two operating sisters. When the ward closed, Marie Wild was in charge and Nancy Wright was the operating sister.

During the 1960s, the urology unit at Christchurch Hospital began to build an international reputation for its work on vesico-ureteric reflux. As early as 1954, Bill Utley began to measure bladder pressure in cases of enuresis and by 1958 he was interested in kidney damage in spinal injury patients due to vesico-ureteric reflux. In 1964, the Spinal Injuries Unit was set up in Christchurch and Bill Utley continued his work with Peter Little (nephrologist), Fred Shannon (paediatrician) and George Rolleston (radiologist). They found that vesico-ureteric reflux was much more common than previously supposed and that the condition tended to run in families. In his notes on the history of the work, Bill Utley wrote:

The reflux can be present for some time causing no renal impairment or scarring until there is a bout of urinary tract infection at which time, during reflux, the infected urine from the bladder is pushed right out into the renal cortex and causes an inflammatory reaction there and the resulting scarring. It is therefore imperative to diagnose vesico-ureteric reflux as early as possible and, if it is gross, then perform anti-reflux surgery before there is any major renal impairment.[4]

In 1972, Colin McRae joined the unit as a registrar. He was appointed as a consultant in 1974 and remained until 1992, when he moved to Auckland. Like Norman Greenslade, Colin McRae played a major role in medical politics and was the first urologist to become President of the RACS. Norman Greenslade retired in 1975 and Bill Utley took over as head of the department. In 1980, Utley was President of the Urological Society and hosted the second ASM of the Society to be held in Christchurch.

Stuart Gowland, son of Humphrey Gowland, joined the Christchurch unit in 1978 and Ted Arnold was appointed as Assistant Professor of Urology the following year. Ted Arnold brought a greater emphasis on academic urology to Christchurch and the profile of the urology unit remained relatively high in international terms. Ted Arnold was President of the Urological Society in 1995, by which date the president was no longer running the ASM and the meeting that year was run by Russell McIlroy in Auckland.

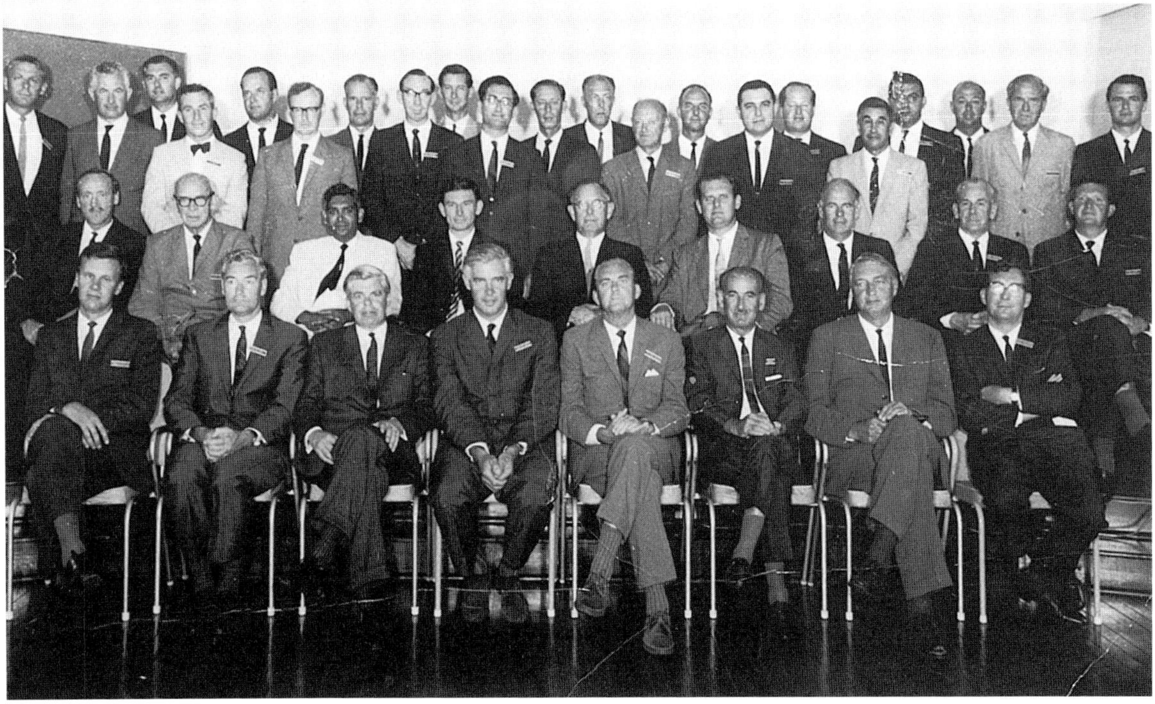

Delegates to the 1966 meeting, Auckland, with Warwick Macky (President) centre front.

Auckland Hospital

Frank Macky was the senior urologist in Auckland, but he was never a full member of the Urological Society. Howard Gaudin, who joined him in 1941 and Lesley Parton, who was appointed in 1946, were both full members, but they were not active in the sense of attending meetings in Australia.

Frank's son, Warwick Macky, however, played an active role as soon as he was able to get away for meetings. In 1957, for instance, he went to Sydney for Malcolm Earlam's meeting. In the early years he would go to Australia by ship or the old flying boats and he made a point of trying to get to as many meetings as possible. His father encouraged him and would cover his work while he was away. 'The taxes were so high here, once it was tax deductible you were mad not to travel a bit.'[5] As a result, Warwick Macky became the face of New Zealand urology in Australia.

The other members of the Auckland urology unit seldom travelled. Howard Gaudin was slightly unusual in that he had trained at the Mayo Clinic and was an expert with the cold punch. He had bilateral congenital cataracts and wore thick glasses which gave him an owlish appearance. In the days before fibreoptics, he would not have been able to see much through the tube anyway and may have operated largely by feel. Certainly he was New Zealand's acknowledged expert with the cold punch. As Warwick Macky said 'He could do things with it no one else in New Zealand could do.'[6]

Warwick Macky, after his time with Terrence Millin in London, continued the tradition of open prostatectomy at Auckland Hospital. He also followed his father in becoming involved on a wider medical stage.[7] Where Frank worked hard for the BMA, Warwick Macky worked hard for the RACS and this was helped by the contacts he had made whilst studying medicine at Melbourne University. He was Vice-President of the RACS in 1976-78.[8] He was President of the Urological Society a decade earlier and the first meeting of the Society in Auckland was in 1966. In 1987, Warwick Macky was made a Fellow of the Urological Society.[9]

Leslie Parton also trained in England, a few years before Warwick Macky, and was appointed as assistant urologist to the Auckland Hospital in 1946. He wrote a urology text book for nurses and another on urology in general practice. He was a great lover of Shakespeare and managed to find room for quotes from the bard in both his books on urology. Following his retirement in 1973, Parton joined the editorial team of the *ANZ Journal of Surgery*, which already included Malcolm Earlam and Leonard Murphy.[10]

During the entire period since the war, the population of Auckland has grown very rapidly, but urology has continued to be concentrated in the Auckland Hospital. The growth in the number of urologists, however, has generally not been much greater than the growth in population. Whereas elsewhere in Australasia the trend was for the population per urologist to fall, in Auckland in 1991 it was much the same as in 1951 at just under one urologist per 126,000. Auckland urologists were perfectly well aware of this and had done their manpower sums many times. Still, in 1996 with seven practising urologists, Auckland was the largest centre for the specialty in New Zealand.[11]

The greatest period of growth in numbers was the late sixties and early seventies. In the late 1960s, David Beck returned to Auckland from the United States where he had been trained in TUR. Athol Duke was already at Auckland Hospital by that stage. In the early 1970s they were joined by Roger Chambers and Russell McIlroy. Meanwhile, Ran De Castro worked in private practice. Athol Duke specialised in renal transplants but tragically died of hepatitis. Roger Chambers had particular expertise in urethral strictures and Russell McIlroy specialised in bladder tumours. By the time they began their work at the Auckland Hospital the fibreoptics revolution was well under way.[12]

During the 1990s, the number of urologists in Auckland increased to eight with the arrival of Colin McRae from Christchurch. The other members of the team were Warwick Macky, Russell McIlroy, Roger Chambers, John Boulton, Derek Rothwell, Jon Cadwallader and Michael Rice. Derek Rothwell was one of the first to have done his formal urology training in New Zealand and he worked in paediatric urology at the Starship, the children's hospital on the same campus as Auckland Hospital. Jon Cadwallader now works exclusively in private practice, and the trend among the other Auckland urologists is also away from full-time work in the public hospital system. The relative shortage of urologists in Auckland gave them a certain freedom of choice.

The second meeting of the Urological Society in Auckland was also the second run under the new system introduced in 1994 where the meeting convenor and the president were two different people. In 1995, Russell McIlroy ran the meeting, but Ted Arnold was President.

Wellington Hospital

In 1948, the senior urologist in Wellington was Patrick Treahy. He drove vintage Talbot motor cars and could have a sharp tongue. It has been said that he liked to shock the nurses with his language. His assistant was Bruce Rennie who was apparently far more jovial. Like Warwick Macky and Bill Utley, Bruce Rennie had trained with Terence Millin but was the senior of the three and hence pioneered retropubic prostatectomy in New Zealand. Bruce Rennie was active in medical politics and as a returned soldier himself, represented the BMA in negotiations with the New Zealand Government and the Rehabilitation Department.

Patrick Treahy was also active in medical politics and sat on the National Health Insurance Committee of the BMA, set up in 1935 when it seemed the Labour Party was going to win the election (as it did) and introduce a national health service (which it did progressively from 1938-41). In about 1943 this committee was replaced by the Medical Planning Committee of the BMA and Bruce Rennie was the representative of the RACS on that body.

Besides their contribution to medical politics, Treahy and Rennie set up the urology unit at the Wellington Hospital and Don Urquhart-Hay, who worked in the unit from 1964, thought they did a good job. 'They designed the urology department at Wellington Hospital in the 1950s and it has stood the test of time. They did well.'[13] Unfortunately the Wellington Hospital suffered from the problems of a cramped site and a hospital that grew in stages. Although the intention was to locate renal dialysis, kidney transplants and urology together, the stops and starts of the building program kept urology and nephrology apart.

Humphrey Gowland and Fergus Ferguson both joined the department in 1960 when Patrick Treahy retired. Humphrey Gowland was a larger than life sort of character, son of the Professor of Anatomy at Otago University. Roy Towers, who joined the staff of the Wellington Hospital as an office boy in the 1920s and remained for the rest of his working life, remembered: 'You would hear this voice booming through the corridors ...' Gowland was President of the Urological Society in 1973 and the James Cook Hotel was duly taken over in March while he entertained the mem-

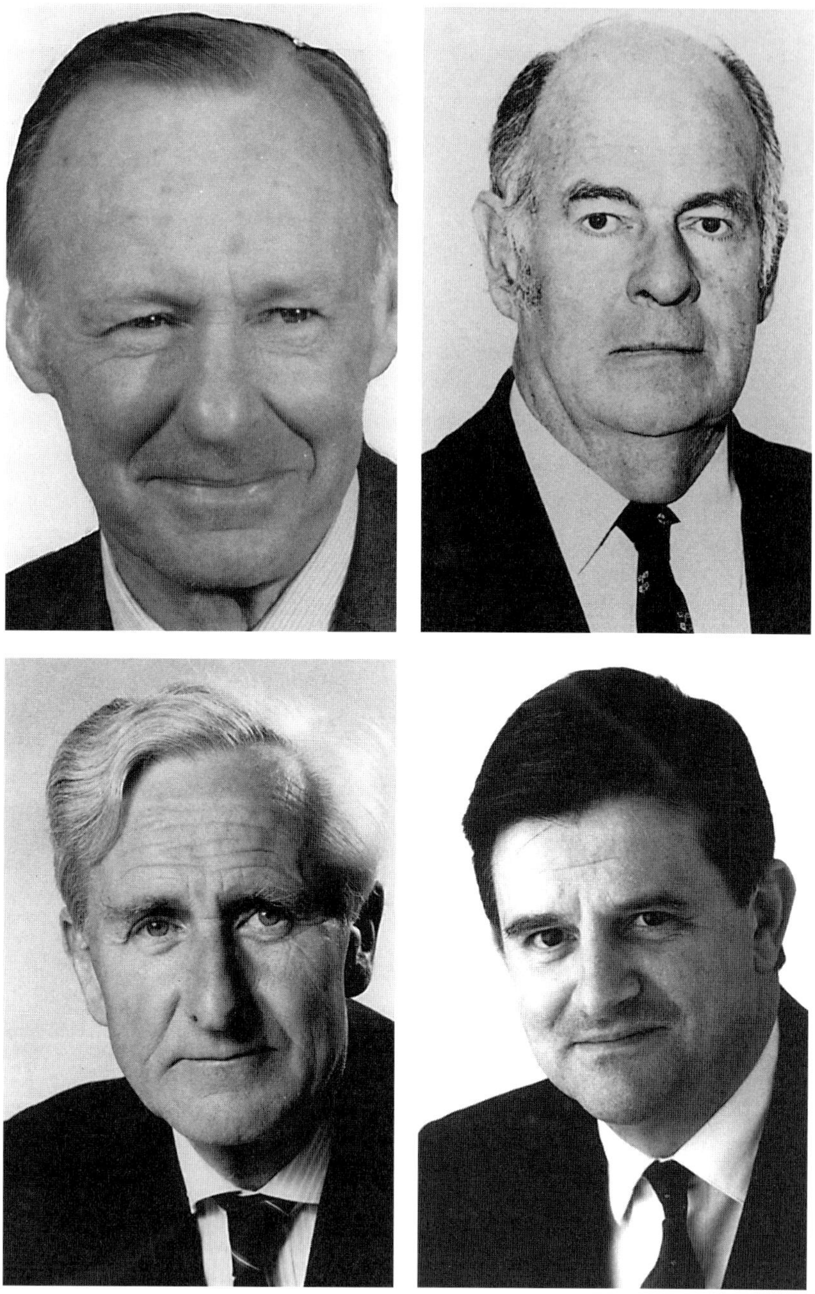

Urologists at Wellington Hospital, A. F. Ferguson, 1960-90, H. W. Gowland, 1960-81, D. Urquhart-Hay, 1965-95, A. G. S. Tulloch, 1983-84. (*Source:* Don Urquhart-Hay)

bers of the Society at their twenty-sixth Annual Scientific Meeting. He died suddenly in 1980.[14]

Humphrey Gowland was one of the first Wellington surgeons to break away from Kelvin Chambers, The Terrace. During the 1990s, the move away from Kelvin Chambers was almost complete and by 1997 there were virtually no doctors left with offices in the building, but from the 1930s until the 1980s it was the favoured place for surgeons, and the trend was started by Campbell-Begg, New Zealand's very first urologist. He was an important figure in the syndicate which built Kelvin Chambers and set up his offices there. Patrick Treahy took them over when he left for South Africa in 1937. Kelvin Chambers was not a convenient location for the Wellington Hospital, but it was convenient for everything else, including the Wellington Club and it became the favoured location for surgeons for over half a century.[15]

Don Urquhart-Hay joined the Wellington Urology team in 1966. He had trained in London, including some time at the Institute of Urology. He established the Renal Transplant Unit in Wellington, performing the first transplant in April 1968. He retired in 1995. Other urologists in Wellington included Alastair Tulloch for a year, before returning to Perth in 1984, John Nacey, who had an academic appointment, Richard Robinson and Grant Russell.

Hamilton

E. T. Dick, an associate member of the Urological Society, was practising in Hamilton from at least 1958. Jim Gray, who had trained with Lesley Pyrah in Leeds, joined him in the early 1960s and Dick disappeared from the scene soon afterwards. Jim Gray was a full member of the Urological Society and carried on alone in Hamilton for many years. A. D. Mee was there briefly in the mid-1970s, but it was another decade before Bill Wright arrived from Dunedin. Jim Gray and Bill Wright worked together until early 1991, when Jim retired and his place was taken by Pat Bary. Michael Vaughan joined the team in 1995.

In the early years, working alone was the norm for country urologists in New Zealand and the pattern experienced by Jim Gray would have been fairly typical. He was on call 24 hours a day, seven days a week and the general surgeons at the Waikato Hospital made it clear that they were not keen on having a specialist urologist in their midst. 'Once it was established they unbent, so others would help a bit.'[16] One of the ways to counteract the isolation was to attend meetings. The first he managed to get to was in Canberra in 1963 and for the next thirty years he attended all except two meetings.

Pat Bary began his urological training as a registrar in Christchurch Hospital before going to Britain for five years. 'Urology in New Zealand started off in three or four centres ... they all had dominant pioneers ... the old boss Bill Utley was like a second father.' Rivalry between Christchurch, Auckland and Wellington was a key feature of the fifties and sixties. 'Their ability to talk to each other has improved over the years.'[17] To a certain extent, the growth of urology in the smaller centres helped to balance the rivalry between the major cities.

Dunedin

The first associate member of the Urological Society to be based in Dunedin was Stanley Wilson, a general surgeon who was very active in College affairs and President of the RACS in 1961-62. Wilson was followed by Ted Arnold who spent a few years in Dunedin teaching at the University of Otago before going on to Christchurch and a combined teaching/surgical role there. He in turn was followed by Bill Wright, who didn't stay long either before going to Hamilton. From the mid-1980s the situation was more stable with Reynold Noronha and Jerry Walton, later joined by Kampta Samalia.

Rotorua

The earliest recorded urologist in Rotorua is A. H. Hackett, who arrived in the early 1960s and stayed for more than twenty years. He worked alone until the mid-1970s when Munir Kadri arrived. Kadri was one of the few full members of the Society in country New Zealand and Mike Cresswell was another, joining the Rotorua team during the 1980s when Hackett retired.

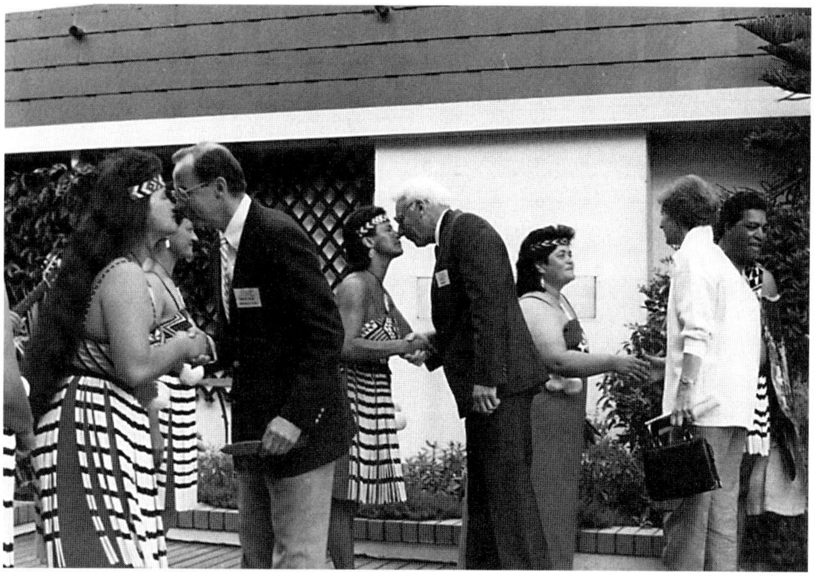

Pat Walsh, Jim Gray and Pam Gray, Maori welcome at Rotorua Meeting, 1987. (*Source:* Jim Gray)

Palmerston North

A. W. Douglas was the first member of the Urological Society in Palmerston North and he retired in the mid-1970s. It seemed likely John Coutts would take over from him. Coutts had had a long association with Palmerston North Hospital, but in 1969 he went to Leeds to spend a year brushing up on his urology. When he returned he ordered the latest fibreoptic equipment, bringing prostatic resection at Palmerston completely up to date. In 1973, a renal dialysis unit opened and in 1975 the hospital offered John Coutts the position of specialist urologist. He declined, wanting to continue to do some general surgery, but remained an associate member of the Urological Society.

Jerry Walton was appointed as a specialist in 1976, later moving to Dunedin to the lectureship in urology. He was replaced by Mano Ranjan Rajaratanum and the department averaged about 500 operations a year during the 1980s, with an increasing number of endoscopic procedures as the telescopes improved. Robin Smart was appointed when John Coutts retired and in 1990, John Chrisp brought the Palmerston North team up to three. Despite this, Robin Smart noted that there were still not enough urologists in Palmerston North and as a result they worked 60-70 hours a week.

New Plymouth/Hawera

Harold Thomas, an associate member of the Urological Society, worked in New Plymouth for a while during the 1960s, before moving to Sydney and an active role in the Urological Society. Meanwhile, L. Neri was working around the coast at Hawera. Then in 1977 Paul Cooke began practising in New Plymouth and remained there into the 1990s.

Nelson

Peter Meffan began in Nelson in about 1965 after training in Britain, including some time as registrar to Richard Turner-Warwick. Working solo was lonely and he was dependent on the general surgeons for cover while he was away. He kept up to date by maintaining his overseas contacts and prided himself on providing an innovative urology service, despite being the sole urologist in a small town. He was the first urologist in New Zealand, for instance, to introduce PSA testing, in 1988. He also worked with Alastair Tulloch on penile prostheses when these were still novel devices. Tulloch came from Western Australia to spend some time based at Wellington Hospital, before returning to Perth. Peter Meffan was also amongst the first to try laser prostatectomy in New Zealand, after seeing Tony Costello's work in Melbourne in 1994. Patrick Meffan, his son, also trained as a urologist and joined him in practice in Nelson. 'I tried to dissuade him, but he liked Nelson and wanted to stay.'[18]

Tauranga

Harry Watts began in Tauranga in 1961 as an associate member, but by 1971 he was a full member of the Urological Society. Mark Fraundorfer started at Tauranga in the mid-1980s and in the 1990s, Peter Gilling joined the team.

Blenheim

John Inder, an associate member, started in Blenheim in 1969 and was still there in the mid-1990s. There was no full-time urologist.

Invercargill and Whangerei

Bruce Wells has been in Invercargill even longer. He began in practice in 1961, and ever since then, he has been the only representative of the Urological Society in the far south. He retired in 1989. George McGirr has played the same role in the extreme north since 1978.

Overview of Country New Zealand

The general pattern was for urology to be mainly in the hands of associate members of the Urological Society, who did some general surgery and persuaded the general surgeons to stand in for them when they went on holiday.

Jim Gray was the senior full member of the Society from country New Zealand and when he became President of the Society in 1987, he decided to hold the meeting in Rotorua. As a major tourist centre it had more to offer, including a suitable hotel, than Hamilton. All the urologists from the surrounding country towns helped, so that it was a joint effort from a number of centres rather than the result of work by urologists in one town. Mike Cresswell from Rotorua was the secretary, Bill Wright from Hamilton was the treasurer and Mark Fraundorfer from Tauranga and Munir Kadri from Rotorua were also heavily involved.[19]

Perhaps co-operation from this wider constituency was behind the idea to buy a lithotripter for Hamilton.

New Zealand Lithotripters

The development of lithotripters revolutionised the treatment of stones, but the process of adopting the technology has seldom been untroubled. The major problem was the cost of the machines, starting at around $3 million. This meant that a population of about a million people, depending on the incidence of stone, was required to cover the costs of a lithotripter. From the early 1980s there were what Don Urquhart-Hay describes as 'desultory discussions' at urological section meetings of the RACS. Some urologists favoured a machine in Auckland, because it had the largest population; others favoured Wellington, on the grounds that it was accessible to a wider area of the country. 'Costings would probably have said Auckland'.[20]

In the event, the first hospital in New Zealand to have a lithotripter was the Waikato, in Hamilton. This was not a popular move in the other centres. In Auckland, for instance, John Cadwallader already had experience of working with lithotripters in England. Jim Gray persuaded the Waikato to organise the funds to buy the machine outside the public hospital system. The money was borrowed from the bank with the hospital as guarantor. Jim Gray believed there was

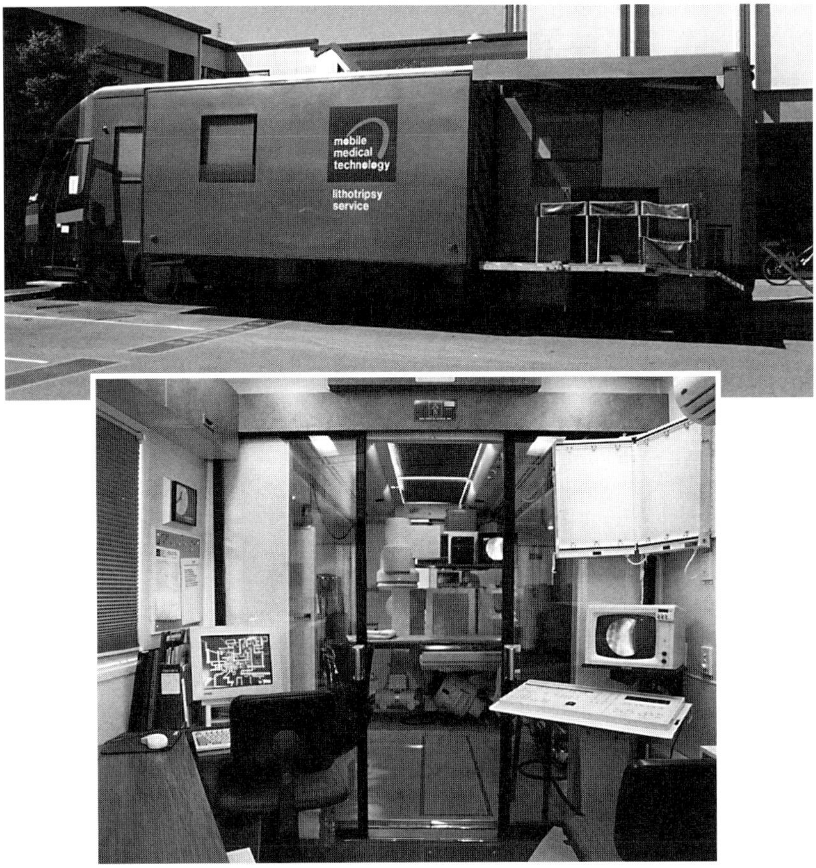

The lithotripter bus, registration 'BBBang', and a view of the inside of the bus. (*Source:* Stuart Gowland)

resentment from the other centres and Christchurch and Wellington sent them very few patients. Some came from Auckland, but most of the patients for the Hamilton lithotripter came from the Bay of Plenty and Palmerston North.

Besides a lack of co-operation from the major cities, the Hamilton lithotripter also suffered from the view of the Southern Cross insurance company that the machine was within the public hospital system. They therefore refused to pay for patients insured with them. The other insurance companies covered patients using the lithotripter, and so did the hospital boards, but Southern Cross was the biggest private insurer.

Meanwhile, on the South Island, Stuart Gowland came up with a novel solution to the problem of insufficient cases of stone in one centre to support a lithotripter. They bought a machine and put it on a purpose-built bus so that the lithotripter could be driven around from hospital to hospital. Initially, the hospital administrators were sceptical. Why should the Auckland Hospital, for instance, pay for it to go to the South Island? Stuart Gowland was able to convince the doubters that sharing the machine made it cheaper for everybody and in June 1995 the bus went on the road.[21]

The New Zealand Section of the Urological Society of Australasia

Urologists in New Zealand have generally had a closer relationship with the RACS than was the case elsewhere in Australasia. It is no accident that both the first urologists to be Vice-President of the College (Warwick Macky) and the first to be President (Colin McRae)were from New Zealand. For many years, the main gathering of New Zealand urologists was at the urology section meetings attached to the meetings of the College. These generally consisted of two half days of papers, in a separate venue from the College meeting. Urologists attended because it was a good opportunity to get together and help educate the general surgeons.[22]

This pattern changed in the early 1980s with the changes to training. New Zealand urologists began to get together once a year under the auspices of the Urological Society for a section meeting to interview and select trainees. The candidates would each present a paper and the committee would interview them. The committee consisted of representatives from the centres that had training posts: Auckland, Christchurch, Dunedin and Wellington, plus one member representing the smaller centres. The meetings would take place at one of the hospitals and the local urologists would organise a social gathering of some kind, thus continuing the Society's tradition of turning scientific meetings into social occasions.

At about the same time, the North and South Island urologists began to develop a tradition of social/scientific meetings once a year on their respective islands. The North Island meeting—NUTS—was in summer and involved sailing. The South Island meeting—STUF—was in winter and involved skiing.

'Everybody on the North Island sails, or jolly near it ... the most beautiful sailing waters in the world—shelter every ten miles, no heavy currents ... people only drown when they're drunk ...'[23] The social side of the NUTS meeting also involved the NUTS oration, supposedly a black tie affair, but generally interpreted as bow tie with shorts.

South Island meetings tended to be better attended, possibly because independent minded surgeons could ski in some freedom and didn't have to spend the weekend squashed together in a boat. The 1987 Southern Travelling Urological Forum, for instance, was held on the Wanaka ski fields and designed as a preliminary to the RACS meeting in Dunedin. The guest was Professor Villis Marshall from Adelaide, but the publicity warned 'As always, science to a minimum, skiing to a maximum.' The STUF meeting involved five days of skiing before three days of science at the New Zealand Section of the Urological Society's meeting in Dunedin, in conjunction with the RACS Annual Scientific Meeting.[24] There was also the Central Urological Travelling Society (CUTS), based in Wellington.

Trainees were expected to attend these meetings and the scientific side was not neglected, even if it did generally occupy less time than the serious business of skiing and sailing.

C H A P T E R 8

Urology in Queensland

~

Introduction

In Queensland, the State and municipalities shared funding for hospitals, but by the 1950s there was a rapid decline in the proportion of funds and contribution to management provided by the latter. Attendance at public hospitals was free and Queensland was the only State without a system of honorary appointments. However, there was a system of intermediate beds in public hospitals, similar to that in New South Wales. In 1950, there were 115 public hospitals administered under the auspices of the State Government through a system of District Hospital Boards. This number grew slowly to about 145 by the 1970s and remained at about that level, despite continued population increase. In 1950, there were also 67 registered private hospitals, 27 of which were in Brisbane.

Queensland's Six Pioneering Presidents

In 1950, only three Queenslanders were full members of the Urological Society: Stanley Roe at the Mater Misericordiae Hospital, and Jack Power and Pip Lukin at the Brisbane General Hospital. Three other men played an important role in the early years of Queensland Urology: Mick Hogg, Alex Inglis and Peter Row. These three were associate members in 1950, but became full members shortly afterwards. All six of these early Queensland urologists became Presidents of the Urological Society in the years when the presidency rotated between Sydney, Melbourne and Brisbane. Once New Zealand, and subsequently the other States, were added to the rotation, the chance of a Queenslander becoming President fell dramatically and there were only three others in the next 35 years.

As at 1996, the full list of Queensland presidents was:

Jack Power 1938, 1946-47, 1952-53
Stanley Roe 1941
Pip Lukin 1950-51
Peter Row 1955-56
Mick Hogg 1959-60 (died in office)
Alex Inglis 1960 (stepped in after Hogg's death and ran the 1960 meeting)
Jeff Watson 1971-72
Ros Parisi 1982-83
Graham Holmes 1990-91

The first six full-time Queensland urologists therefore take on a particular importance. Together with Mordo Sutton, a part-time urologist who also practised in gynaecology at the Brisbane General Hospital, and Paul Hopkins, a part-time urologist who pioneered country urology in Queensland, at Mackay, they had a strong influence on the early years of the Society. In particular, those annual meetings which were held in Queensland helped to set an expectation of combining fun with hard work in a relaxed atmosphere. Jack Power tended to be formal, but his strong horse racing background brought an added dimension to his meetings, while both Hogg and Roe made their mark on the Society through informality.

Mick Hogg was the first to persuade the Executive to allow women to attend the Annual Dinner, although he died before the 1960 meeting and Inglis was persuaded to revert to the men only tradition. Stanley Roe's major contribution was the tradition of gathering at Roe's Kamp on Stradbroke Island at some time during the meeting, and Keith Kirkland seems to have enjoyed the informality that went with such gatherings, even if Bobby Silverton did not:

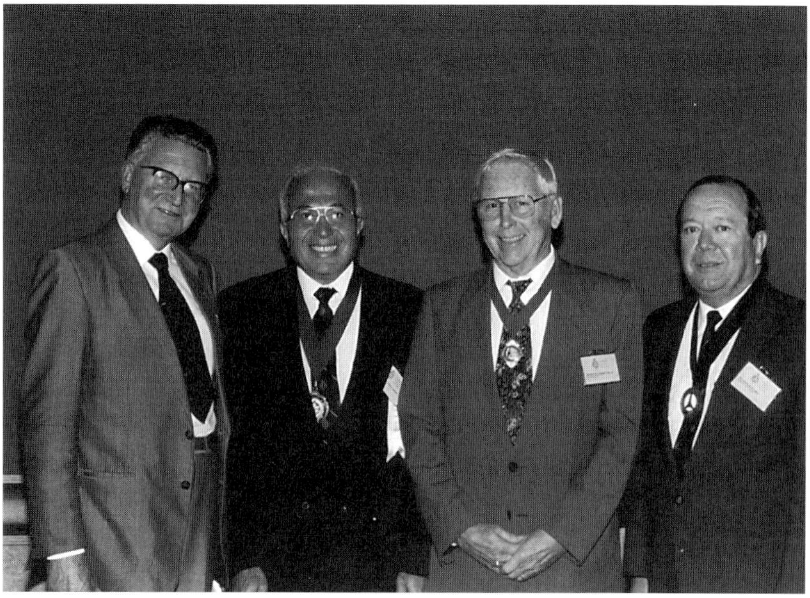

Left to right: Richard Turner-Warwick (President British Association of Urological Surgeons), Said Awad (President Canadian Urological Association), Guy Leadbetter (President American Urological Association) and Graham Holmes (President Urological Society of Australasia), Vancouver, July 1990. (*Source:* Graham Holmes)

In the Nineteen Forties and Nineteen Fifties, whenever it was Queensland's turn, the meetings were held in Brisbane, and the Sunday Outing preceding the clinical sessions was usually a trip to Roe's Kamp. The urologists, their wives and their friends spent the day surfing, swimming or walking on the ocean beach, with a large smorgasbord lunch served on the trestle tables set out in front of the Kamp.

I remember at one of these Outings watching Keith Kirkland, who had been a champion swimmer in his youth, showing magnificent body-surfing skills. Other members of the party surfed with Keith, waded in the shallows or sunbaked; while Bobby Silverton, dapper in immaculate cream slacks, dark coat and tie, walked briskly down the beach into the middle distance.[1]

In the period 1953-55, John Phillips was the Urology Registrar at Brisbane General Hospital. By that stage, Jack Power and Stanley Roe had more or less retired. Their contribution to the beginnings of the Urological Society is described in Chapter 2. However, Phillips remembers Power as a rather formal man, devoting more time to his commitments to Queensland racing than to urology. John Phillips also remembers Mordo Sutton. He was brother of the Professor of Surgery at the University of Queensland and a gentle soul, but never on time. Sutton pioneered retropubic prostatectomy at the Brisbane General Hospital. He also designed a number of instruments. Jeff Watson remembers him as inventive and a very good surgeon. 'If as an energetic resident you tried to assist too much, he would say, "I'll do this operation Doc."'[2]

From 1947, Pip Lukin was the senior urologist at the Brisbane General Hospital. Pip Lukin was in the Australian Flying Corps during WWI before completing his studies. He began as a general practitioner before turning to urology in the 1930s. Lukin was very active in medical politics and his record included twenty-three years on the Council of the BMA. From 1958 to 1964, he was President of the Medical Defence Society of Queensland and from 1948 to 1973 (the year before his death) he was the BMA/AMA's representative on the Medical Board of Queensland. He has been described as generally kind and occasionally peppery, but a more than competent surgeon.[3]

The next Queensland President of the Urological Society after Lukin was Peter Row. He came from a medical family and gained his FRCSEng before joining the AIF as a medical officer. On returning to Brisbane, he was a junior urologist at the Brisbane General until August 1957, when he was appointed the first senior urologist at the newly opened Princess Alexandra Hospital. He is generally remembered with considerable affection. Jeff Watson joined him in setting up the urology unit at the Princess Alexandra:

Dr Peter Row was a quiet, unassuming surgeon with a very good judgement and when he was assessing a very poor risk patient he would say, "let's circle him for a while before we decide". If the patient was too poor a risk for surgery he would say, "why don't we fan him with our hat".[4]

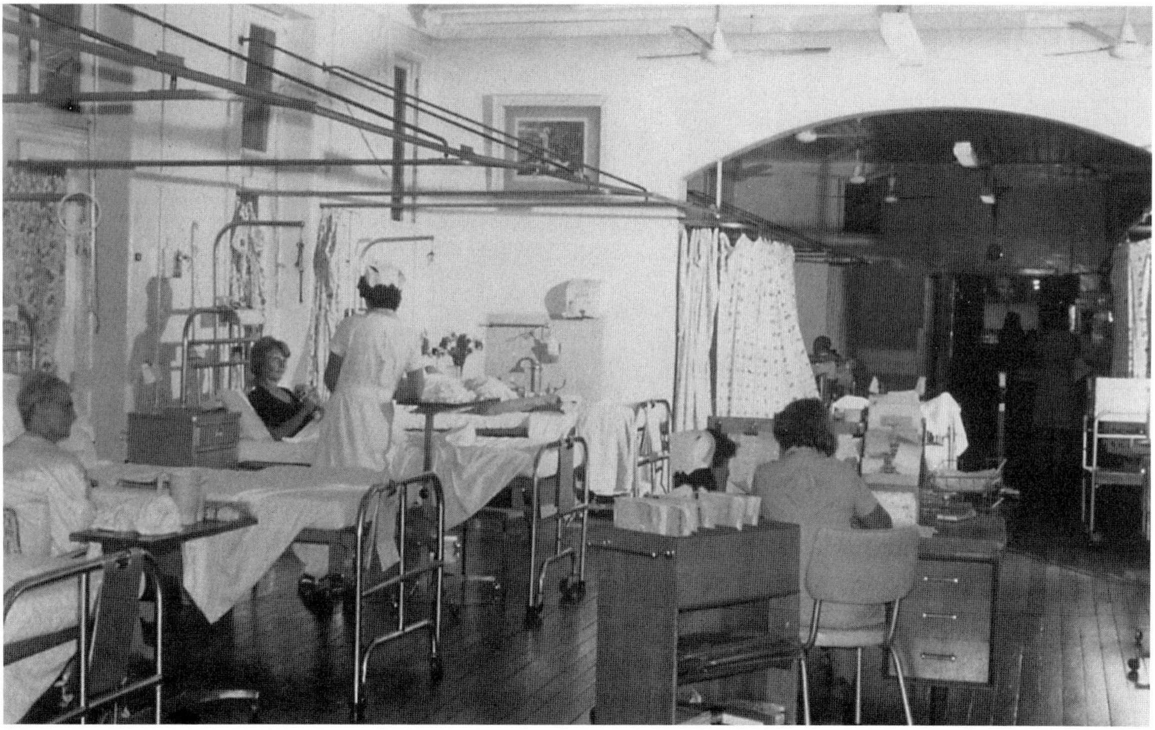

Adult surgical ward, Mater Hospital, Brisbane, c. 1970. (*Source:* Mater Misericordiae Hospitals)

Like Pip Lukin, Peter Row was active on a much wider stage than Brisbane urology. He was elected to the Council of the RACS in 1962 and remained on Council until 1966, when ill health forced him into semi-retirement. The Peter Row Department of Urology at the Princess Alexandra was named in his honour. He died in 1973.

Mick Hogg was President of the Urological Society in 1959. Hogg was of the older generation of Queenslanders who took their MB BS at the University of Sydney before it was possible to do so in Queensland. He obtained his FRCSEd in 1937 and followed Pip Lukin as the Senior Urologist at Brisbane General Hospital. He was not always an easy man to work with, although he could be kind to his juniors. Cricket was one of the fields where he excelled, but he had a lung problem and died at the early age of 49, before the 1960 annual meeting.

Alex Inglis, who had succeeded Stanley Roe as the Senior Urologist at the Mater Misericordiae Hospital, stepped in to run the meeting in his place. Like Mick Hogg, Alex Inglis did his initial training in Sydney. He began his university career as an engineering student, transferring to medicine after the first year. This was during the 1920s and he was a Registrar at St Vincent's, Sydney, in 1931. He then moved to Queensland and joined Stanley Roe at the Mater and succeeded him when Roe first retired in 1938. He spent the war years in the army and returned to the Mater in the mid-1940s. Charles Roe remembers him as a great storyteller who 'often had the surgeon's room at the Mater enthralled and highly amused by his stories.'[5]

The Growth of the Specialty in Brisbane

Between 1950 and 1958, the number of full members of the Urological Society in Queensland grew from three to seven (besides the six Presidents already discussed, the seventh full member was Jeff Watson, President 1971-72) and the number of associate members grew from six to nine. Of the associate members, Steve Ferguson practised in Toowoomba for many years and was not a full-time urologist, but the other new associate members were young urologists beginning their careers and all subsequently became full members of the Society. John Phillips has already been mentioned. The others were Peter Grant, a paediatric surgeon with an interest in paediatric urology, Barney Moy, Alex Splatt, Ron Yaxley and Stanley Roe's son, Charles.

This represents an increase of more than 75 per cent in the number of urologists in eight years. Growth in numbers continued during the 1960s and 1970s but was never again that rapid. In addition, new arrivals were balanced by retirements so that in 1971 there were twelve full members and five associates, a total of seventeen, compared with sixteen in 1958.

This expansion in the number of urologists was associated with the growth in population south of the Brisbane River and along the Gold Coast. The opening of the Princess Alexandra Hospital in 1956 reflected this increased population south of the river and provided an increased number of public hospital appointments. It began taking medical students the following year.

The other teaching hospitals of this era were the Brisbane General, the Mater Misericordiae and the Repatriation General Hospital at Greenslopes. All had urology departments.

Brisbane General/ Royal Brisbane Hospital

In the early 1950s, the hospital had two urology wards. Ward Seven was built of stone with canvas blinds enclosing the verandahs and also had a number of little pavillions with canvas blinds all around. Ward Four was even more rustic. There was a tap in the kitchen but the only source of water on the ward itself was a jug in a large china bowl. Both wards were very busy.[6]

This was a major public hospital with more than 1000 beds by the end of the 1960s. In 1960 Sid Cantamessa, who had played rugby for Queensland, joined the team at the Royal Brisbane Hospital. When Mick Hogg died in 1960, Alex Splatt succeeded him as the Senior Urologist and remained in that position until the 1980s. He has been described as taciturn but with a dry sense of humour and a large repertoire of jokes. He was known as a neat, competent surgeon and he was in private practice with Pip Lukin. Like most Brisbane surgeons until the 1970s, they had rooms in Wickham Terrace.

When Alex Splatt started his urological career, prostatectomy, which was usually performed as an open two stage procedure, had a very frequent association with urosepsis, so much so that bilateral vasectomy at the time of prostatectomy was a routine practice. With Sid Cantamessa and John Phillips, Alex introduced the idea of including hibitane together with lignocaine in catheterisation lubricant gel to lessen the likelihood of catheter associated urinary infections.[7]

Splatt was the first in a line of urologists to occupy what was effectively the position of Urological Registrar at the Brisbane. The official title in 1949 was Senior Resident Medical Officer, Department of Urology. He was followed by John Phillips (1953-55) who had trained at St Peter's in London, Barney Moy (1955-59), Bill Cadzow (1964-66) and Stephen Stening (1969-71).

Stephen Stening was originally from New South Wales, but decided he liked Queensland after a holiday at Surfers Paradise. He spent some time as surgical registrar at the Royal Brisbane Hospital before going to Melbourne to work in paediatric urology with Douglas Stephens and Durham Smith and then to England for four years. In 1969 he returned to Queensland. That was the first year that positions for senior registrars in urology were advertised at the Royal Brisbane Hospital, the Princess Alexandra and the Repatriation General Hospital, under the new training scheme. Robin Spork was appointed at Greenslopes, Stephen Stening at the Brisbane and Graham Holmes at the Princess Alexandra. They had all spent some time in England and returned to the RACS-approved positions to work for their FRACS. 'It was never an approved training program really', recalled Graham Holmes. 'We all sort of looked after ourselves.' He and Stephen Stening studied together and both passed in November 1970.[8]

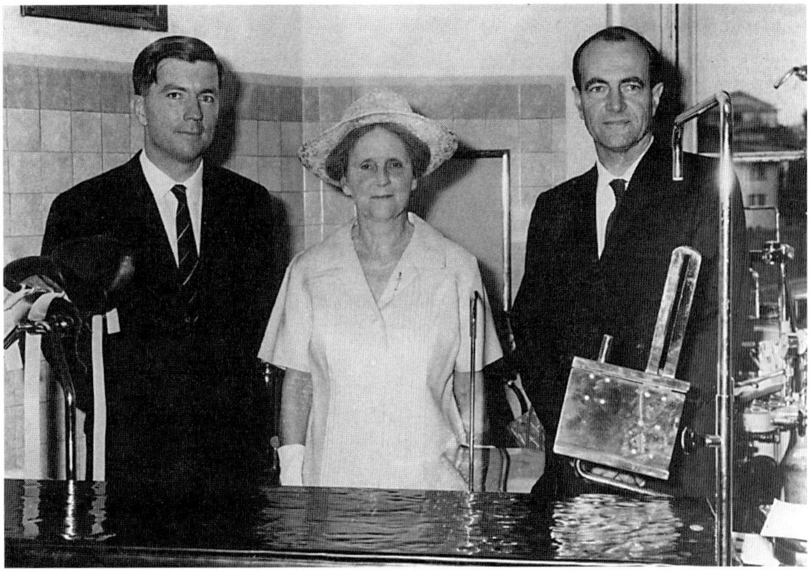

Dr D. O'Callaghan (Medical Superintendent), Mrs Emily Roe and Dr Charles Roe on the occasion of the presentation of an operating table to the Mater Public Hospital in memory of Dr Stanley Roe, October 1968. (*Source:* Charles Roe)

Jim Pye also had an appointment at the Royal Brisbane during the early 1970s. He was the son of Aubrey Pye, a well-known local character who was Superintendent of the Brisbane Hospital for many years. Jim Pye died in 1976, aged only 41 and Stephen Stening returned to the Brisbane after two years at the Mater. In 1980, Frank Gardiner returned to the Brisbane Hospital after several years in London. In 1996, the urologists at the Royal Brisbane Hospital were John Phillips, Sid Cantamessa, Stephen Stening, Robin Spork, Frank Gardiner and Anthony James.[9] Several played an important role in the Society. Alex Splatt was Queensland's representative on the Executive for much of the 1970s. Frank Gardiner was editor of *Prospectives*. Stephen Stening was heavily involved in training and accreditation as a RACS Examiner in Urology and Robin Spork was the convenor of the Society's 1997 ASM in Port Douglas.

Princess Alexandra Hospital

In 1971, the Princess Alexandra had forty-four urological beds plus twenty paraplegic beds, four urologists (Jeff Watson, Barney Moy, Bill Cadzow and Lionel Lukin) and two training posts, one of which was RACS approved. It had grown from its small beginnings in 1957 to be the largest urology department in Queensland.

The leading figure in Brisbane urology in the 1970s was the head of the unit, Jeff Watson. After a period as resident in urology at the Brisbane he went to England, where he joined the long line of eminent Australasian urologists who spent time as RSO at St Peter's. There he began research on bladder carcinoma and won a fellowship to the University of Michigan. In Ann Arbor, he worked with Reed Nesbit and Jack Lapides and was impressed with the size of the urology department: seventy beds, fourteen trainees, two associate professors and one professor. In 1957 he returned to Brisbane as the first fully trained resectionist in town. After a brief period at the Royal Brisbane, he and Peter Row moved to set up the urology unit at the new Princess Alexandra Hospital.

Geof Hirst was an RMO there in the late 1960s and remembers that Jeff Watson made his presence felt.

> *He wandered about the hospital doing consults and would walk into a ward with a handful of blue consultation slips. Because he never wore a suit, a prerequisite for attention in those days, the nurses ignored him. It infuriated him and he would stand on his 'dig' demanding attention. Created quite a scene.*
>
> *In those days we had a cystoscopy room just outside the urology ward which was M3. We had a funny guy who would prepare the patients on two cystoscopy tables with all the rest sitting outside in the corridor. Jeff would be there doing cystoscopies under local and the resident, me at times, would scribe as he yelled out the findings. Those who worked there will always remember those times. He was a good surgeon and really the only one in those days who could really do a TURP.*[10]

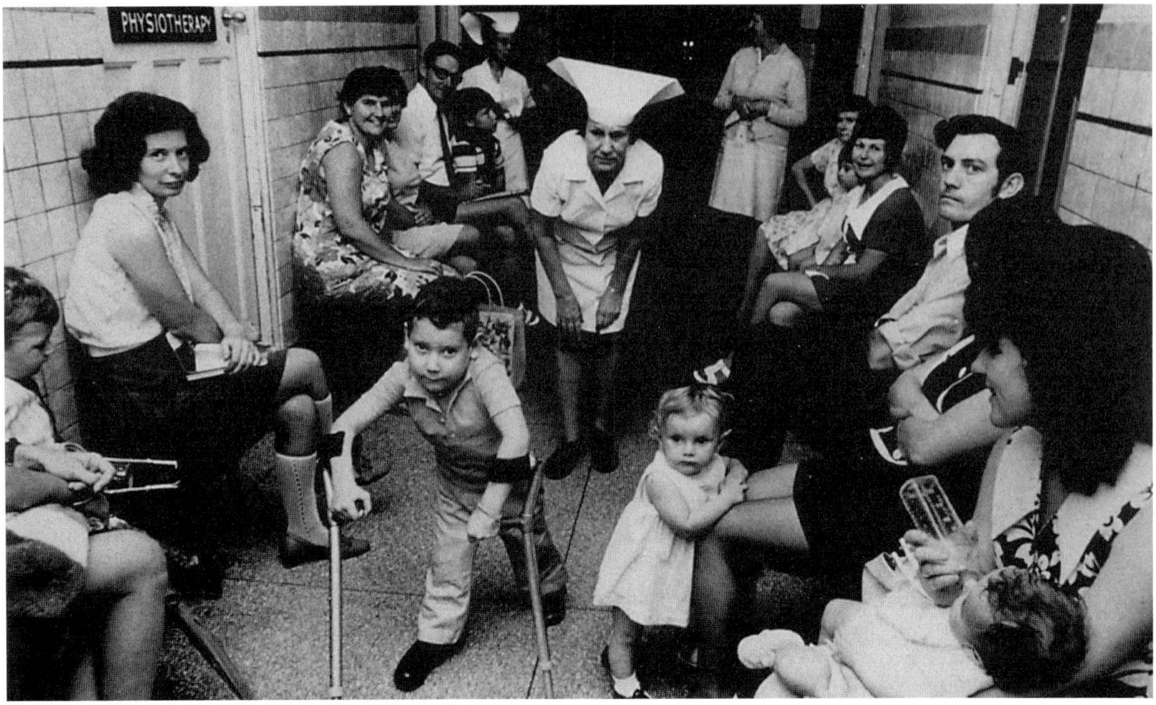

Outpatients Department, Mater Children's Hospital, Brisbane, c. 1970. (*Source:* Mater Misericordiae Hospitals)

The other urologists in the 1960s were Barney Moy and Lionel Lukin, son of Pip, who both trained in Brisbane and Bill Cadzow, who spent time at St Thomas' in London. Graham Holmes also trained in England, including some time in Edinburgh with Professor Selby Tulloch, father of Alastair, and a year as Urology Registrar at the Institute of Urology. He returned to Brisbane in 1970, initially to the position of Urology Registrar at the Princess Alexandra. He was appointed as Visiting Urologist in 1973. Graham Holmes played a particularly active role in the Urological Society and was the first Chairman of the Queensland Section of the Training, Accreditation and Education Committee. After eight years of work on T, A & E, he went on to the Executive and was President of the Society in 1990-91.

Ray Que Hee was the Urology registrar in 1972 and was based at the Princess Alexandra for most of the 1970s. Ross Cartmill did some of his early training at the Princess Alexandra before spending time in London and Houston. He returned to the Princess Alexandra in 1978 with expertise in urodynamics and also initiated the program of implanting penile prostheses. In 1996, the urologists at the Princess Alexandra were Bill Cadzow, Graham Holmes, Ross Cartmill, Peter Heathcote, Les Thompson, David Nicol, Roger Hinsch and Peter Mactaggart.

Perhaps fittingly for the largest urology department in Queensland, the Princess Alexandra has provided the Society with two presidents, Jeff Watson and Graham Holmes.

Jeff Watson was the Queensland representative on the Executive in the 1970s and from 1971 the Queensland regional advisor on training. Graham Holmes took over and played an important role in training during the 1980s. He was President in 1990-91.

The Mater Misericordiae Public Hospitals

The Mater was a complex hospital, or rather group of hospitals, with adult and children's sections, public and intermediate beds and also private maternity and general hospitals. In contrast to other hospitals in Queensland, all the doctors at the Mater were appointed under an honorary system until 1965, when it was fully incorporated into the public hospital system. Alex Inglis succeeded Stanley Roe as the Senior Urologist, although Roe remained as a consultant into the 1960s. Charles Roe was appointed as Honorary Assistant Urologist in 1951, but neither he nor Inglis had a senior surgical qualification at the time, although Charles Roe obtained his FRACS in 1977.

Ron Yaxley, who had both the English and Edinburgh fellowships, joined them as an Honorary Urologist in 1960 and remained to become the Senior Urologist to both the adult and the children's hospitals at the Mater in the1970s. He was a forthright character who said what he thought and his relationship with the paediatric surgeons was frequently somewhat strained. He could, however, be very kindly and attracted the loyalty of his patients. One of his sons, John Yaxley, also became a urologist and became a provisional member of the Urological Society in 1995.

John Lynch had a visiting appointment at the Mater in the 1970s. He had trained at the Institute of Urology in London and returned to Brisbane as the Government Medical Officer with a limited urological practice. Interestingly, he had one eye, but this does not seem to have affected his operating skills. It did, however, affect his choice of urology as a specialty.

> *I had always only ever considered doing medicine and becoming a surgeon. The loss of my left eye did not distract me. However, when a Resident at the Mater Hospital I saw that other Doctors might be reluctant to send their patients to a one-eyed Surgeon, and felt they may be more disposed to recognise a one-eyed Urologist.*[11]

John Lynch found his work as Government Medical officer took up more and more of his time and from 1988 he ceased working as a urologist to concentrate on his court work with drunk drivers. He wore an eye patch and brought an exotic touch to Brisbane's courts. One defendant said he looked like a Spanish pirate.

In 1976, Geof Hirst joined Ron Yaxley at the Mater. He had been a surgical registrar at the Princess Alexandra in 1969-72 and then went overseas for three years. He spent a year at the Institute of Urology in London, where he worked with David Innes Williams, and then spent two years in Toronto, where he continued to train in both adult and paediatric urology. When he returned to Brisbane, he

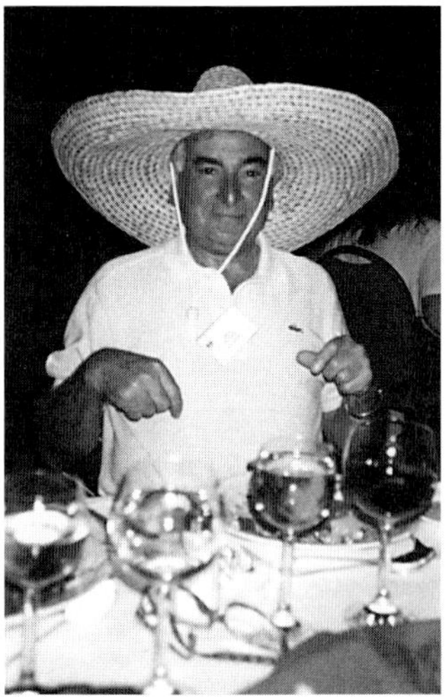

Michael Rosen in relaxed mood at the Annual General Meeting, Surfers Paradise, 1991. (*Source:* Graham Holmes)

brought with him the first major influx of North American ideas since Jeff Watson. His appointments at the Mater were to both the adult and children's hospitals and Jeff Watson believed his main influence on Brisbane urology was in the paediatric field. The pattern in Brisbane has been for the integration of adult and paediatric urology and Geof Hirst was the first with specialised training in both areas from both Britain and the United States.

Soon after his return, Geof Hirst became involved in the use of chemotherapy for testicular tumours, initially importing cisplatinum through his contacts in Toronto:

> *I first became involved with cisplatinum I think in 1978. I had a young guy with very advanced non-seminomatous germ cell tumour. He went off to the Cook Islands [for treatment] ... he returned ... worse for wear. A guy I trained with in Toronto was involved in a National Cancer Institutes trial with cisplatinum and took a bottle out of his fridge and sent it to me ... The next patient who hoved into sight got the drug from the same source, although by then I always kept a spare bottle. The Customs said that once a patient was started on treatment they could not refuse importation of more! Subsequently I was made a Phase 2 participant in the trials and everything became easier.*[12]

Geof Hirst and Martin Tattersall, an oncologist, were among the pioneers of this treatment in Australia, one of the major success stories in the treatment of cancer.

After Ron Yaxley's death Lionel Lukin moved to the Mater from the Princess Alexandra. David Winkle joined the Mater team in the late 1980s. Like Geof Hirst, he had a background in both adult and paediatric urology, including training in paediatric urology in London, and he held appointments to both the adult and the children's hospitals on the Mater campus. The other urologist at the Mater in 1996 was Roger Watson, son of Jeff, who had spent time training in both London and Miami.

The urologists at the Mater played an important role in the Urological Society. Ron Yaxley was active, for instance as the Society's representative on the Electro-surgical subcommittee of the Standards Association. Geoff Hirst was on the Executive from 1984 to 1996 and Chairman of ANZAUS in 1988-91. He was also Chairman of the Society's ESWL Committee, in 1986-88, and the inaugural Chairman of the Society's Continuing Medical Education Committee from 1992 to 1996.

Repatriation General Hospital, Greenslopes

Besides his appointment at the Mater, Ron Yaxley was also associated with the Repatriation Hospital, taking over from Pip Lukin. Sid Cantamessa, Raymond Que Hee and Lionel Lukin also had visiting appointments at the Repat. Ray Que Hee was RMO there in 1965, before there was an accredited training post. He went on to the post of surgical registrar at the Princess Alexandra.

I can always remember Peter Row asking me to do a check cystoscopy as he was having difficulty bending to see up the cystoscope. I told him I could not see anything. He agreed with me as he felt there should be no recurrence. In reality I meant that I could not ***see*** *anything.*[13]

In 1969 Que Hee went to England and spent three years learning 'something about the subject'.

One of the memories that sticks is of D. I. Williams operating in great Ormond Street. He was so slick I could hardly believe it. I saw him do a bilateral reimplantation and a nephrectomy on different patients in ninety minutes. Making conversation, he asked me if stones were common in children in my country. He seemed a little nonplussed when I told him that stones were very uncommon in children in Australia. I also watched Tricky Dicky do a few operations and tried to understand what he was talking about when he discussed this new science of urodynamics.[14]

Ray Que Hee returned to the Princess Alexandra Hospital in 1972. He was appointed as Visiting Urologist at the Repatriation Hospital, Greenslopes, in 1981. In the 1990s, the Repat. became a private hospital and lost its status as a teaching hospital. The early 1990s were a turbulent period for the hospital with rows over the contracts for Visiting Medical Officers. From 1997, there was once more an accredited training post at Greenslopes. In 1996, the urologists were Andrew Gallagher, Ray Que Hee, Terrence Farrell and David Nicol.

Country Queensland

Until the 1970s, between 80 and 90 per cent of Queensland's urologists were Brisbane based. In 1950, a little over 40 per cent of the population of Queensland lived in the greater Brisbane area and by the 1990s the figure was around 45 per cent. Since the 1960s, the most rapidly growing area of Queensland has been the Gold Coast and Brisbane urologists also covered that area until Dan Kleinig began practising in Southport. He was a Consultant at the Gold Coast Hospital from 1975.

By the 1980s, about two-thirds of the population of Queensland was concentrated in the south-east corner, around Brisbane and the holiday and retirement centres along the coast. Elsewhere, the population is also concentrated in the coastal fringe and the population of outback Queensland has tended to decline since the 1950s. Mining towns such as Mount Isa are the exception. The population there grew rapidly in the 1950s and 1960s, but has declined since. Tony Paul, later the flying surgeon, was the urologist at the Mount Isa Base Hospital in 1974, but he was not a member of the Society.

Few centres apart from Brisbane and the Gold Coast have a population large enough to support one or more urologists, but distances are so great between towns along the north coast that each serves a very wide hinterland.

Urology in country Queensland was pioneered by Paul Hopkins at Mackay. He was the son of Brisbane surgeon George Herbert Hopkins and, unusually, did his medical degree in Melbourne, not Sydney. In 1925, he was appointed as Medical Superintendent at Mackay Base Hospital and from the 1940s also held the post of Visiting Urologist. He was an associate member of the Society and regularly attended meetings. In the late 1960s he was succeeded by Stan Duke.

The pioneer urologist in Toowoomba was Steve Ferguson, who trained in Sydney and England. In 1954, he was appointed Honorary Consultant Urologist to the Toowoomba General Hospital. 'As Urologists also had a general surgical degree I was expected to take my turn with any Surgical Emergencies after hours including major trauma and orthopaedics.' He found problems in both the standard of equipment and facilities. On windy days, dust came up between the floorboards causing wound infection. 'Expensive items like Foley catheters, ureteric catheters and stone baskets had to stand repeated use ...' The hospital had no diathermy machine and Steve Ferguson used a cold punch, but without diathermy. ' Haemostasis was left to nature.'[15]

In 1974, John Sander became an associate member of the Society and, as was the pattern in country Queensland, also combined his urology with general surgery in Toowoomba.

Ros Parisi, in Townsville, was probably the first full-time country urologist and appropriately he was the first Australian urologist from outside a capital city to become President of the Society (1982-83). Ros Parisi's career was very much concentrated in North Queensland. He was RMO in Townsville in 1956-57, Registrar at Broken Hill in 1957-58 (in obstetrics and gynaecology), Registrar in Townsville in 1959-60, and obtained his Edinburgh Fellowship in 1962. He was apppointed Consultant Urologist at Townsville General Hospital in 1971. He recalls that until 1963, complex problems were referred to Brisbane. Between 1963 and 1969 he was in practice as a consultant general surgeon-urologist and progressively more of the urological cases were referred to him. By 1969, he was able to confine his practice to urology.

In 1974, there were five members of the Society at hospitals outside Brisbane: Steve Ferguson and John Sander in Toowoomba; Ros Parisi at Townsville General Hospital; Stan Duke at Mackay Base Hospital and Richard (Ginger) Marsden at Bundaberg Hospital. As was the case elsewhere in Australasia, country urologists tended to stay in the same area for a particularly long time. Twenty years later, Richard Marsden was still at Bundaberg and Stan Duke was still in Mackay but Steve Ferguson and Ros Parisi had retired.

During the 1980s, the proportion of Queensland urologists based in Brisbane fell from 78 per cent in 1981 to 67 per cent in 1986. David Splatt, son of Alex, began practising in Cairns as a private specialist in 1984. Dan Kleinig, the first urologist based on the Gold

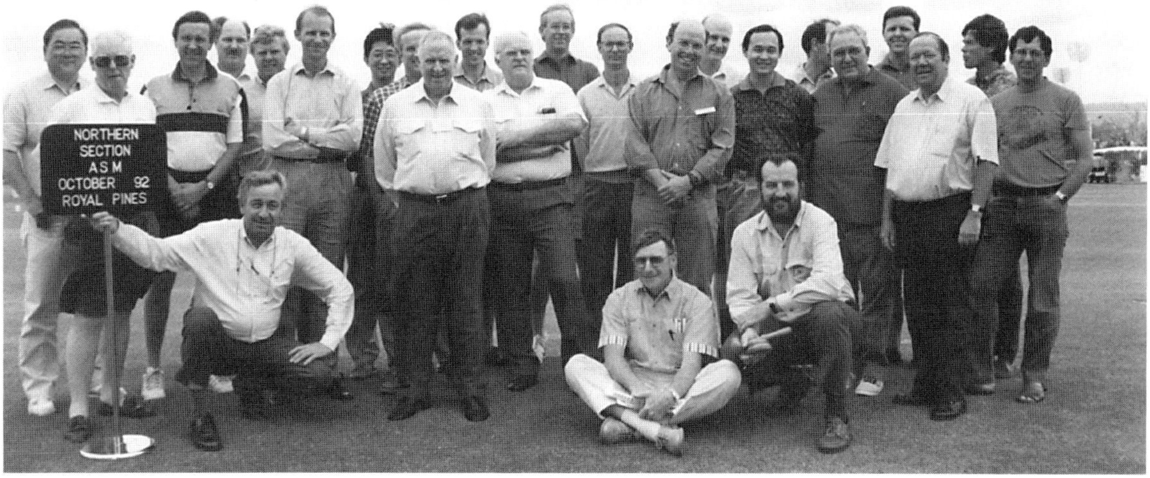

Northern Section Meeting, 20 November 1992. *Standing, left to right:* Ray Que Hee, Richard Marsden, Ross Cartmill, Malcolm Boyle, Geof Buckham, Professor Chris Woodhouse, Ken P'ng, Tony James, Jeff Watson, David Nicol, Terrence Farrell, Philip McDougall, David Splatt, David Kerle, Frank Gardiner, Steven Lun, Roger Hinsch, Ros Parisi, Roger Watson, Graham Holmes, David Winkle, Geof Hirst; *Kneeling, left to right:* Robin Spork, Graeme Heap, Peter Heathcote;

Coast, had been joined by Philip McDougall. From 1977 he was a private specialist based in Southport. In Toowoomba, Steve Ferguson and John Sander were joined by Geoff Buckham who pioneered laser surgery in the area.

By 1996 there were urologists in six centres outside Brisbane: one in Bundaberg; one in Cairns; one in Mackay; three in Nambour; five on the Gold Coast and three in Toowoomba. This expansion was reflected in a proposal for a training position at the Gold Coast Hospital. Rockhampton did not get a urologist until 1994 and coverage of country Queensland remained a problem, for instance in areas such as Mount Isa and the far north. This problem of distance had long been recognised in Queensland, the birthplace of the flying doctor service, and Tony Paul, the flying surgeon based in Roma, did a fair amount of urology.[16]

The Northern Section of the Urological Society

The development of State sections of the Urological Society began in Queensland, with a proposal early in 1958. In March, the Executive set up a sub-committee to consider State branches and the Northern Section first met on 27 May 1958. Mick Hogg was the first Chairman. Queensland was also a pioneer in setting up a Journal Club. This was independent of the Northern Section and began meeting in 1961.

The Northern Section was not very active during the 1960s, but there were an increasing number of meetings during the 1970s, including regular Saturday morning Clinical Meetings. In the 1980s, like other State sections, activity was stimulated by increased involvement in the selection and monitoring of trainees. In 1983, for instance, the Annual Clinical Meeting was in Noosa Heads and in 1984 it was Toowoomba. The committee at this stage consisted of Ros Parisi, Graham Holmes and Stephen Stening.

TABLE 8.1 NORTHERN SECTION ASMs, 1981-1996

1981	Kooralbyn Resort, visitor Dermot O'Flynn, convenor Graham Holmes
1982	Surfers Paradise, visitor John Wickham, convenor Graham Holmes
1983	Noosa, visitor Bruce Pearson, convenor Graham Holmes
1984	Toowoomba, visitor John Maddern, convenor Graham Holmes
1985	Greenmount Resort, visitor Stuart Taylor, convenor Graham Holmes
1986	Stradbroke Island, visitor John Kearsley, convenor Lionel Lukin
1987	Noosa, following ICUC meeting, large international faculty, convenors Graham Holmes and Geof Hirst
1988	Byron Bay, visitor Don Moss, convenor Stuart Sillar
1989	Coolum, visitor Michael Lieber, convenor Robin Spork
1990	Sanctuary Cove, visitor Tony Costello, convenor Robin Spork
1991	Sanctuary Cove, visitor Villis Marshall, convenor Robin Spork
1992	Royal Pines, visitor Chris Woodhouse, convenor Robin Spork
1993	Twin Waters, visitor Reg Hall, convenor Robin Spork
1994	no meeting, SIU meeting, Sydney
1995	Kooralbyn Resort, visitor Stan Wisniewski, convenor Peter Heathcote
1996	Twin Waters, visitor Nick Bruchovsky, convenor Peter Heathcote

As with the rest of Australasia, Queensland had its fair share of rivalries but the introduction of lithotripters to Queensland seems to have caused fewer conflicts than in the other States and New Zealand. Tony James negotiated with the Queensland Government to pay urologists treating patients using the machine at the Holy Spirit Hospital.

In 1997, Philip McDougall from the Gold Coast was Chairman of the Northern Section. The pattern was for a meeting in Brisbane every month. These were held in Brisbane at the Holy Spirit Hospital on Saturday mornings. They grew out of X-ray meetings started by Frank Gardiner and Philip McDougall when they were both registrars in Brisbane in the mid-1970s. The idea was to get people from the hospitals south of the Brisbane River together with the people from the north. There was always a degree of rivalry between the Royal Brisbane Hospital and the hospitals south of the river and this seems to have intensified after the opening of the Princess Alexandra.

By the 1990s, the Saturday morning meetings were well attended, not only by the Brisbane urologists, but also by people from further afield, including northern New South Wales, the Gold Coast, Toowoomba and Bundaberg, and sometimes even north Queenslanders. They combined business and educational components.

The Annual General Meetings were held in country centres, generally some time in Spring, and the guests usually included the President of the Society, plus one or more other interstate urologists. Overseas urologists were invited when available, for instance with the assistance of RACS or drug company funding.[17]

CHAPTER 9

Urology in South Australia and the Northern Territory

~

Introduction

The population of South Australia is particularly concentrated in the area around Adelaide. In 1947, more than 59 per cent of the population of the State lived in the capital and by 1986 this had risen to more than 68 per cent. However, this measure of the City area alone underestimates the concentration of population. If outer Adelaide is included, 79 per cent of the population lived in the Adelaide area in 1989 and only about 300 000 people lived in the whole of the rest of the State. In 1986, there were no other major towns and only two towns with populations greater than 20 000: Whyalla with 26 900 and Mount Gambier with 20 813.

Urologists have been similarly concentrated in Adelaide. All the South Australian members of the Urological Society have lived in the Adelaide area.

Specialist medical services of all kinds, including urology have historically been concentrated in Adelaide's major teaching hospitals. Of these, the Royal Adelaide Hospital was the first and remains the largest.

The Royal Adelaide Hospital

Until the 1970s, the Royal Adelaide was not a free public hospital. Treatment was means tested for out patients and fees were charged for in patients. For many years it was the only teaching hospital for the University of Adelaide and the hospital where most of Adelaide's first generation of urologists received their earliest clinical experience. Strongly following the general Australasian pattern of working in their home town, they grew up in Adelaide, went to the University of Adelaide, travelled to England, or the United States, or both, to learn their urology, and returned to practise urology in

Adelaide. The first Adelaide urologist to take this path was Noel Bonnin and he began at the Royal Adelaide. He lists his Public Hospital Appointments as follows:

> *1947: Hon. Assistant Surgeon (General Surgical Staff)*
>
> *1948: Awarded Carnegie Travelling Fellowship. Spent some six months overseas getting updated in urology. Some two or three months with Reed Nesbit at Ann Arbor, and then at other clinics in America and England. Returned via Canada where I obtained a resident appointment in Kingston, Ontario, with Nathan Berry who believed his main mission in life was to teach the technique of transurethral resection.*
>
> *1950: Appointed Hon. Surgeon in charge of newly formed Urological Unit. There were the usual troubles with some of the general surgical staff and restricted referral rules were applied to the unit. I got fed up with this and eventually applied for a general surgical appointment at the new Queen Elizabeth Hospital.*
>
> *1959: Appointed Hon. Assistant Surgeon at Q.E.H. becoming Surgeon 1961 to 1969. There I did mainly urology but now with full access to the work I wanted.*
>
> *1969: Retired to private practice and full-time urology...*
>
> *A major trouble which I encountered was that my surgical appointment precluded me from becoming a full member of the Urological Society of Australasia. However, on leaving the Q.E.H. I became a full-time urologist and in 1976 the Society honoured me by electing me a Fellow.*[1]

Noel Bonnin's move to the Queen Elizabeth coincided with John Maddern's arrival at the Royal Adelaide. John Maddern gradually built up the unit and eventually achieved direct referral, but it took many years. His attitude to change at the Adelaide was that he wanted evolution, not revolution. John Maddern was the first full member

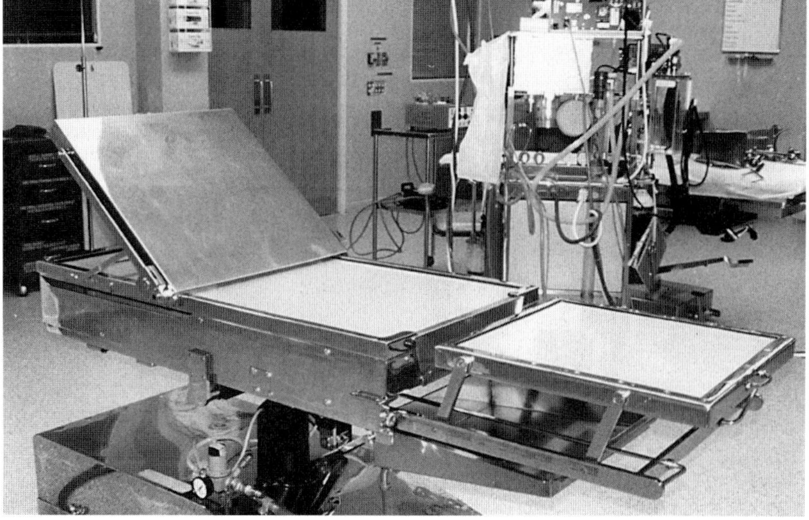

Noel Bonnin was noted for his technical innovation. He adapted features of the Harris and Millin prostatectomy operations and made a number of modifications to instruments, sometimes in conjunction with Edward and Donald Both, instrument makers. In 1954 he also designed a series of urological tables, a number of which were still in use in hospitals around Adelaide in the 1990s.

of the Society in South Australia and despite his problems with referrals in his public hospital work rapidly built a busy private practice on direct referrals from GPs. In 1969-70 he was the first South Australian President of the Urological Society. He also found time to act as an examiner for the RACS and in the 1980s played a leading role in developing the training scheme for urologists.

In 1965, John Jose joined him and found that patients still had to be referred by a general surgeon. John Jose is the son of Sir Ivan Jose. During the 1930s and 1940s Sir Ivan was one of the more notable Adelaide surgeons to have an interest in urology. John Jose spent some time at Cambridge but returned to Adelaide for his clinical years and was a house surgeon at the Royal Adelaide in the mid-1950s. He took his FRACS in 1960 and then returned to London to take his FRCSEng. This was unusual at the time, the general pattern being to take a British fellowship before the FRACS. Jose spent two years in London as a senior registrar in urology, returning via Los Angeles. Even as late as the 1960s, TUR was regarded as being still in its infancy in England and he joined the long tradition of Australasian urologists learning their TUR in the United States.

On returning to Adelaide in 1965, John Jose went into partnership with Noel Bonnin, rather than John Maddern. He was on the Executive of the Urological Society for many years and President in 1984-85, besides being active on the Board of Management of the Royal Adelaide Hospital.[2]

Graham Sinclair began his urological training at the Royal Adelaide in 1971 and remembers that the general surgeons did more urology than the urologists. 'The general surgeons were the power brokers. They would send us cases when they didn't want to deal with them.'[3] At that stage, the urologists at the Royal Adelaide were John Maddern, John Jose and Michael Hamilton. Michael Hamilton was known as an anglophile and never attended many meetings of the Urological Society of

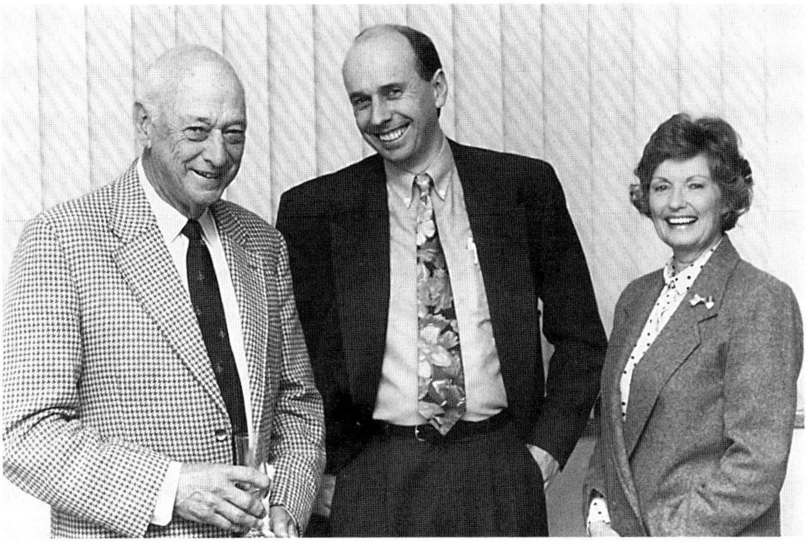

John Maddern with his wife Betty and his son Guy at the time of Guy's appointment as Professor of Surgery at the University of Adelade, 1993. (*Source:* John Maddern)

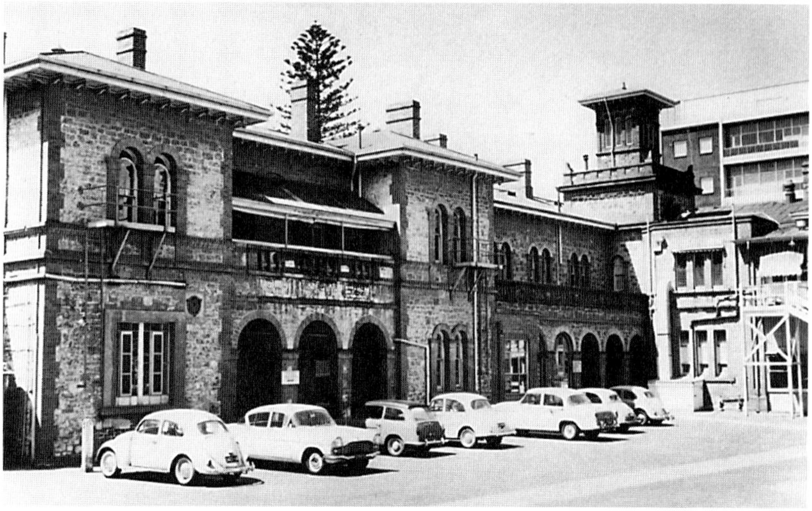

Royal Adelaide Hospital, the old hospital c. 1963, since demolished

Australasia, but he travelled to Britain to the BAUS meetings. He did, however, attend South Australian State Section Meetings. In 1976, Chris Switajewski joined the urologists at the Royal Adelaide, and in 1983 John Jose succeeded John Maddern as Director of the Urology Unit.

For much of the period since its formation, the Urology Unit at the Royal Adelaide has not been an easy place to work. Relationships between the three senior urologists at the hospital tended to be strained to such a degree, that some younger urologists felt that they and their careers suffered because of the intense rivalry between the members of the triumvirate. To a certain extent, this tension extended to relationships with urologists at the Queen Elizabeth Hospital, particularly in the early years.

The Queen Elizabeth Hospital

The Queen Elizabeth opened in 1954 as a 55-bed maternity hospital. In 1957 and 1959 new blocks were opened and it became a (free) public general hospital. Noel Bonnin's appointment was as a general surgeon, but in the mid-1960s he was joined by Peter Harbison. Harbison was the second full member of the Urological Society in South Australia and in 1967 he was appointed as the first Urological Surgeon at the Queen Elizabeth. At that stage it was a university teaching hospital with about 530 beds, less than half the size of the Royal Adelaide.

Peter Harbison followed the pattern of leaving Adelaide for urological experience overseas and spent time in England, obtaining his FRCSEng in 1957. He was an active member of the Urological Society and President in 1977-78. Soon afterwards, he began visiting Alice Springs and Darwin and moved to the Northern Territory in 1989. In 1992 he retired back to Adelaide.[4]

In 1971 Geoffrey Burfield joined the unit as the second urologist. He had a special interest in transplants and was head of the transplant unit. He remembers that until the early 1980s, the senior general surgeons had all worked with Noel Bonnin and thought they knew urology. Geoffey Burfield has the distinction of being awarded the Urological Society's first ever travelling fellowship. In 1968 he was in London as a houseman at St Peter's and heard of the new fellowship. He recalls that it upgraded his income in 1969. He returned to Adelaide via Los Angeles and was a consultant at the Repatriation Hospital as well as the Queen Elizabeth, where he was apppointed Director of Urology in 1989, when Peter Harbison left for the Northern Territory.[5] Kim Moretti was appointed to the Queen Elizabeth Hospital in1987 and became Head of the Unit in 1998.

Repatriation General Hospital

This was a military hospital during World War II and it was taken over by the Repatriation Commission in 1947. As with other Federal repatriation hospitals, free treatment was available to returned service personnel and their eligible dependents. By the 1970s the beds were seldom full and eventually arrangements were made to treat patients with no repatriation entitlements. In 1976, links were established with the new Flinders University and the Repat. became a teaching hospital. In 1995, it became a general hospital under the State system, integrated with the Flinders Medical Centre.

In the early years, Sir Ivan Jose and Geoffrey Verco did the urology at the Repat. Verco was an associate member of the Urological Society from the mid-1950s. Peter Harbison began attending the Repat. from about 1964 and he was joined by John Jose, Geoffrey Burfield, Graham Sinclair and later Adrian Porter. Alan Stapleton was head of the unit from July 1997. Like all repatriation hospitals, the clientele of increasingly elderly men provided a particularly large amount of clinical work for urologists and from the 1980s this clinical base was integrated with the research work at the Flinders Medical Centre.

Flinders Medical Centre

The centre is an integrated teaching hospital and medical school on the campus of Flinders University. It first admitted patients in 1976 and had 471 beds in use by 1980. Villis Marshall was appointed initially as Associate Professor and in 1984 became Professor of Surgery. Graham Sinclair was also appointed to the urology unit in 1976 and they were later joined by Adrian Porter and, in 1984, by Peter Sutherland. The unit had an enormous impact on academic urology around Australasia. Villis Marshall's research interests included the causes of growth in stones and growth in the prostate, whether benign or cancerous. He was also interested in urodynamics.

The Urology Unit at the Flinders Medical Centre acquired a reputation for excellent research in all these areas. However, the unit not only introduced academic urology to South Australia. It also changed

TABLE 9.1 OFFICE BEARERS OF THE SOUTH AUSTRALIAN SECTION OF THE UROLOGICAL SOCIETY

1976	Peter Harbison, President, Graham Sinclair, Secretary
1977	John Jose, President, Graham Sinclair, Secretary
1978	Geoff Burfield, President, Graham Sinclair, Secretary
1979	Villis Marshall, President, Graham Sinclair, Secretary
1980	Chris Switajewski, President, Adrian Porter, Secretary
1981	Saeed Ahmed, President, Adrian Porter, Secretary
1982	John Maddern, President, Adrian Porter, Secretary
1983	Graham Sinclair, President, Zenon Herzberg, Secretary
1984	Michael Hamilton, President, John Maddern, Secretary
1985	Adrian Porter, President, John Jose, Secretary
1986	Zenon Herzberg, President, Peter Sutherland, Secretary
1987	Agnelo De Sousa, President, Peter Sutherland, Secretary
1988	Peter Sutherland, President, David Elder, Secretary
1989	Peter Harbison, President, Kim Moretti, Secretary
1990	Geoff Burfield, President, Kim Moretti, Secretary
1991	John Jose, President, Kim Moretti, Secretary
1992	John Bolt, President, Hilary Boucault, Secretary
1993	Kim Moretti, President, Hilary Boucault, Secretary
1994	Adrian Porter, President, Hilary Boucault, Secretary
1995	Paddy Dewan, President, Hilary Boucault, Secretary
1996	Brian Landers, President, Denby Steele, Secretary
1997	Zenon Herzberg, President, Denby Steele, Secretary

Chairmen of the South Australian Branch of the Training, Accreditation and Education Committee:

1982-84	John Maddern
1985-88	Villis Marshall
1989-94	Peter Sutherland
1995-97	John Bolt

the atmosphere of urology in Adelaide with an alternative focus to the tensions at the Royal Adelaide and the Queen Elizabeth Hospitals. 'Flinders defused a lot of it because of the very benign nature of Villis and the enormous respect that everyone has for him.'[6]

Like the majority of Adelaide urologists, Villis Marshall was a graduate of Adelaide University. He took his FRACS in 1971 and went on to London, where he specialised in urology at the London Hospital, working with John Blandy, becoming a lecturer before returning to Adelaide in 1976 to the new position at Flinders. He subsequently served as an examiner for the RACS and was Chairman of the South Australian RACS State Committee. He also played an active role in the Urological Society. He was chairman of the T, A & E Committee in 1986-88, President in 1991-92 and made a Fellow of the Society in 1995.

Adrian Porter followed the general Adelaide pattern of doing his initial training in Adelaide before going on to Britain. He spent time in Edinburgh and Cambridge and at the London Hospital with John Blandy. He returned to the position of senior registrar at the Royal Adelaide for two years before being appointed as a consultant at the Repat. and Flinders.

The two hospitals were geographically close and the visiting consultants were the same at both centres for many years before they amalgamated in the 1990s.[7]

Adelaide Children's Hospital

Geoffrey Verco was the first member of the Society involved at the Children's Hospital and was still the specialist attached to the Urology Unit in 1980. He specialised in ileal loop diversions for spina bifida cases. From the 1970s, Saeed Ahmed was the Director of the Urology Unit. Saeed Ahmed was originally from Pakistan but had trained in England and was the first fully trained paediatric urologist in Adelaide. In the late 1980s he moved to King Faisel Hospital in Saudi Arabia. The members of the Society associated with the Children's Hospital since then have been Paddy Dewan and Hilary Boucaut, the first female full member of the Society. In 1996, Paddy Dewan moved to the Royal Children's Hospital in Melbourne.

Modbury General Hosiptal

Modbury, in Adelaide's north-eastern suburbs, opened in 1973 with 134 beds, rising to 214 over the next few years. Zenon Herzberg was the first member of the Urological Society associated with the hospital and in the 1990s he was joined by Denby Steele.

The Northern Territory

In 1966 the population of the Northern Territory was only just over 56 000, but by 1981 it had grown to more than 123 000. In theory this is a large enough population to support a full-time urologist, but the two major urban centres of Darwin and Alice Springs are well over 1000 kilometres apart and the rest of the population is scattered over an area greater than New South Wales and Victoria put together. The problems of providing specialist services to the Northern Territory are therefore considerable.

Urological services have traditionally been provided from Adelaide. From the late 1970s, Peter Harbison visited Alice Springs and Darwin on a regular basis and between 1989 and 1992 he was based full-time in Darwin. Since then, a visiting service has been provided through the Flinders Medical Centre. Initially, Villis Marshall, Adrian Porter and Graham Sinclair took it in turns and provided a

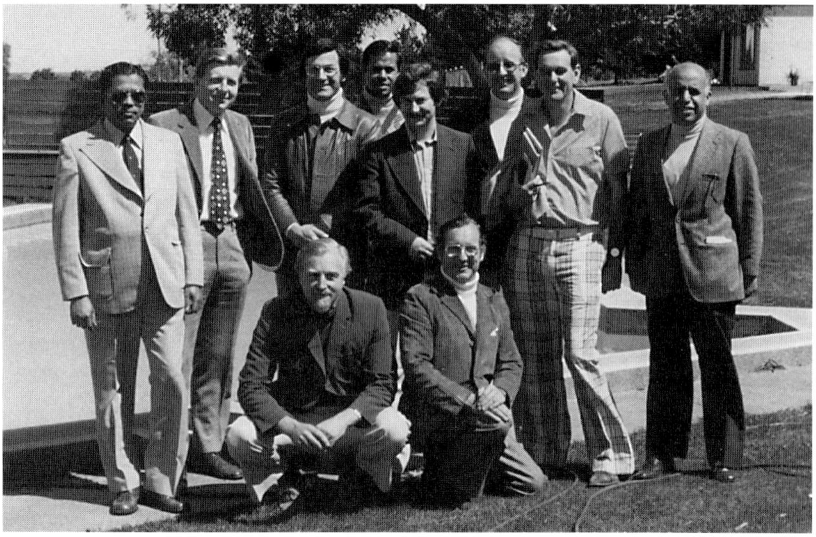

Inaugural meeting of the South Australian State Section, Renmark Golf Club, 1976. *Back row, left to right:* A. S. Naryan, Villis Marshall, Graham Sinclair, Agnelo De Sousa, Adrian Porter, Geoff Burfield, Peter Harbison, Saeed Ahmed; *Front row:* John Jose and Joe Murnaghan. (*Source:* Peter Harbison)

monthly service between them. However, for various reasons, Marshall and Porter have dropped out, as Graham Sinclair notes:

> *I have been the only one going now on a three monthly basis. Although I started in June 1992, I have still not been able to convince the Royal Darwin Hospital to buy a urodynamic machine, but I have convinced them to set up an Impotence Clinic with the use of prostaglandin and introduced the concept to local practitioners. Generally I have shown the Gynaecologists how to perform anti-incontinence procedures and several of the local surgeons percutaneous pyelolithotomy.*
>
> *There are a lot of unusual problems in Darwin, such as retained stents in Aboriginal people who disappear after surgery and don't come back causing major problems, prostatic abscesses and advanced diseases.*
>
> *I find it a pleasure to treat the Aboriginal people and that is the reason I continue to go there.*[8]

The South Australian Section of the Urological Society

The inaugural meeting of the South Australian State section was in 1976. As with other State sections, the changes in the training program in the 1980s gave it a sharper focus. Regular meetings were arranged at the teaching hospitals, including the Adelaide Children's, and trainees presented papers. This also provided a useful forum for the discussion of difficult or interesting cases. The Annual General Meetings were usually held somewhere pleasant in October and often included a lighter side, in addition to the serious papers. At the 1983 AGM at Wirrinna, for instance, John Jose posed as a visiting naturalist to the Galapagos Islands.[9]

CHAPTER 10

Urology in Tasmania

~

Urology in Tasmania before 1957

There were no full members of the Urological Society in Tasmania before 1964 and no associate members until the mid-1950s. Urological procedures were performed by general surgeons and the earliest to develop an interest in urology seem to have been Tom Giblin in Hobart and Bill Woodward in Launceston. Tom Giblin did very little resection work but did do open prostatectomies. By 1958, H. B. Gatenby in Launceston was an associate member of the Society. Bill Woodward at Launceston also maintained his interest in urology and associate membership of the Society until the late 1960s, when he went to England and took up orthopaedic surgery.[1]

The population distribution in Tasmania is different to that in the mainland Australian States, where the urban population is overwhelmingly concentrated in the capital cities. Launceston has been an important centre to rival Hobart since the earliest days of white settlement and more recently the population of the Burnie/Devonport area has grown to provide a third major centre. The development of Tasmanian urology in all three centres reflects this balance.

Tasmania is the smallest State in both area and population but the relatively small distances involved mean that urologists in Launceston and Hobart effectively served most of the island. The population was 257 000 in 1947, rising to 419 000 in 1981. Over the same period, the number of urologists rose from none to four, including one at Burnie in the north-west.

Proximity to Victoria has also meant that it has been relatively easy for specialist services to be provided from Melbourne. This is in contrast to the Northern Territory with a population about one quarter the size of Tasmania's, but more than ten times the area, creating far greater logistical problems for the provision of urological services to a small population.

Launceston 1957–1997

Alan Holmes did his initial training at the Royal Prince Alfred Hospital in Sydney. In 1953, he moved to Launceston General Hospital as Surgical Registrar and recalls that the general surgeons did all the urology in Launceston at that time. He began to develop an interest and went to England, where he spent eighteen months with Harry Graham at the Preston Royal Infirmary. Preston had a relatively large urology unit with forty beds. In 1957, he returned to Launceston, initially as outpatient surgeon and then as inpatient surgeon, but maintained his interest in urology. Late in 1963, Alan Holmes moved to Hobart.

D. I. Roberts was an English-trained general and urological surgeon, who trained in urology at All Saints Hospital, London and passed the FRACS in urology on arrival in Australia in 1957. Like Alan Holmes, he began as outpatient surgeon and was subsequently inpatient surgeon at Launceston General Hospital so that both of them were general surgeons with an interest in urology at the same hospital. D. I. Roberts found that Bill Woodward had set up the Launceston General Hospital for endoscopic work:

> *In 1957, urological instruments at the Launceston General Hospital were adequate and a full set of ACMI endoscopes was available—largely due to the foresight of Bill Woodward. These scopes were*

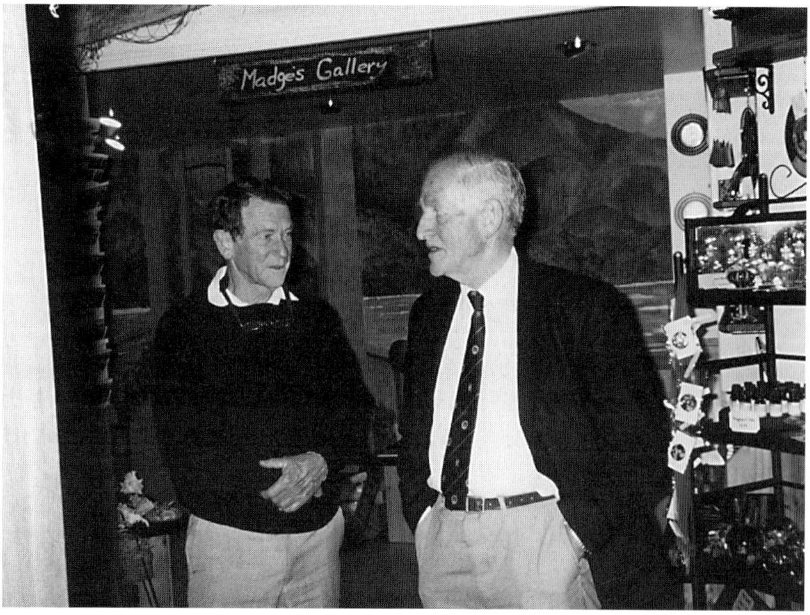

Alan Holmes (left) and 'Robbie' Roberts at the 1997 ASM of the Tasmanian Section of the Urological Society. (*Source:* Terry Morgan)

steadily upgraded and replaced by Storz equipment. In 1957 a cobalt 'bomb' was installed at the Peter MacCallum Clinic at the Launceston General Hospital, and many cases of carcinoma of the bladder were treated with radiotherapy by this unit. A teaching eyepiece was available from early on, so that registrars who were interested could follow endoscopic procedures and eventually perform simple ones themselves. As a result, 10 urologists have commenced their career discipline in Launceston.[2]

In 1967, D. I. Roberts was appointed to the new post of Sessional Urologist at Launceston General Hospital. By 1971 he was the only member of the Society left in Launceston and remained so until Ian Hill joined him in 1985. In 1989, Hill moved to Western Australia. He was succeeded by Michael Monsour and in 1992 by Rob Jensen, both of whom had developed their interest in urology as registrars at the Launceston General Hospital. Mike Monsour trained in Brisbane and Rob Jensen trained in Perth, both subsequently spending time in Britain.[3]

Urology in Hobart 1964–1997

Before 1963, Tom Giblin did most of the urology in Hobart, plus general surgery. When he retired, the general surgeons thought it was time to set up a urology unit. Part of the deal when Alan Holmes took up the position at the Royal Hobart Hospital was that he would become a full-time urologist and the general surgeons would stop doing any urology. Unlike the position in many other hospitals, it was an amicable arrangement.

Alan Holmes arrived to find fairly primitive instruments and they still had red rubber catheters, but he was given the freedom to equip the unit with reasonable instruments. Initially, he worked full-time at the Royal Hobart with only one private session per week, but later cut back his public sessions and increased his private practice.

In the 1960s and 1970s the unit at the Royal Hobart was very busy and understaffed. Problems were covered by co-operation with Melbourne. For spinal injury work, for instance, Alan Holmes liaised with the Austin Hospital in Melbourne and for paediatric urology he liaised with Douglas Stephens at the Royal Children's Hospital. Over time, however, this changed. 'The paediatric surgeons are in the box seat because they have the children referred to them and gradually they take it over.'[4]

Terry Morgan joined Alan Holmes at the Royal Hobart in 1977 and became a full member of the Urological Society in 1983. He was originally from Hobart, but spent three years in Adelaide as a general surgical trainee before going to Wellington, where he worked with Humphrey Gowland, and then on to two years at the Institute of Urology in London. Ian Middleton joined Alan Holmes and Terry Morgan in 1990.

Burnie

In 1996, there were only seven members of the Urological Society in Tasmania, three in Launceston, three in Hobart and one in Burnie. John Kille was an English-trained surgeon who had been at the Hull Royal Infirmary since 1968. In 1974 he moved to Tasmania to the position of general surgeon, and from 1977, urologist, at the North West General Hospital, Burnie. Initially, he was an associate member of the Society, but became a full member in 1983. He remained the only registered urologist in Burnie until he retired in 1993 to concentrate on cattle breeding.[5]

Tasmania and the Urological Society

From 1964, Alan Holmes was the first, and until 1983 the only, full member of the Urological Society in Tasmania. He replaced Bill Woodward as the Tasmanian representative on the Executive and remained there until the 1980s. Once D. I. Roberts was elected a full member, he relieved Holmes on the Executive until 1990, when Terry Morgan took over. In 1994, he was succeeded by Michael Monsour.

The small number of urologists in Tasmania meant that it was not a viable group to have an independent section and during the 1980s, Tasmanian urologists belonged to the Victorian section. A Victorian State section meeting was held in Launceston in 1988.

Small numbers also meant that it was very difficult for a Tasmanian to take on the job of President, especially when the President ran the ASM—there were simply not enough urologists in Tasmania to help run the meeting. The other problem was the lack of a suitable venue. The only possibility was the University in Hobart and that was not available during the autumn when the Society ran its ASMs. Alan Holmes therefore turned down the suggestion of becoming President. However, by 1993 a building was available and Warren Johnson held his meeting in Hobart at the Sheraton Hotel.[6] By then, Tasmania had a separate State Section. Ian Middleton was the driving force behind the move to separate from Victoria. Meetings alternated between the Hobart and Launceston areas and they were entitled to financial support form the Society for a paid visitor every other year.[7]

CHAPTER 11

Urology in Victoria

~

Introduction

Victoria is the most densely populated State in Australia, with one quarter of the country's population living on just under 3 per cent of the land area. In the mid-1990s, the population was about four and a half million, about three million of whom lived in the greater Melbourne area.

Despite this concentration of population in Melbourne, there are a number of other significant population centres in Victoria. Geelong is the largest of these, with a population approaching 150,000 in the 1990s. No other centre had a population over 100 000, but since the 1960s, Albury-Wodonga, Ballarat and Bendigo have all had populations well over 50 000 and in 1990, the Shepparton-Mooroopna district had a population of about 40 000. As a result, there have been fewer problems in providing a reasonable level of specialist services in country Victoria than in the rural areas of the larger States.

Victorian public hospitals evolved as independent institutions, each with its own board, but by 1948 the level of State Government regulation and funding support was already considerable. In 1948, the Hospitals and Charities Act increased this level of Government co-ordination and supervision through the Hospitals and Charities Commission. By the 1960s about 65 per cent of public hospital revenue was provided by the State Government and a substantial proportion of the rest was provided by patients. Victorian public hospitals were not free. Patients were means tested and either paid about half the cost of their accommodation, receiving free medical care through the honorary system, or paid the higher intermediate or private hospital rates, plus medical fees.

In 1975, the introduction of Medibank brought the end of the honorary system. Specialists were paid sessionally or on a fee for service

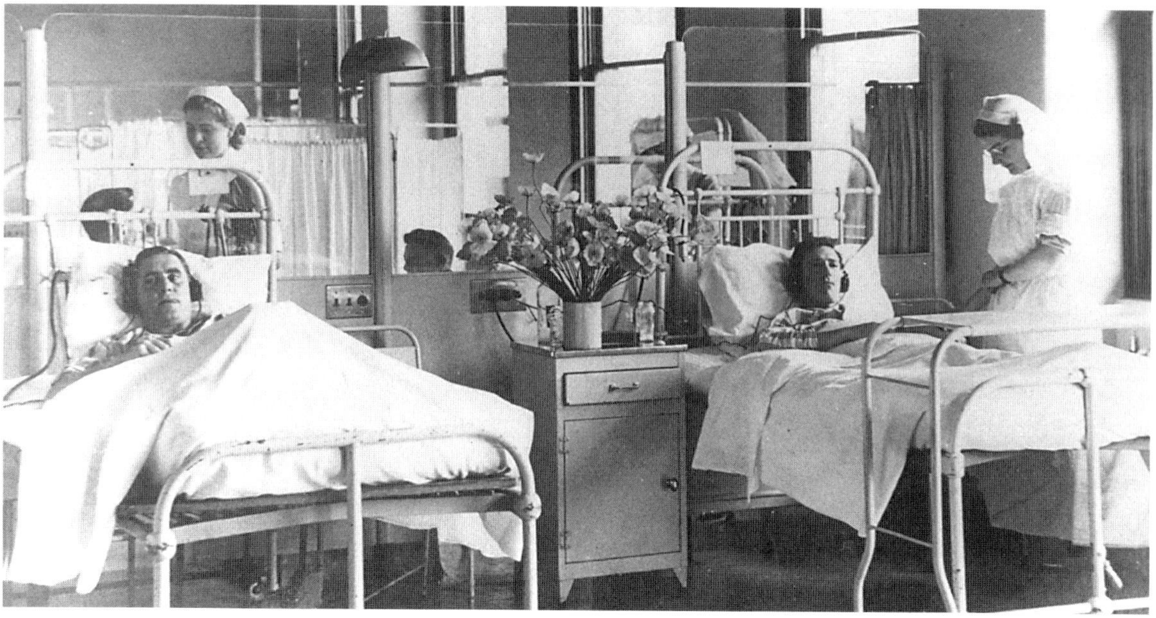

Surgical Ward, Royal Melbourne Hospital, 1950s. (*Source:* Royal Melbourne Hospital Archives)

basis and between 1975 and 1981 the State and Federal Governments shared hospital operating costs. Under this system, uninsured patients were treated free of charge.

In the 1990s, Victoria had about 170 public hospitals and about 110 private hospitals. The private hospitals were generally small, and in 1992 only 14 had more than 100 beds. Country public hospitals also tended to be small. In contrast, the average size of Melbourne's public hospitals was over 200 beds. However, private hospitals played a significant role in the Victorian hospital system.

Since 1947, the population of greater Melbourne has doubled and this growth has been associated with a sustained process of suburbanisation. The area covered by the city has grown enormously in the west and the north, but it has grown particularly markedly to the east and south-east. At the end of World War II, the area now occupied by Monash University was on the eastern fringe of the built-up area. By the mid-1990s, it was more or less the geographical centre of greater Melbourne.

There have been a number of developments in hospital building that reflect this population shift, including the Monash Medical Centre, but on the whole, as in Sydney, there has been a considerable time delay between the growth of population and the development of specialist medical services in suburban areas.

Over time, Victorian urologists have adjusted to this process of suburbanisation and it has particularly affected those who have commenced their practice since the 1950s. Most have held more than one public hospital appointment and been involved in more than one private practice, and as many as two-thirds of them have changed the area in which their practice is based. Melbourne's older generation of urologists were far more likely to spend their entire career based in the same area.[1]

Over time, urologists spread out from the major teaching hospitals. A pattern emerged of adding attendance at one or more suburban hospitals to an appointment at a metropolitan hospital and this pattern seems to have begun with Bowie Somerset at the Royal Melbourne Hospital.

The Royal Melbourne Hospital

The current buildings of the Royal Melbourne Hospital at Parkville, adjacent to the University, were completed in 1942 but were then occupied as an American Military Hospital for two years. Patients were moved from the old city centre site in December 1944. By 1962, the hospital had 630 beds and was an adult general hospital. Paediatric and obstetric services were provided by the Royal Children's Hospital and the Royal Women's Hospital.

David Webb has suggested three phases in the history of the hospital. The first phase was strongly influenced by non-conformist religious principles—dour, serious, god-fearing. The second phase was clubbish and concerned with prestige and making money, while the most recent phase is modern, academic and less self-centred. He suggests that developments in the urology unit have reflected these three phases.[2] While it is not clear that all the urologists associated with the Royal Melbourne Hospital fit this pattern, the changing styles of the heads of the unit can broadly be categorised in this way.

The first head of the unit was John Thompson Tait, a foundation member of the Urological Society. In 1947, he was succeeded by William Harold Moore, who had been his assistant since 1928. Warren Johnson has described Moore as a 'quiet Baptist gentleman'.[3]

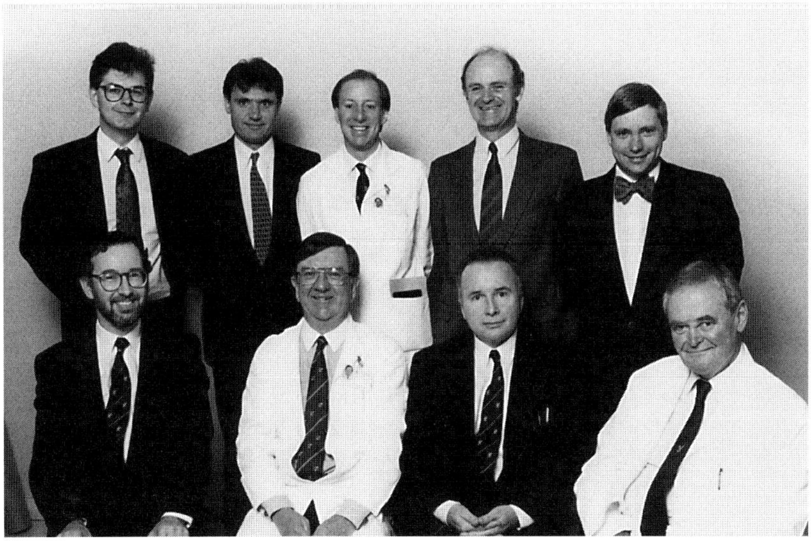

The Royal Melbourne Hospital Urology Unit, 1992. *Standing left to right:* Nick Redgrave, Greg Neerhut, David Webb, Laurence Cleeve, Doug Travis. *Seated:* Alan Crosthwaite, Warren Johnson, Laurence Harewood and Ian Nunn. (*Source:* Laurence Cleeve)

His grandfather was a Baptist Minister and his father, the distinguished surgeon William Moore, was President of the Baptist Theological College.

Besides his appointment at the Royal Melbourne Hospital, from 1937 to 1953 Harold Moore was Honorary Urologist to the Women's Hospital, where he held a weekly clinic. In 1953 he retired to private practice from his Collins Street consulting rooms.[4]

Harold Moore was succeeded as head of the urology unit by John Bowie Somerset, often known as Bowie Somerset. Warren Johnson has described him as:

> *hard working, energetic ... enjoyed the good things in life. Spent a lot of time at the Melbourne Club. Suspicious of academics and was not one himself. Wonderful lecturer and post graduate lecturer.*[5]

Bowie Somerset built up the unit to a commanding position in Melbourne urology through appointments at other hospitals.[6] He himself had an appointment at the Repatriation Hospital and his assistants had appointments at suburban hospitals: Douglas Duffy at the Royal Women's and Box Hill; Ian Nunn at Footscray; Harold Story at the Austin; Peter Tuckfield at Preston and Northcote Community Hospital and Peter Bruce at Sandringham Hospital. Peter Bruce shared Somerset's fondness for a way of life very different from Harold Moore's:

> *Perhaps my happiest moments in the urology team at the RMH were spent with John Somerset duck shooting in the wetlands of Northern Victoria and Southern New South Wales. We were both very keen on this blood sport and explored the swamps near Benalla, Moulamein and Geelong. John had a vast knowledge of European royalty and in a most entertaining way was able to recount who slept with whom and who didn't.*[7]

Bowie Somerset learned his urology at St Peter's Hospital for Stone in London, continuing the tradition of British training begun by Tait. The next head of the unit, Douglas Duffy, had also trained in London, working for a while with Terrence Millin, but he went on to learn TUR in the United States. On returning to Melbourne, he began to build a large private practice, at its peak the biggest in Victoria. Duffy has been described as a very private person with exceptional technical skills and superlative judgement in patient selection, timing and technique. He was not always popular and it has been said of him that when he walked into a room the temperature fell by five degrees. Certainly he was a considerable contrast to Somerset 'whose pugnacious charm, ginger hair and chain smoking endeared him to many'. Douglas Duffy was head of the unit at the RMH from 1969 to 1977.[8]

In 1977, Ian Nunn took over as head of the unit and the atmosphere changed again. Nunn continued the tradition of British training, having worked with Sir Eric Riches at the Middlesex Hospital. On returning to Melbourne, he did research in paediatric urology

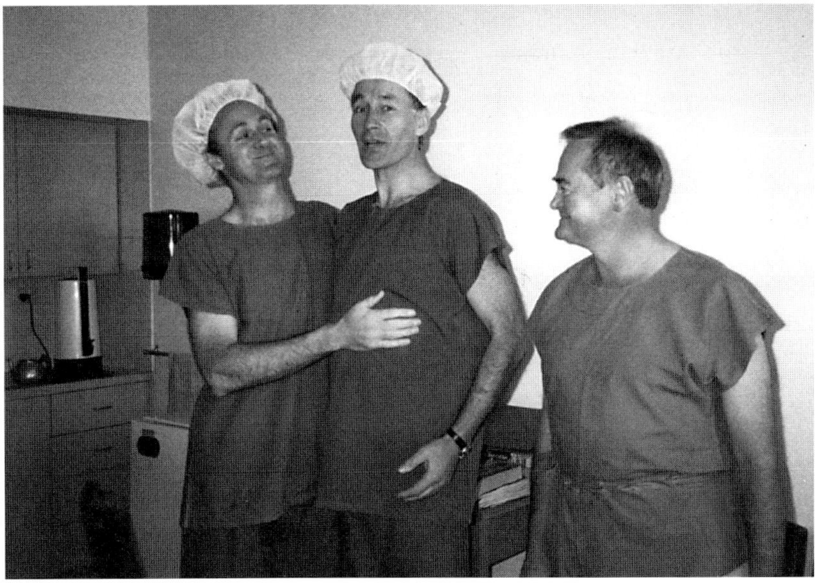

Laurence Cleeve, Joe Marich (anaesthetist) and Ian Nunn, Freemasons Hospital, Melbourne, 1987. (*Source:* Laurence Cleeve)

with Douglas Stephens at the Royal Children's Hospital. This taste of academic urology brought a new element to the RMH. Warren Johnson describes Ian Nunn as a conservative surgeon but with a flare for new techniques. With his colleague Professor Bill Hare, he performed the first percutaneous nephrolithotomy in Australia.

In 1987, Warren Johnson became head of the unit. He broke the tradition of British training at the RMH, having done a full three years training in urology at the Cleveland Clinic, Ohio. He returned to Melbourne in 1969 and became involved in the renal transplant program. This was set up by Professor Maurice Ewing, in conjunction with the Walter and Eliza Hall Institute which was working on problems of rejection. The first successful transplant was in 1965 and Bowie Somerset declined the offer to become involved in this first experimental phase.

From 1968, Vernon Marshall worked on setting up a Department of Surgical Metabolism for intensive care. Priscilla Kincaid-Smith was the nephrologist on the project and urologists began to take part—first Peter Bruce and then Warren Johnson. At a later stage Peter Lawson, Laurence Harewood and Alan Crosthwaite were also involved.

In 1996, Laurence Harewood succeeded Warren Johnson as head of the urology unit at the RMH. He began as a resident at the RMH in 1972. In 1971, when the RACS training scheme began, the RMH had a urology registrar, but it was not a RACS-approved position. This led to considerable competition between the RMH and St Vincent's, which did have an approved training post. Apart from the issues of prestige, there were substantial advantages to the unit in having an advanced trainee, providing considerably greater skills, for instance in diagnosis of emergency admissions, than could be expected of a junior resident.[9]

The RMH had an accredited training post from 1974, but a formalised program with rotation through other posts was not set up until 1983-84.

> *The unit has set itself very high standards and attracted the best people ... the last ten years has been a period of development from nineteenth century style to twentieth century style ... Warren Johnson was driving the change.*[10]

Despite its prominence, the urology unit at the RMH had a relatively small number of beds. In 1971, for instance, the unit had 12 beds, but two urologists, two assistant urologists and two associates. Over the years, many Melbourne urologists began their careers at the RMH and moved on to senior positions at other hospitals. Harold Story was the first of these, moving on to become head of the unit at the Austin Hospital. Peter Bruce moved to the Queen Victoria, and later to Shepparton; Rod Syme moved to the Austin; Ron Brown moved to the Alfred; Peter Lawson left for Box Hill; Don Moss went to Ballarat.

This spin-off of urologists to other hospitals, in conjunction with a continuation of the pattern of multiple public hospital appointments, helped maintain the RMH's influential position in Melbourne urology. Within the Urological Society, the RMH has also been influential. Laurence Cleeve was Chairman of ANZAUS during 1991-94 and all the heads of the unit, up to and including Warren Johnson, have been presidents of the Society. The only other Melbourne Hospital to rival this record is St Vincent's.

St Vincent's Hospital

At the end of World War II, St Vincent's had a capacity of about 320 beds, but there was considerable expansion during the 1950s, bringing it up to over 500 beds and the hospital had an important clinical school, opened in 1910. Hospital policy favoured the development of the specialties and a number of autonomous clinics were set up during the 1930s, including the urology unit, with 22 beds.

Henry Mortensen, the first urologist at St Vincent's, was the only Victorian to be President of the Urological Society more than once. He was a big man with a big personality and he had a major impact on urology in Victoria as a whole, not just at St Vincent's. However, not all his relationships with his peers were amicable. James Peters joined the St Vincent's clinic in 1948, but the two did not get on and Peters left for Prince Henry's Hospital. In 1949 Leonard Murphy, who had done his early training at St Vincent's, returned from his study tour on the Gordon Craig Travelling Scholarship. Initially, he got on well with the Mortensens, but in later years relationships became strained. Henry retired from St Vincent's in 1955 to devote more time to his private practice, and his son, generally known as Jim, joined Leonard Murphy at St Vincent's in the same year.

In the early years, Henry Mortensen had consulting rooms at 33

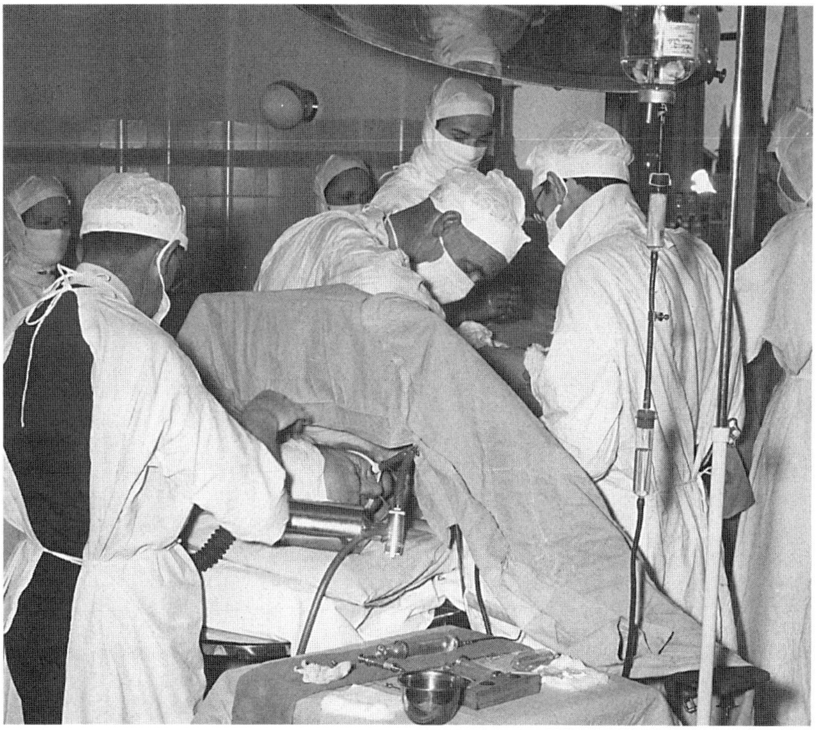

Dr John Catarinich (anaesthetist), W. Leadbetter (visiting American Urologist) and Dan Lenaghan operating, third floor theatre, St Vincent's Hospital, 1964. (*Source:* Christine Lenaghan)

Collins Street, but in the 1950s he moved to 254 Albert Street, a site that became known as the 'Palace of Urology'. At the time, it was quite novel to move from Collins Street and Harold Story relates that Mortensen was asked how his patients would get to him without a car, to which he replied that if they didn't have a car, he didn't want them as patients.[11]

In 1957, Dan Lenaghan joined Leonard Murphy and James Mortensen and between 1959 and 1961, Michael Salvaris was also attached to the hospital. Dan Lenaghan did his initial clinical training at St Vincent's before going to England for four years, where he worked at a number of hospitals, including St Paul's and the Bradford Royal Infirmary. On returning to Melbourne he was involved in research work at the Royal Children's Hospital with Douglas Stephens, besides his work at St Vincent's. The unit was very busy with long waiting lists and Leonard Murphy arranged additional operating lists on Saturday mornings. Dan Lenaghan remembered that era with some affection:

> *A feature of the Clinic since its establishment was the weekly ward round which, during L. Murphy's appointment, was carried out on Wednesday mornings and which all members of the Clinic attended. This custom of a formal round served as a unit meeting, enabled discussion on special problems encountered on the round, student teaching, and finally tea and fresh scones in the surgeons lounge. Everything, even the elegant plated containers on the examination tray so admired by M. Salvaris, seemed to stress the*

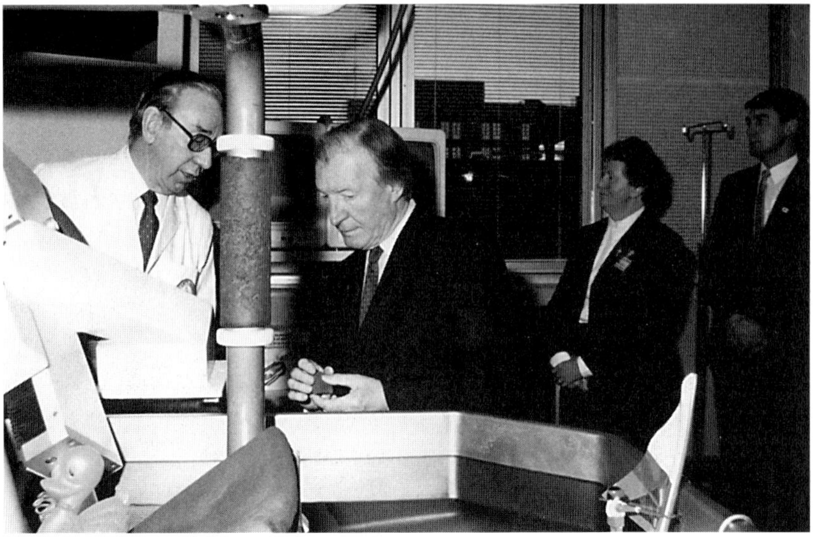

Dan Lenaghan, Charles Haughey (Prime Minister of the Republic of Ireland), Sister Anthea Groves (Sister Administrator), St Vincent's Hospital Lithotripsy Unit, 1988. (*Source:* Christine Lenaghan)

importance of the occasion. Not only the appearance of cafe-bars and disposable gloves but also the inexorable demands of time on the other members of the Clinic have long since put an end to this form of sociable and educational round.[12]

In 1966, Leonard Murphy retired from St Vincent's in unhappy circumstances. There were a number of contributing factors, including ill health and the pressure of work on his monumental *History of Urology*, which was published in 1972. Jim Mortensen succeeded him as head of the unit and relationships between the two families were strained at this time.

The *History of Urology* was very well received and Leonard Murphy continued in private practice for many years, besides following his interest in medical history. He was a member of the RACS archives and library committees and a sub-editor of the *Australia and New Zealand Journal of Surgery*. He was President of the Urological Society in 1958-59, made a Fellow in 1972 and awarded the RACS medal in 1987. His collection of books on medical history was purchased by the Urological Society and is housed at the College of Surgeons building on Spring Street.[13]

In 1963, the urology unit began a training program for urologists. Initially, the position was funded by Smith, Kline and French. Gerry Joyce was the first trainee and remembers that: 'Dan Lenaghan devoted a great deal of time and effort to my training and to each of the succeeding trainees. He remained friends with and kept in touch with all of them.'[14] Gerry Joyce did three years at St Vincent's and then went to Sydney for a final year with Joe Murnaghan before returning to the staff of St Vincent's.

In 1971, the unit had twenty beds and was by far the largest in Victoria, with a RACS-approved training post. Over the years, the unit trained a number of urologists from overseas, who returned to

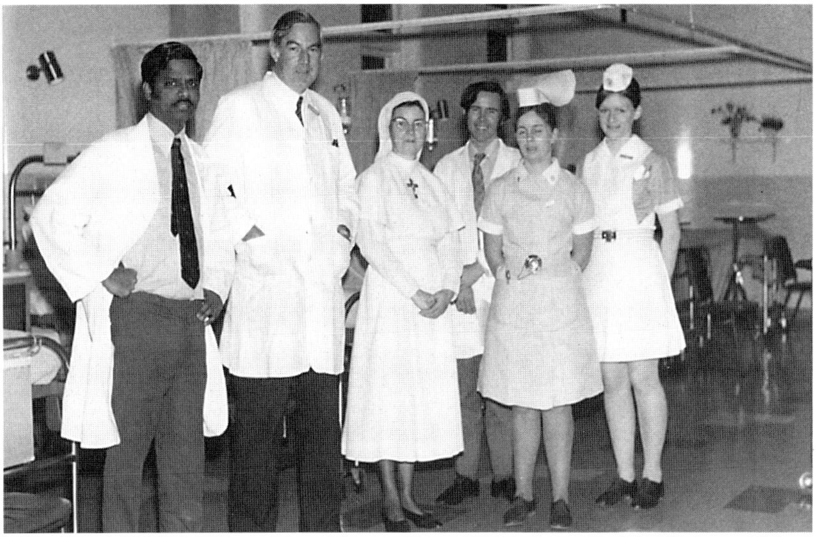

Ward round, St Vincent's Hospital, Melbourne, 1971. *Left to right:* N. Subbiah, P. J. Mortensen, Sister Justine, David Westmore, unknown

their countries of origin, plus several who joined the staff of St Vincent's, including Tony Costello, Justin Peters (son of Jim Peters) and Peter Mortensen (son of Jim Mortensen). The selection of trainees could cause problems, and Jim Mortensen resigned from his position as Chairman of the Victorian Training and Accreditation Committee when there was a disagreement about an appointment.

In 1988, Jim Mortensen retired as head of the unit and was succeeded by Dan Lenaghan, who remained as head for only two years before retiring. Meanwhile, Gerry Joyce had not been in the best of health and supported Tony Costello's application to become the next head of the unit. Tony Costello was a St Vincent's-trained urologist, but he also spent time in London with John Blandy and in Houston, where he worked with Doug Johnson of the Houston Cancer Institute, who was developing the use of lasers. When Tony Costello returned to St Vincent's he became the principal Australasian pioneer of the technique of laser surgery of the prostate. There was considerable publicity surrounding this new technology and he was a controversial figure for some years.[15]

St Vincent's has a strong tradition of involvement with the Urological Society and this is reflected in the number of presidents from the hospital. Besides Henry Mortensen and Leonard Murphy, Jim Mortensen was President 1968-69 and Dan Lenaghan in 1983-84.

The Alfred Hospital

The Alfred was Melbourne's second teaching hospital, the clinical school opening in 1880. Initially, it was purely a public hospital, but private and intermediate beds were opened in 1933. In 1963, there were 450 public beds and 90 private and intermediate beds.[16]

Compared with the Royal Melbourne and St Vincent's, the hos-

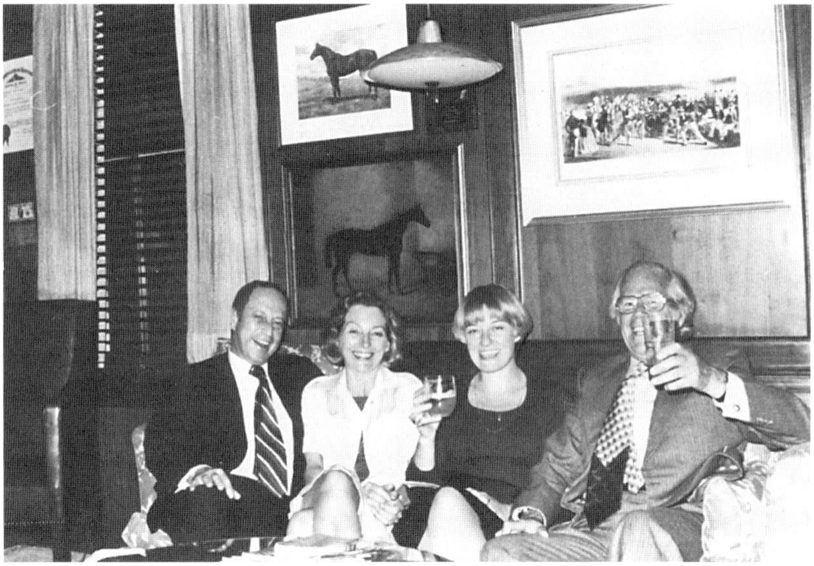

Left to right: Jim and Gale Glenn, and Beverley and Kennedy Burnside at the Glenns' home, Durham, North Carolina, 1977. (*Source:* Beverley Burnside)

pital was very late in setting up a urology unit. Kennedy Burnside was appointed as a general surgeon to the out patients department shortly after his return from Singapore, where he was a POW in Changi gaol. He developed a strong interest in urology and in 1955 toured England and the United States to see the urology units there. On his return, he submitted a detailed proposal for the formation of a urology unit, which the Board of Management accepted in 1956.[17]

Kennedy Burnside had already performed a considerable number of prostatectomies and adopted a rather unusual approach to TUR. He went to great pains to minimise the use of catheters. David Gunter, David Kennedy and Alex Wood have all written about the enormous impact of Kennedy Burnside on the unit at the Alfred. Of Burnside's technique, Gunter wrote:

> *To avoid infection, acute retentions were operated on prior to catheterisation. The admitting officers knew this and would admit anything up to five or six patients with acute retention on Ken Burnside's receiving day and most of them would have a TUR that night ... To avoid urethral stricture, Ken introduced post-operative management of TUR without an indwelling catheter ... The resident or the urological assistant would have to pass a Tieman catheter to empty the bladder whenever it filled.*[18]

David Gunter, who had trained as a general surgeon, was the first assistant urologist, joining the unit when it opened in 1956. He remembered the pathology conferences on Tuesday mornings, 'with a review of all the sections and specimens from the week's work, together with post-mortems.'[19] David Kennedy remembers these as twice weekly, after out patients. 'These meetings are still held today and are the most rewarding of all the activities of the Urology Unit.'[20] Kennedy Burnside also made a deep impression on Alex Wood:

Following X-ray and pathology conferences, ward rounds of all patients were made with great vigor of discussion. They were not for the faint hearted or frail bodied as Kennedy Burnside a fit lover of boating and fishing led his group rapidly, and often this would include up the stairs to the 8th floor which was the gynae ward. To be able to speak on arrival was a feat, but Sister Stalker filled the pauses most ably with a perceptive detailed summary of the patient's problem.[21]

The 1960s had a Fellow in Urology. Henry McCoy, Alex Wood, Alex Cass and Bill Straffon were among those to hold the position. In 1964, David Kennedy joined the unit as a fully trained urologist, having worked at St Paul's in London and with Roger Barnes, among others, in the United States.

Ken Burnside and David Gunter both retired in 1972, the latter to private practice. Ken Burnside was President of the Urological Society in 1973-74. Ron Brown from the Royal Melbourne Hospital was appointed as the new head of the unit. He persuaded the hospital to set up a full registrar position, and in 1975 Douglas Druitt was appointed as the first full-time Urology Registrar on the same basis as other training posts under the RACS-Urological Society training scheme.

Ron Brown was particularly interested in training and in 1986 followed John Maddern as Chairman of the Training and Accreditation Committee of the Urological Society. He was President of the Society in 1988-89 and resigned from his position at the Alfred in 1991, when David Kennedy took over as head of the unit.

Many of the assistant urologists associated with the Alfred moved on to suburban and country positions. Bill Straffon went to Prince Henry's, Alex Wood went to the Royal Melbourne and later the Southern Memorial and David Yoffa, who also had an appointment at Prince Henry's, went to Dandenong Hospital. Don Macdonald went to Gippsland Base Hospital in Traralgon. Alex Cato went to the Caulfield General Medical Centre but he and his colleague Gabriel Reisner were associated with the Alfred again when Caulfield became part of the same Regional Health Care Network.[22]

Prince Henry's Hospital

Prince Henry's began in 1869 as the Melbourne Homeopathic Dispensary at 153 Collins Street and in 1876, the Homeopathic Hospital began treating inpatients at the site on St Kilda Road. Over time, the hospital grew and more and more of the staff came from a conventional background in allopathic medicine. Balfour Wishart, the first urologist at the hospital, reflected this transitional stage. He came from a New Zealand family with a background in homeopathy but was himself conventionally trained. In 1935, the name was changed to Prince Henry's, to reflect the Royal visit and the change to a conventional hospital. By 1964, the hospital had 432 beds, 44 of them intermediate.[23]

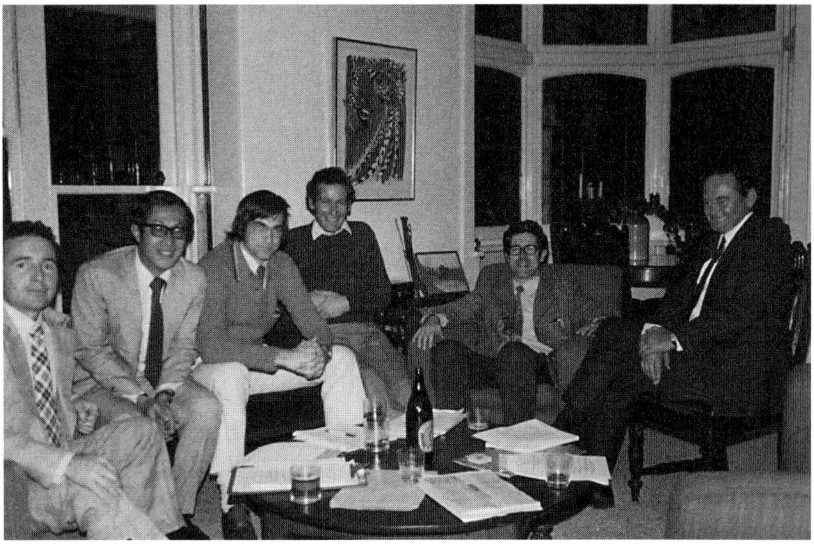

Urology Journal Club, Melbourne., 1975. *Left to right:* Laurence Harewood, Jimmy Beng (who went on to practise as a urologist in Singapore), David Young, Peter Lawson, John Wheelahan and Ian Nunn. (*Source:* Peter Lawson)

In 1948 there was a substantial turnover of staff. Bill Straffon describes it as a 'spill' designed to accommodate surgeons returning from military service. It would also have removed the last staff links with the homeopathic past. Balfour Wishart was replaced as urologist by John Bowie Somerset and his assistants were Jim Peters and I. J. Weyman. While Bowie Somerset was head of the unit, Prince Henry's became an undergraduate teaching hospital for the University of Melbourne. This was a period of expansion for Prince Henry's, but the Royal Melbourne Hospital had higher status and when Harold Moore retired, Somerset was appointed to replace him at the Royal Melbourne and resigned from Prince Henry's.

Jim Peters was head of the unit at Prince Henry's from 1954 to 1973 and the unit as it emerged was substantially his creation. He trained in Britain and America, including spending some time at the Mayo Clinic. Jim Peters has emphasised that in this era, established urologists were keen to encourage young surgeons to take up urology, and help them get a start in their careers. 'The people who started the Urological Society were very very fair to people who were back from training ... exchanged patients ... went out of their way to help them.'[24]

Not all of the next generation of urologists would agree with this, but for Prince Henry's, Bill Straffon substantially agrees with the man who was his boss for nearly ten years: 'Jim Peters ... did much to develop the unit and in particular was a great support and encouragement for younger urologists.'[25]

During the rest of the hospital's life, about fifteen other urologists spent some time at Prince Henry's. Two of the appointees—Alex Alder and Peter Tuckfield—died young. In 1965 Michael Salvaris became head of the unit at the Queen Victoria Hospital. Most of the others moved on to suburban hospitals. Robert Leggett went to Geelong. David Yoffa went to Dandenong. Joseph Sinha went to the western suburbs and David Ellis also spent an increasing amount of his time on his western suburbs practice. Gabriel Reisner shifted his focus east to a practice based around the Caulfield area and the south-eastern suburbs. James O'Collins, Jim Peter's brother-in-law, also attended at Frankston and Dandenong, but remained an Assistant Urologist at Prince Henry's until it closed.[26]

In 1965, Bill Straffon joined the team at Prince Henry's and remained to become head of unit when Jim Peters retired in 1973. He saw the unit through the turbulent years of the 1980s, when it was first amalgamated with the Queen Victoria, which in turn moved to the Clayton site as part of the Monash Medical Centre. From the early 1990s, the St Kilda Road site was the Monash Medical Centre, Prince Henry's campus, and the urology unit amalgamated with that on the Clayton campus. Bill Straffon had long had an association with the West Gippsland Hospital in Warragul and in 1994 he moved out to West Gippsland, returning to Melbourne weekly to his private practice.[27]

The Austin Hospital & Repatriation General Hospital, Heidelberg

The Austin only really became a general hospital in the 1960s. It began in 1882 as the Austin Hospital for Incurables, specialising in facilities for long-term patients, including those with tuberculosis, cancer and, from the 1930s, poliomyelitis. In 1939 an air-conditioned block was opened for private and intermediate patients and by 1948, the Austin Hospital, Heidelberg, had grown to 474 beds.

The major change came in 1959 when the hospital opened a casualty and out patient department and began to make beds available for general medical and surgical patients. However, the hospital retained a number of special units and the most important of these for the urology department were the Tuberculosis Unit and the Spinal Injuries Unit.[28]

The first urologist at the Austin was Bernays Melville, who had previously held an appointment at the Alfred. Harold Story believes Melville had spent some time at the Mayo Clinic and learned to use the cold punch for resection of the prostate. Harold Story joined him in 1957 from the Royal Melbourne Hospital. He had trained at St Peter's Hospital for Stone in the mainstream of British urology and believed that TUR was mainly suitable for smaller prostates. However, most of his work was connected to the Austin's special units.

> *In my early years the work of the Urologist was mainly related to the growing Spinal Unit. The Spinal Unit was started in about 1956, and its development received impetus with the visit of … Dr Ludwig Guttmann, in 1957 and the appointment of a Director in 1959. Much of the State's surgical tuberculosis was concentrated at the Austin as a consequence of the Commonwealth State financial agreement for the treatment of tuberculosis. The period 1957-1967 saw a rapid change in the character of the Austin Hospital with the aim of developing toward an acute general hospital.*[29]

Developments in the urology unit were also rapid. Melville retired in 1961 and Harold Story replaced him as head of the unit. Peter Tuckfield joined the unit that year but died in 1968 of heart disease. In 1965, the Austin became a teaching hospital for Melbourne University and in 1967 a Renal Unit was set up, to develop home dialysis. A transplant program began in 1974. Later developments included urodynamics from 1976, run by Stephen Clarke and percutaneous renal surgery from 1987. Harold Story retired in 1989 and was succeeded by Rod Syme.

Rod Syme was appointed to the Austin in 1968. He had worked at both the Royal Melbourne Hospital and St Vincent's and found the atmosphere at the Austin to be very different.

> *The atmosphere at the Austin was wonderful ... Harold Story allowed the people working with him to develop urologically. Harold kept a benign eye on things ... I do the same now. People grow under that kind of environment. It worked extremely well.*[30]

The Austin and the Repatriation General Hospital are relatively close to each other. Until the 1970s there was no unit as such at the Repat. but Jim Peters, Harold Story and Ian Nunn visited independently. As with other repatriation hospitals, there was a large volume of clinical material and Jim Peters organised a training post from about 1968. Michael Wong, David Ellis and Peter Lawson were the first three registrars at the Repat.[31] In 1971 Warren Johnson began at the Repat. as a locum and then became a junior consultant. He said he found the clinical experience mouthwatering and worked there half time. Over the next decade, the Austin and the Repat. came to have the same urologists.

When Harold Story retired in 1989, it was clear that a merger between the Austin and the Repatriation General Hospital was likely. The three urology staff at the Austin all had appointments at the Repat., so a joint unit was set up. Initially, Rod Syme was acting head while there was a lot of political manœuvring and he was appointed head of the unit in 1990. With the amalgamation of the two hospitals in 1995, the unit expanded and the urologists were Rod Syme, David Angus, John Rogerson, Michael Chamberlain and Stephen Clarke. In 1993 when Stephen Clarke moved to Newcastle, Damian Bolton joined the team.

Before amalgamation, there had been too much work for one registrar at the Repat. and not enough for one at the Austin. The merger allowed for two full training posts, giving the trainees experience in spinal injuries, transplants and the large volume of urodynamic work, plus the prostatectomies at the Repat.

The Queen Victoria Memorial Hospital & Monash Medical Centre

The hospital began in 1896 as a free out patients clinic for women and children. In 1897, it was named the Queen Victoria Memorial Hospital and a building in Little Lonsdale Street was acquired with the proceeds of a public appeal. From the beginning, the hospital was run by women for women. In 1946, the Queen Vic. moved to the buildings vacated by the Royal Melbourne Hospital, across Little Lonsdale Street from the State Library and the Museum of Victoria.[32]

Lorna Sisely joined the staff of the Queen Vic. in 1948. She was a general surgeon who did her initial training at St Vincent's Hospital before spending time in Britain and America on a Gordon Craig Travelling Fellowship. She remembered that it was very hard to find any female urology. She spent four months in England and then four months in America, including time working at Johns Hopkins with Houston Everett. The gynaecologists did the urology at Johns Hopkins and she was taught to perform air cystoscopy in the knee-chest position.[33]

Lorna Sisely was the first Victorian woman to become a FRACS and only the second Australasian woman. When she joined the staff of the Queen Vic., most of the other surgeons had an MS, but no fellowship and they began to send her most of the urological work. At that time, male surgeons were not acceptable to the Queen Vic. but Lorna Sisely persuaded Dame Mabel Brookes (President of the Hospital Board) to appoint Leonard Murphy as a consultant. He and Henry Mortensen proposed and seconded Miss Sisely for Associate Membership of the Urological Society and she duly became the first, and for many years the only, female member of the Society.

In 1963, in line with the other major changes in the hospital at that time, the Queen Vic. appointed its first male members of the medical staff, including an orthopaedic surgeon. In 1965, Michael Salvaris was appointed as Urologist and Lorna Sisely went back to general surgery, subsequently becoming a noted breast surgeon. Over the next decade or so, Ron Brown, Bill Straffon and Gabriel Reisner all spent brief periods assisting Michael Salvaris at the Queen Vic. His wife, Mary Irvine, was an anaesthetist there and her appointment predated his. In 1977, they retired to the Greek Islands and John Wheelahan took over Salvaris' private practice.

Peter Bruce, who had held an appointment at the Queen Vic. since 1975, succeeded Salvaris as head of the unit. In 1986, he moved to Shepparton and Richard Fletcher took over. By then, the Queen Victoria was on the move again, this time to a new 450-bed hospital at Clayton, the urology unit subsequently moving to Moorabbin in 1993. The amalgamation of the Queen Vic., Moorabbin Hospital and Prince Henry's produced the Monash Medical Centre and most of the old Queen Victoria/Royal Melbourne Hospital buildings were demolished.[34]

The Royal Children's Hospital

In 1876, the Royal Children's Hospital opened in Rathdowne Street, Carlton, in what had been the private house of a wealthy politician and businessman. By the 1950s, the hospital was bursting at the seams to accommodate 270 beds in far too little space and in

1957 work began on new buildings west of the Royal Melbourne Hospital. HM the Queen opened the new hospital on 25 February 1963.[35]

Before the 1950s, most urological procedures were performed by the general surgeons, including Harry Douglas Stephens, although first Thompson Tait and then Harold Moore from the Royal Melbourne Hospital acted as consultants. Harry Douglas Stephens' son, Frank, graduated MB BS in 1936 and seems to have been a resident at the Children's Hospital when war broke out. He returned from military service and then went to England for further study.

> *After the war, Ginger Burston arranged for thirty doctors who had served in the war to go to England as Nuffield Foundation Fellows. I was one of them ... went to England to study three things: congenital urethral obstruction; Hirschsprung's disease and portal hypertension.*[36]

Douglas Stephens spent three years at the Great Ormond Street Hospital for Sick Children, where he worked with Denis Browne, Twissington Higgins and the pathologist, Martin Bodian. He recalls that it was while working on autopsies with Martin Bodian that he was first inspired to study congenital abnormality, especially of the uro-genital tract. 'It's taken a lifetime to work it out.' He was eventually to publish four major books on the subject.

In 1950, Douglas Stephens returned to Melbourne to the position of Research Surgeon at the Royal Children's Hospital. In 1958, he became Director of the Department of Surgical Research. During this period, he made a considerable contribution to the Urological Society, especially at the Annual Meetings. Several times, when these were held in Melbourne, they included half a day at the Children's Hospital.

In 1962, the principal guest was Frank Hinman and the President was Jim Peters, a war buddy of Stephens'. The half day at the

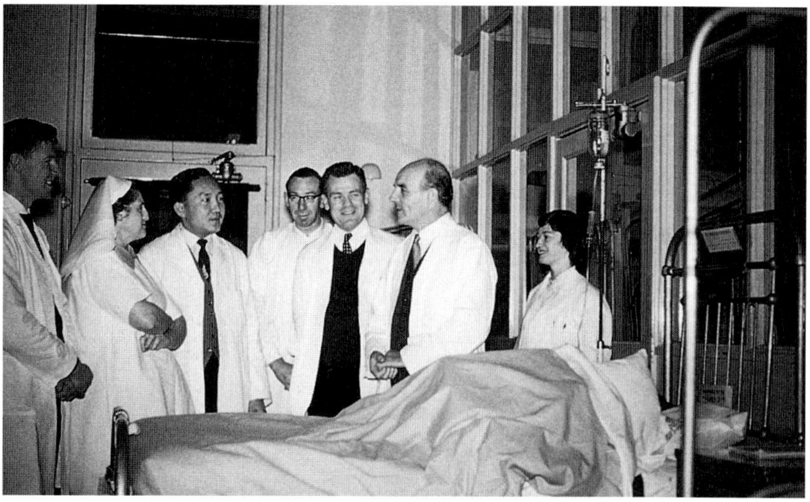

Robert Fowler, Kiti Tayakkavonta from Thailand, Dan Lenaghan and Douglas Stephens at the Royal Children's Hospital, July 1960. (*Source:* Kiti Tayakkavonta)

Children's Hospital was devoted to poster presentations held in a school hall opposite the hospital.

> *Each research worker would prepare this poster board, very large boards, very large print, very little information. These days they overdo the wording ... There was a table in the middle with a gong ... everybody was given ten minutes ... twelve to fifteen posters, chairs in front of each one ... when the gong sounded, you moved to the next. Each poster was manned. It was an innovation in those days. Then numbers got too big and they didn't ask me to do it any more. The international people thought the method was good and the content international standard ... Frank Hinman Jr was there and he went back to California and told them of the method we used.*[37]

The pattern which developed in Melbourne was for paediatric urology to be in the hands of paediatric surgeons, and this was in contrast to Sydney and Brisbane, where paediatric urology was largely in the hands of urologists. The system at the Royal Children's Hospital was made possible by the payment of surgeons. Paediatric surgery is not usually lucrative and so under the honorary system, surgeons often combined their paediatric work with adult surgery. The Children's was the first Melbourne hospital to end the honorary system and begin sessional payments. 'Once we were paid, we all specialised.'

This pattern meant that Melbourne's paediatric urologists were not eligible for full membership of the Urological Society and this caused problems in 1975 when Douglas Stephens went to Chicago as Professor of Urology and Surgery at the McGaw Medical Center. The Executive of the Urological Society wanted to make him a Fellow, but Associate Members were not eligible to become Fellows. Instead, they made him an Honorary Member, an honour normally reserved for distinguished overseas visitors. In 1986, he returned to Melbourne and was made a Fellow of the Urological Society in 1988.

There were a number of other notable paediatric urologists at the Children's, including Robert Fowler and Durham Smith, and later Justin Kelly, Alan Woodward, Hock Lim Tan and John Hutson.

Over the years, there was considerable discussion of the relationship between paediatric surgeons engaged in paediatric urology and urologists engaged in paediatric urology. In the early 1980s, each group produced a position paper on training requirements and they were unable to agree, although there was no rancour on either side. The issue was put on one side as too hard to resolve, but then in1986 a group including Alan Woodward as foundation Secretary-Treasurer met in Adelaide to found the Paediatric Urology Club. Members included Saeed Ahmed and Hilary Boucaut from Adelaide, Dennis Arnold, Bob Farnsworth and Ralph Cohen from Sydney and Alan Woodward, John Hutson and Robert Fowler from Melbourne. Since then, the Club has met annually, bringing together all those interested in paediatric urology in an amicable atmosphere.[38]

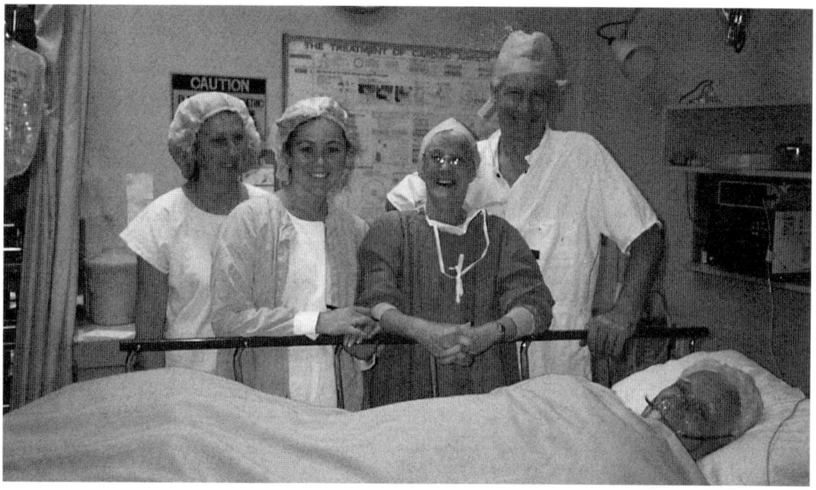

Left to right: Heather Hyden, Leanne Hindez, Dawn Giltinan (anaesthetist) and Peter Lawson after a TURP at Allendale Hospital, Melbourne, 1993. (*Source:* Peter Lawson)

Other Melbourne Hospitals

Mention has already been made of a number of Melbourne's suburban hospitals. Most are relatively new, opened since the 1940s to serve Melbourne's growing population. At least a dozen provide specialist urological services. Initially, these were generally provided by visiting urologists who also held inner city public hospital appointments, but since the 1970s, there has been an increasing trend for Melbourne urologists to move their practices to the suburbs.

One of the largest suburban public hospitals is Box Hill. Until the 1970s, the hospital had a Consultant Urologist, but he was rarely called. Jim Mortensen was the consultant during the 1960s, and in 1971, when he was proposing to retire, he complained about the situation to the Executive of the Urological Society, asking for their co-operation in trying to persuade the hospital to provide better urological services. At the time: 'The urology is almost entirely performed by the general surgeons. Consultations are rarely requested and are usually for elderly people in acute retention, presenting hopeless or near hopeless surgical risks.'[39]

In 1979 Peter Lawson was appointed as Urologist and in 1982 he invited Alan Crosthwaite to join him. By 1992 there were four urologists on the Box Hill team: Peter Lawson, Alan Crosthwaite, Geoffrey Wells and Ravi Asopa. Between them they made a substantial contribution to the Urological Society. Peter Lawson served as Chairman of the Victorian State Section and the Society's Honorary Archivist. Alan Crosthwaite was also on the Victorian Executive and from 1992 was Victoria's representative on the Federal Executive of the Urological Society and Chairman of the Therapeutic Devices and New Technologies Committee.

On the whole, the eastern suburbs were probably better served than the west. David Ellis was one of the few who practised in the western suburbs.

Ian Nunn had established a urological practice at the Western Hospital I think in the late 60's, as an extension of the Royal Melbourne Hospital practice. He was replaced by David Kennedy in the early 70's and when I commenced practice in Williamstown in 1972 ... David approached me and asked if I would also be prepared to come and help him at Western Hospital Footscray ... It has always proved difficult to get urologists to drive across the bridge into the West ... more recently Doug Travis ... has provided a service at both Werribee and Footscray. For a short time Tony Costello was also working at Werribee and Footscray ...

At Williamstown Jim Mortensen, from St Vincents Hospital had traditionally provided a urological practice and in the very early days, Dan Lenaghan had provided a urological service at Werribee. Jim was not very keen to operate at the Williamstown Hospital ... he would transfer the patients into St Vincents Hospital or the Mercy. When I arrived on the scene in 1972 prepared to consult in Williamstown and also operate in the local hospital ... then within six weeks I had every general practitioner in the Williamstown and Altona area, referring me all of their urology.[40]

Ballarat

The first urologist in Country Victoria was Ron Davidson at Ballarat. He trained at All Saints in London and set up practice in Ballarat in 1929. He was never a full-time urologist and therefore only an Associate Member of the Urological Society, but he was an active and valued member who regularly presented papers at the ASMs for many years. In 1956, he was joined by Ken Neerhut, who became a full member of the Urological Society in the late 1960s. Ken Neerhut retired in 1985. His son followed in his footsteps and from 1989 practised in Geelong.

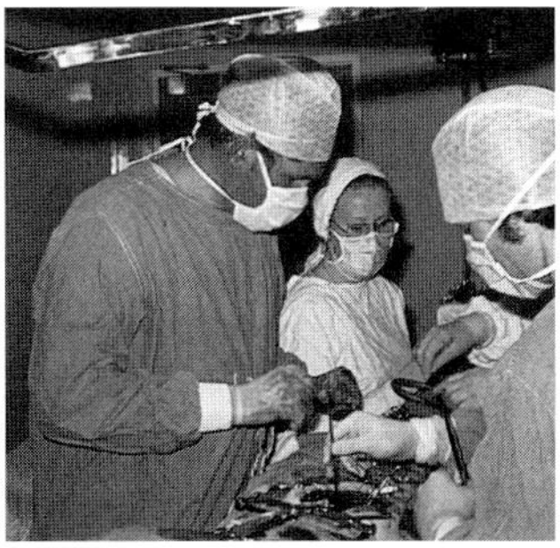

Ken Neerhut, 1982.
(*Source:* Don Moss)

In the mid-1970s Don Moss, who had done his initial training in Adelaide, joined the team at Ballarat. He did pioneering work on impotence in Ballarat. Don Moss also had a considerable involvement in training and from 1994 was Chairman of the Training, Accreditation and Education Committee of the Urological Society. In 1998 he joined the small, but growing, number of presidents of the Urological Society with practices outside the capital cities. In 1998, the other urologists in Ballarat were David Cook, Richard McMullin and Lachlan Dodds.[41]

Geelong

Bob Leggett was the first urologist in Geelong, moving there from Melbourne in 1964. In 1978 he was joined by Don Murphy and by 1989 Greg Neerhut had joined them, plus Karl Breslis from 1995. The Geelong practice covered the area between Geelong and Portland.

Bendigo

Urology in Bendigo was a family affair. Ian Gordon, who initially ran a urology service in Mildura, began practising in Bendigo in 1961, becoming a full member of the Urological Society in 1979. When he arrived in Mildura in 1958 he found:

> *There were a dozen or so old chaps with suprapubic tubes draining into Winchester bottles at the bed side with a few millilitres of formaldehyde in the bottom to compensate for the ammoniacal smell produced by the Proteus organisms. I believe that a few Freyer's operations had been done but no-one had progressed as far as the Harris or Millins procedures and when I said I'd be doing some T.U.R.P.'s and other Urological procedures I might as well have said I was going to hop aboard one of the Sputniks which nightly passed overhead in the clear Mildura skies...*
>
> *Things were not a whole lot better when I arrived in Bendigo on 1st January 1961 ... When the Hopkins lens and the continuous irrigation instruments and fibreoptic illumination became available, urology became a breeze.*[42]

Ian Gordon retired in 1989 and his son Neil took over the practice.

Albury–Wodonga

The first full time urologist in Albury was John Russell. He had trained with William Boyce in North Carolina and set up practice in Albury–Wodonga in 1981. Robert MacGregor, who had trained with Jack Lapides at Ann Arbor, Michigan, joined him in 1983.

The Border Urology Clinic draws its patients from both sides of the border, but the urologists in Albury–Wodonga have tended to play a more active role in the Victorian Section of the Society, rather than looking to New South Wales.

Henry Duncan joined the team in 1992.

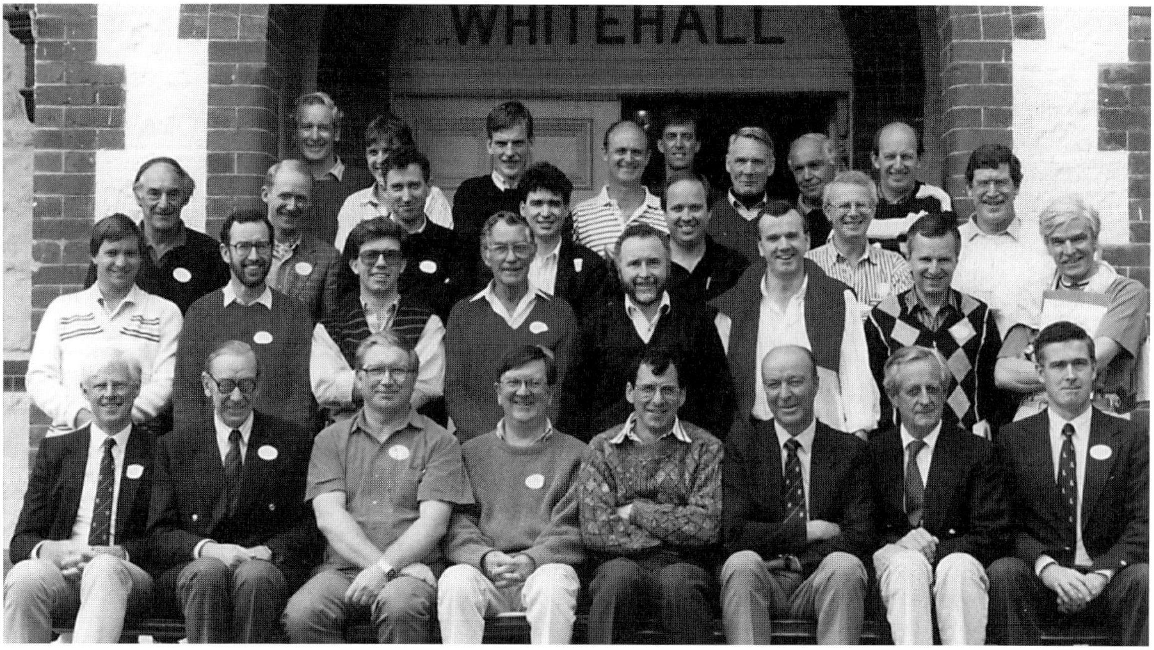

Victorian State Section Meeting, White Hall, Sorrento, October 1989. *Back row:* Peter Lawson, Geoff Wells, David Angus, Laurie Cleeve, Peter Royce, David Gunter, Jim O'Collins, Don Moss. *Second row:* David Yoffa, Richard Fletcher, David Cook, Jeremy Goad, Michael Chamberlain, Ross Snow, Tony Costello. *Third row:* Doug Travis, Alan Crosthwaite, Chris Love, Bob Leggatt, Laurence Harewood, Justin Peters, Gabby Reisner, Rod Syme. *Front row:* Alex Wood, Dan Lenaghan, Bill Straffon, Warren Johnson, Geof Hirst, Ron Brown, David Kennedy, John Wheelahan.

Other Country Centres

The only other country centres to have urologists based there were Hamilton, where S. G. Fitzpatrick practised in the 1950s and 1960s, Traralgon, where Don Macdonald is based and Shepparton where Peter Bruce moved in 1986. Many other centres, however, have been visited on a regular basis. In 1996, the report 'The Urology Workforce in Australia' listed fifteen Victorian country towns visited at least monthly, mainly by Melbourne-based urologists. However, country urologists also visited other centres. Greg Neerhut, for instance, visited Colac and Portland from Geelong and Richard McMullin visited Horsham and Castlemaine from Ballarat.[43]

The Victorian Section of the Urological Society

The first meeting of the Victorian Section of the Urological Society was on 21 October 1958 and Leonard Murphy was the first Chairman. However, there was a considerable period during the 1960s when the section did not meet on a regular basis. In July 1970, fourteen Victorian members of the Urological Society met at the Alfred Hospital to hear the Chairman of the Victorian Branch of the Otolaryngological Society propose joint action by surgeons over fees. Kennedy Burnside arranged a meeting a month later to discuss this proposal and consider 'The desirability of re-establishing the Victorian branch of the Urological Society of Australasia as an active body'. Of the thirty-two Victorian members of the Urological Society, only six turned up and the meeting was abandoned. The Victorian Section was, however, revived in the 1970s by Ron Brown and Warren Johnson. Gerry Joyce remembered the change:

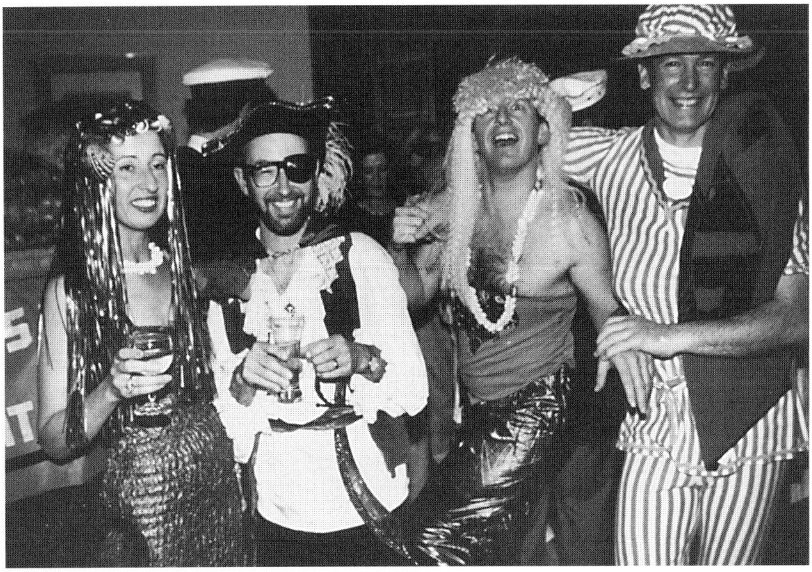

The Victorian Section meeting at Sorrento, October 1989, had a nautical theme. *Left to right:* Rosemary Crosthwaite, Alan Crosthwaite, Don Moss, Peter Lawson. (*Source:* Gwen Pearson)

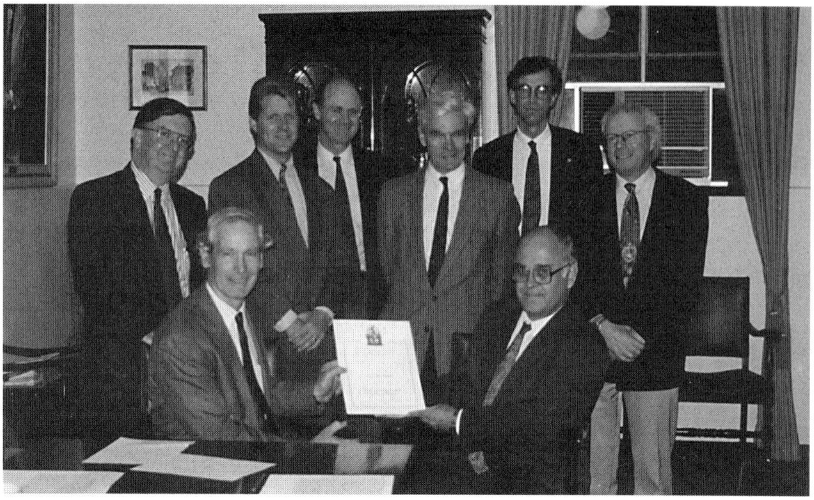

Presentation of a certificate of appreciation from the Victorian Section to ICI, 1994. *Left to right:* Warren Johnson, Daniel Walsh (ICI), Laurie Cleeve, Rodney Syme, Peter Royce, Ross Snow; *seated:* Peter Lawson, Dr Howard Smith (ICI)

I attended my first meeting of the Urological Society in 1959 ... you couldn't crank up a Victorian State meeting ... Warren Johnson and Ron Brown reactivated the Victorian State Section at the ... beginning of the 1970s ... we started to have some good meetings ... the relationships were very good, but the old fellows, none of them got on well. But after Ron Brown and Warren Johnson [started to run meetings] it became very popular. People liked getting together, got along very well.[44]

By the 1980s, there was a regular program of events, including an Annual General Meeting and an Annual Country Meeting. These were great social events. At the 1983 meeting, for instance, held at Erskine House, Lorne, there were twenty-eight urologists, twenty-two wives and twenty children. Fancy dress parties became popular, but serious scientific business was not neglected. During 1983 alone, the Victorian Section managed to arrange lectures by Professors Darracott Vaughan, John Blandy, Pavone Maculoso and Paul Lange, plus a pyelogram clinic with the Texan Urology group.[45]

CHAPTER 12

Urology in Western Australia

~

Introduction

Western Australia is by far the largest State in Australia, covering almost one-third of the total area, but it is very sparsely populated and large areas are more or less uninhabited. Most Western Australians live in the Perth area, and this concentration has increased over time, passing 70 per cent of the State's population by the 1976 census. Despite this and the rapid growth since the 1950s (the population of Perth more than doubled between 1954 and 1976), Perth remains a relatively small city. In the mid-1990s, the total population of Western Australia was about 1.8 million and 1.3 million, or about 72 per cent, lived in the Perth metropolitan area.

There are few towns of any size outside the Perth area. The gold-mining town of Kalgoorlie is the largest, followed by Bunbury, Geraldton and Albany, all of which are sea ports.

In 1957, there were four main public hospitals in Perth—the Royal Perth Hospital, Fremantle Hospital, Princess Margaret Hospital for Children and the King Edward Memorial Hospital for Women, plus the Commonwealth-funded Repatriation General Hospital and the directly State-run Perth Chest Hospital. In the mid-1960s, this last became the Sir Charles Gairdner Hospital. Overall the city suffered from a shortage of beds and nursing staff and the State Government was embarking on a major program to train nurses. In 1957, there were only 309 honorary and 107 salaried medical staff, an indication of the small size of Perth compared with the eastern State capitals.

The 1960s were a period of considerable growth in the Western Australian hospital system, with the opening of a new medical school and the Sir Charles Gairdner Hospital. This growth continued into the 1970s and growth in the number of urologists was particularly rapid in the early 1970s. In 1971 there were only four full members of the Urological Society in Perth, plus two associate members. By 1976, this number had more than doubled to six full members, plus seven associates.

The pioneering phase of Perth urology ended in 1969 with the formation of a joint urology unit between the Royal Perth Hospital and Sir Charles Gairdner Hospital and the beginnings of provision for training.[1] The first official trainee was Tony Low, appointed in 1970.

Urology in Perth before 1969

Of the first five urologists in Western Australia, three did their initial training in Melbourne, one in Adelaide and one in England. Of these the first to be trained in endoscopic work were Stan Watson, in Cardiff, and Ernie England, in the United States. These men were the first two Western Australian Presidents of the Urological Society.

Eric Kyle and Ralph Cato preceded them in urological appointments at the Royal Perth Hospital. They were both more or less self-trained urologists. Gwynne Brockis was very different, an Englishman and the first academic urologist in Perth. However, for many years he held appointments in general surgery which placed him in a slightly awkward position in relation to the other urologists. Perth is a relatively small city and the urologists were able to remain a more or less coherent group, whatever their differences. They all held appointments at the Royal Perth Hospital, plus appointments at one or more of Fremantle, the Perth Chest Hospital/Sir Charles Gairdner and the Repatriation General Hospital, Hollywood.

ERIC KYLE

The first full member of the Urological Society in Perth was Eric Kyle. He became an associate member in 1949, a full member in 1957 and was made a Fellow in 1977. He was a Melbourne graduate who went to Britain for his FRCSEd in 1931. He was appointed to the Royal Perth Hospital when the Urological Unit was established in the late 1940s. In 1949, Norman Robinson, who also held an appointment to the Urological Unit, was appointed Senior General Surgeon. Eric Kyle became the Urological Surgeon and remained the senior urologist at the RPH until his retirement in 1961. He also held an appointment at the Repatriation General Hospital, from which he retired in 1965.

Despite the apparently early date of the Urology Unit at the RPH, there were no direct referral rights until 1974. 'At the biggest teaching hospital, the Royal Perth Hospital, urological cases are referred in the first place to the general surgeon, who refers in turn to a urologist as he sees fit.'[2]

Ralph Cato

Ralph Cato was another Melbourne graduate, but in 1933 he moved to Perth to a position as RMO at the Royal Perth Hospital. He then spent a number of years in outback Western Australia as a flying doctor. He was himself a keen pilot and although he obtained his FRCSEd in 1937, he then went on to a career in the RAF, rising to the rank of Squadron Leader. After the war, he returned to Perth as a GP and it was not until 1949, when he was over forty, that he turned to surgery on a full-time basis. In 1953 he was appointed assistant urological surgeon and from then until his retirement he was associated with the Urology Unit at the RPH, taking over as senior when Kyle retired. He also held an appointment at the Fremantle Hospital. He became an associate member of the Urological Society in 1956 and a full member in 1964.[3]

Stan Watson

Stan Watson was the third Melbourne graduate in the Urology Unit at the RPH. He went on to obtain his FRCSEng in 1951 and was Urological Registrar in Cardiff in 1955-56. He returned to Australia and was appointed Honorary Clinical Assistant Urologist at the RPH, eventually succeeding Ralph Cato as the senior urologist there. In 1962, he was the first urologist appointed to the Sir Charles Gairdner Hospital. He also held an appointment at the Repatriation General Hospital and in 1969 he shifted his focus from the RPH to work in the joint unit at those two hospitals, becoming full-time in this position from 1979 until his retirement in 1989.

He was the first urologist in Western Australia with any endoscopic training and marked the beginning of the establishment of the specialty as an area that general surgeons could not enter at will. This increase in the status of the specialty was given considerable impetus by the development of fibreoptic systems. Patients treated by urologists using the new technology were suddenly seen to be doing much better than patients treated by open surgery. Stan Watson was in private practice with Eric Kyle. Later, they were joined by Ernie England in what became a notable example of a group practice. At its peak there were seven urologists involved but by the 1990s, the number had fallen to four. In 1976-77, Stan Watson was the first Western Australian President of the Urological Society.[4]

Ernie England

Although a Western Australian, Ernie England did his initial clinical training in Adelaide, graduating in 1954. He returned to the Royal Perth Hospital to the position of RMO, working his way up to registrar in general surgery. He obtained his English and Australasian Fellowships in 1958. In 1960, he was Clinical Assistant Surgeon to

Ralph Cato at Fremantle Hospital (both were general surgical appointments). He then spent some time gaining urological experience in the United States and returned to Perth in 1963. At that time, there were three positions in the Urology Unit at the Royal Perth Hospital: Urologist (Ralph Cato); Assistant Urologist (Stan Watson) and Ernie England was appointed as Clinical Assistant Urologist. He maintained an association with the RPH until his retirement in 1990, becoming chairman of the department in 1979. He also returned to the Fremantle Hospital and was the senior urologist there and in the early years also held appointments at the Repatriation General Hospital and Sir Charles Gairdner. It was he who, along with Stan Watson, 'shamed the part timers to stop doing urology'. In 1985-86, he was the second Western Australian President of the Urological Society and in 1994, he was made a Fellow.

The Spinal Cord Injury Department

In 1954, a Spinal Cord Injury Department was set up at the Rehabilitation Hospital, Shenton Park. Three of the four early urologists were involved with this unit, Eric Kyle in 1954-61, Stan Watson in 1961-63 and Ernie England from his return from the United States in 1963. The project was particularly dear to Ernie England's heart. As a Registrar in 1954 he had been involved with the initial establishment of the unit. Over the years, it developed a world class reputation, including for the urological side of the work, and was something of a model for the later and also outstanding unit in Christchurch.[5]

Gwynne Brockis

Gwynne Brockis was born in England. He obtained his FRCSEng in 1949 and did his initial urological training as Registrar to Professor Leslie Pyrah in Leeds. Subsequently he worked in a number of other English urological units, including at St Peter's Hospital for Stone, and developed an interest in academic surgery, particularly academic urology. In 1958, he was appointed as Reader in Surgery in Perth at the new medical school. In 1961, he went to Boston on a Carnegie Travelling Fellowship and became interested in the pioneering transplant work there. On returning to Perth, he carried out research in kidney transplantation, performing the first successful renal transplant at the RPH in 1967. At this time, his appointments to Perth's hospitals, both the RPH and the Repat., were as a general surgeon, but in 1969 he was appointed as a urologist at the Royal Perth Hospital and joined Stan Watson and Ernie England in the new joint unit that had just been set up with the Sir Charles Gairdner Hospital.

During the 1970s, most of Gwynne Brockis' research was concerned with the aetiology of kidney stones, including a project run in conjunction with Sumatra, Indonesia, on changes in diet to prevent kidney stones in children. Most of the members of Perth's new

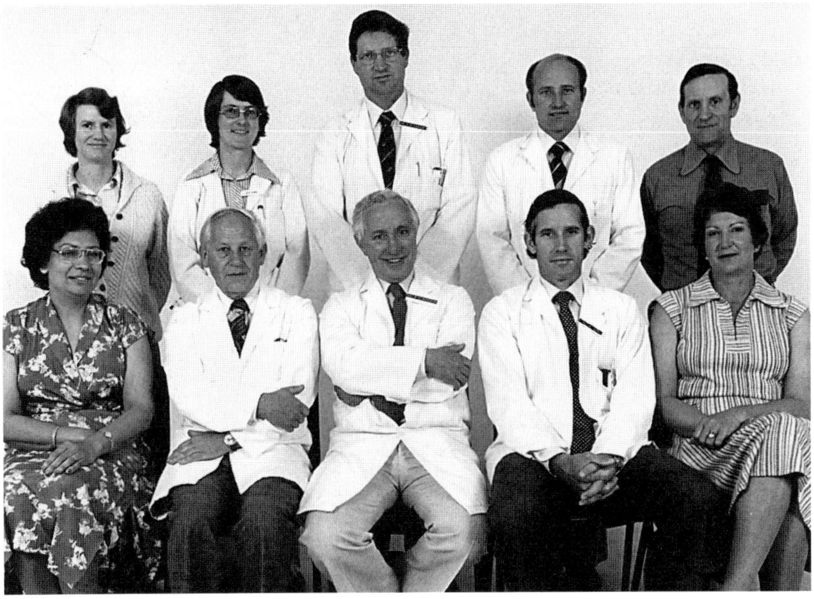

Royal Perth Hospital Urology Department, 1980. *Back row, left to right:* Jill Sturcke (cystoscopy theatre head nurse), Helen Stokes (resident), Tony Taylor (clinical assistant), Stan Wisniewski (registrar) and Charles Tong (cystoscopy theatre organiser). *Front row:* Daphne Coehlo (secretary), Gwynne Brockis, Ernie England (head of unit), Tony Low and Shirley Zazula (typist). (*Source:* Royal Perth Hospital)

generation of young urologists worked with him at one stage or another, including Tony Low, Tony Taylor, Stan Wisniewski and Pat Bary. In August 1979 he convened the first International Conference on Stone Disease in Perth and in 1983 he was involved in the introduction to Perth of percutaneous ultrasonic stone disintegration. He retired in 1984. Because his university work long involved some general surgery, he did not become a full member of the Urological Society until 1979.[6]

General Surgeons with an Interest in Urology

Throughout this period, Phillip Goatcher was an associate member of the Urological Society. Don Fleming spent some time with Terrence Millin in London and in the 1960s he joined Goatcher as an associate member of the Society. Both had general surgical appointments at the Royal Perth Hospital, but were interested in urology. Fleming actually held a position as a urologist at the King Edward Memorial Hospital for Women, but he was assistant surgeon at the Princess Margaret Hospital for Children. He was active in College affairs and a member of the Council of the RACS from 1969 to 1981.[7]

Urology in Perth Since 1969

There were three main stages in the history of the urology unit at the Royal Perth Hospital. Up to 1969, there were three urologists, but only a small number of beds and no direct referral rights. Between 1969 and 1974 a joint unit between the RPH and the Sir Charles Gairdner made possible the provision of a training position.

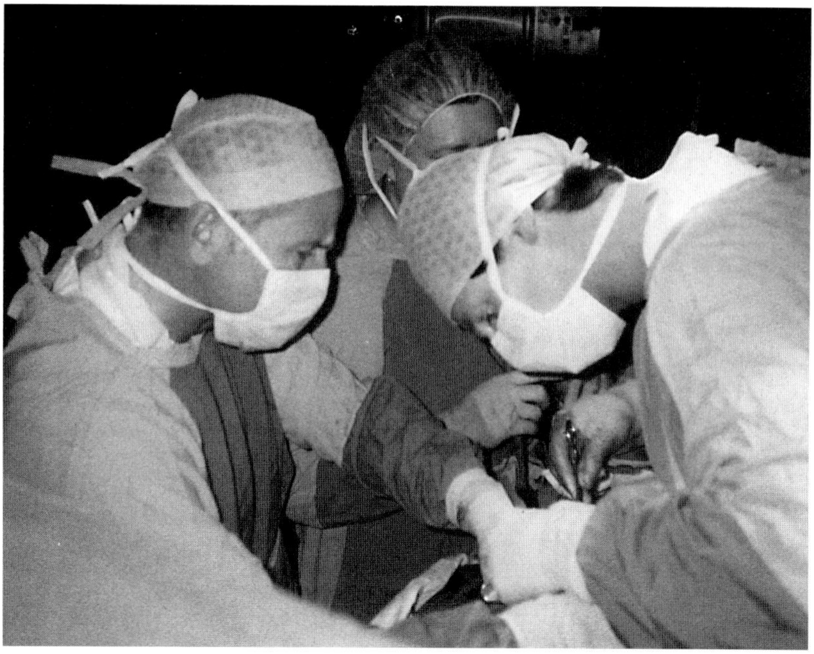

Stan Wisniewski and John Stanley operating in about 1989. (*Source:* Stan Wisniewski)

In 1971, the RPH unit had fourteen beds, the Sir Charles Gairdner unit twenty-four, and the adjacent Repatriation Hospital twenty. The Registrar in the RACS-approved position was Tony Low and he gained his FRACS in Urology in 1972. He then spent time in further training overseas and returned to the RPH in 1974. In 1996-97, Tony Low was the third Western Australian President of the Urological Society. Alastair Tulloch, son of Selby Tulloch, a well-known Edinburgh urologist, and Brian McGregor from New South Wales, followed him through the training position and both were subsequently appointed to the Sir Charles Gairdner.[8] Brian McGregor was a particularly active member of the Society and Chairman of ANZAUS in 1994-96.

The third stage of the unit at the RPH began in 1974. Both hospitals were expanding and the units separated, with the unit at the Royal Perth Hospital enjoying direct referral rights for the first time. Stan Watson remained the senior urologist until 1979, when Ernie England succeeded him and Tony Taylor joined the team in 1980. Pat Bary from New Zealand was appointed in 1984 when Gwynne Brockis retired and Paul McRae was appointed in 1988.

Meanwhile, the unit at the Sir Charles Gairdner Hospital continued to grow. A joint service was provided with the Repatriation Hospital on its adjacent campus and between them they provided a large volume of clinical experience for the registrars, who included Stan Wisniewski. In 1984, the training position was fully approved as a part of the Society's accredited training scheme. In 1983, Alastair Tulloch left the unit for New Zealand and Stan Wisniewski was appointed in his place.

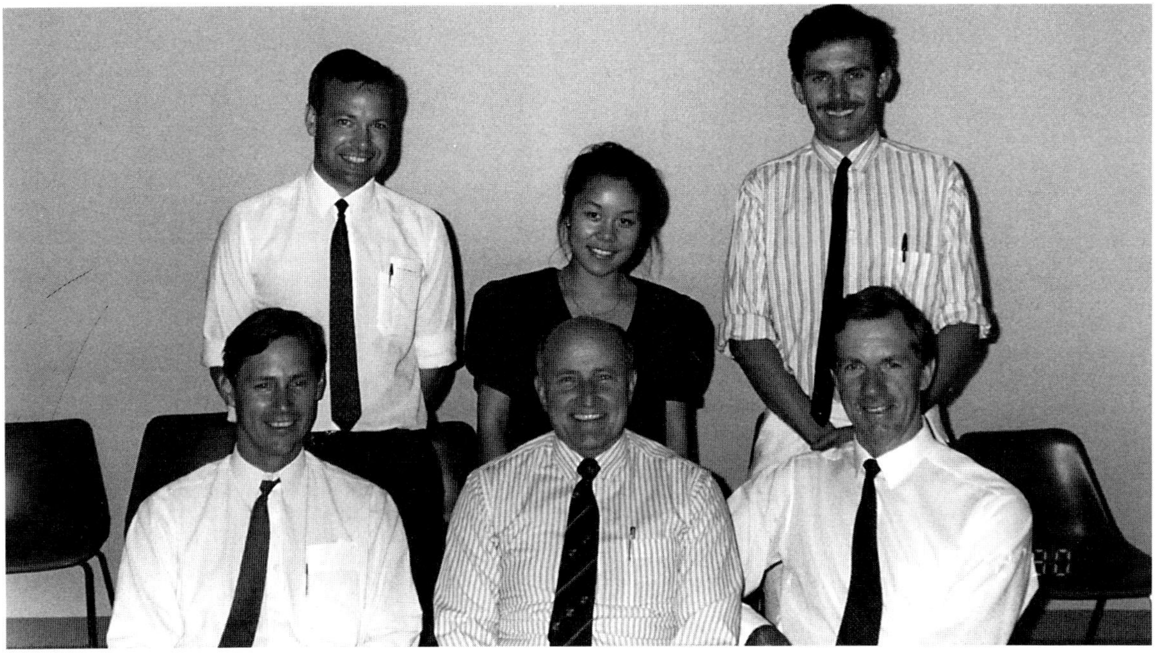

Sir Charles Gairdner Hospital Urology Unit, 1992 *Back row, left to right:* Robert Flynn (service registrar), resident, and Richard McMullin (registrar). *Front row:* John Stanley, Stan Wisniewski (head of unit) and Ian Hill. (*Source:* Stan Wisniewski)

Despite the small number of urologists in Western Australia, they managed to provide a comprehensive range of urological services. Besides the specialised work of the spinal unit, the first penile implant in Australia was performed in Perth by Alastair Tulloch, and from the 1980s reconstructive surgery was also available. In addition, Western Australia was something of a pioneer in group practice, Ernie England setting up what was one of the few genuine partnerships. The first professor of urology in Australasia was in Western Australia. During the early 1990s, funding for the position was raised by public appeal and the concerted efforts of many, especially Alastair Tulloch and Sid Corser, who was Chairman of the Perth Urological Research Centre campaign. In 1993, Keith Kaye was appointed as Professor of Urology. He advocated population screening for prostate cancer. This policy was controversial within the Urological Society and debate on the issue continued for some years.

From the 1980s, Perth had a third training position at Fremantle Hospital. Although the population per urologist ratios remained higher than elsewhere in Australia and comparable to those in New Zealand, the supply of urologists did begin to improve.[9]

Country Western Australia

Apart from John Swinney, an English urologist who practised in Bunbury during the 1970s, there were no urologists based outside Perth. However, there was a well developed system of visiting outback towns and during the 1990s, urological services were provided to all the towns of any size. Stan Wisniewski, for instance, spent four

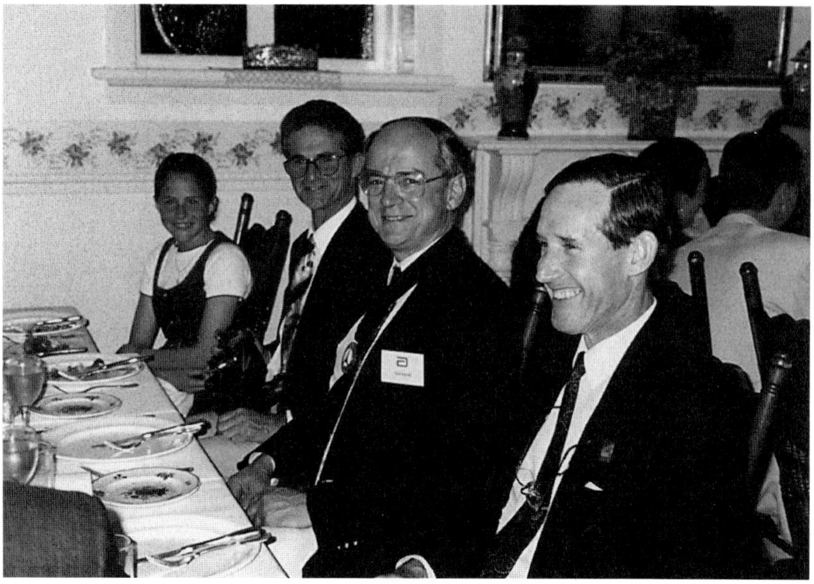

Busselton, October 1994, WA State Section Meeting. *From right to left:* Tony Low, Ted Arnold, Keith Kaye and Maxine Joscelin Kaye. (*Source:* Stan Wisniewski)

days a month in Albany, consulting and operating in the local public hospital. Less than 5 per cent of patients had to be flown to Perth for more specialised treatment and there was enormous community support for this kind of service. When John Swinney returned to England in the late 1970s, Ernie England began providing a visiting service to Bunbury. He was succeeded by Brian McGregor and Paul McRae. Brian McGregor also provided a similar service to Kalgoorlie, Tony Taylor to Geraldton, Tony Low to Northam and Alastair Tulloch (after his return from New Zealand) to Mandurah and Busselton.[10]

The Western Australian Section of the Urological Society

As might be expected, given the small numbers involved, the Western Australian State section was relatively late in beginning to meet regularly. However, geographical isolation has advantages as well as disadvantages and Perth urologists have always been a relatively cohesive group. As Tony Low and Tony Taylor put it:

> *We've managed to not let the obvious differences between us become a running sore ... it would be very destructive in Perth ... so ... we worked on pacifist principles ... we all trained through the same three hospitals ... we've all grown up with each other.*

The Western Australians have always been strong supporters of the Urological Society. Eric Kyle began trying to persuade the Executive to hold a meeting in Perth almost as soon as he became a member. He failed, but the pressure helped bring about the first meeting in the

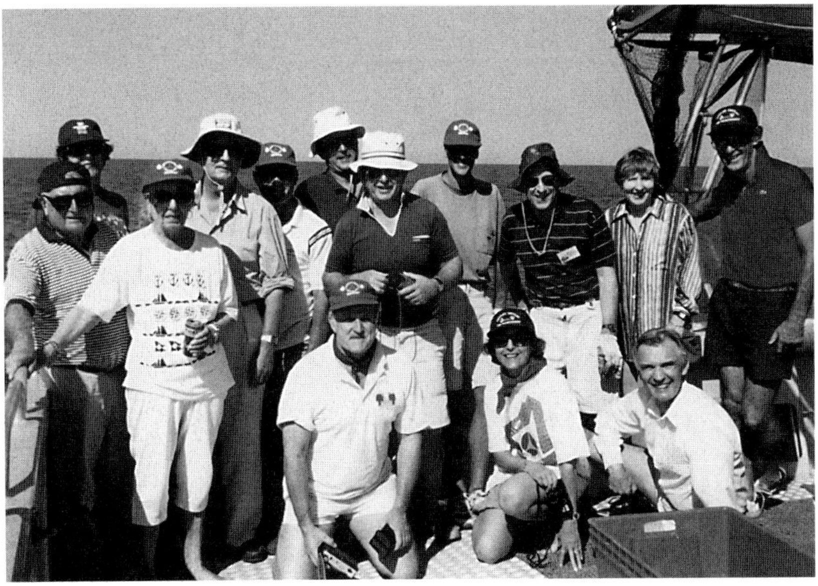

Fishing trip, in conjunction with the Broome ASM, June 1994. *From left to right standing:* Michael Rosen, Nina Saalfeld, Joan Rosen, David Kennedy, John Saalfeld, Professor Holmtag, Bob Wines, Mark Fraundorfer, Helmut Madersbacher, Chirsty Hendry, John Taylor. *Kneeling:* Stan Wisniewski, Melli Madersbacher, Bill Hendry. (*Source:* Stan Wisniewski)

other remote area—New Zealand—and State representation on the Executive. Over the years, Stan Watson, then Ernie England, John Taylor, Brian McGregor, Tony Low and Tony Taylor have represented Western Australia on the Executive.

The reduced costs and increased speed of air travel were the factors which helped break down the isolation. 'Robert Menzies used to say we were three years behind the rest of Australia. Now we are three hours behind.' During the 1970s, the new generation of Western Australian urologists began to attend the ASMs on a regular basis, but it was still difficult to persuade international guests to go to Perth.

Meanwhile, the urologists began running a monthly journal club. Like so many of the State-based activities, in Western Australia as elsewhere, the focus was on the trainees. Initially, the journal club met in people's homes, but from 1994 it began meeting in the university department where Keith Kaye was based. Annual State meetings began in 1982 and were generally held in an attractive country venue. The 1984 gathering, for instance, was in Bunbury, at the Lighthouse Motel and the 1988 meeting was held at the Rottnest Island Resort Lodge. Guests included Ron Brown, Frank Gardiner and Warren Johnson from Australia and John Nacey from New Zealand, plus Anne Jequier from Britain.[11]

NOTES

~

CHAPTER 1

1 Sir Henry Simpson Newland, 'The Archibald Watson Memorial Lecture', the *Medical Journal of Australia*, vol. II, no. 13, 27 September 1947; Julian Orm Smith, *The Archibald Watson Memorial Lecture;* also *Stones, Diamonds, Coronets, Kings and their Surgical Custodians,* Thomas Peel Dunhill, Melbourne, 1967; R. G. Elmslie, 'The Archibald Watson Memorial Lecture: Our honoured anatomists', *Australia and New Zealand Journal of Surgery,* 51, 1981; Dr Earle Hackett, 'The Body Programme: Archibald Watson', ABC radio broadcast, June 1984; Owen H. Wangensteen and Sarah D. Wangensteen, *The Rise of Surgery,* Minnesota, 1978.

For the early development of anaesthesia in Australia see Gwen Wilson, *One Grand Chain: The History of Anaesthesia in Australia 1846-1962,* vol. 1, 1846-1934, Australian and New Zealand College of Anaesthetists, Melbourne, 1995.

There have been a number of articles on the introduction of 'Listerism' to Australia, see for instance, David M. O'Sullivan's masterly article, 'The introduction of antiseptic surgery to Australia' in *Medical Journal of Australia,* 1967, vol. 2, pp. 896-901. In 1989 three papers on Listerism were presented to the First National Conference of the Australian Society of the History of Medicine: Julius S. Rocca, 'The introduction of Listerism to New South Wales'; John C. Murray, 'Thomas Fiaschi and Listerian Antisepsis in Sydney 1880-1900'; and Susan Hardy, 'A note on the historiographical significance of the correspondence on "Listerism" in New South Wales, 1867-1868'.

Brief summaries were published in H. Attwood, R. Gillespie and M. Lewis, eds, *New Perspectives on the History of Medicine,* Melbourne, 1990; Thomas B. Hugh, 'The beginning of antiseptic surgery in Australia' in *Australia and New Zealand Journal of Surgery,* 65, 1995, pp. 887-9; Knut Haeger, *The Illustrated History of Surgery,* London, 1988, p. 223; John C. Murray, 'Thomas Fiaschi and Listerian Antisepsis in Sydney 1880-1900', p. 30; and James A. Ross, *The Edinburgh School of Surgery after Lister,* Edinburgh, 1928.

2 Archibald Watson, notebooks, p. 1/2/20, 28 May 1909, St Vincent's, case 4, RACS archives.

3 W. G. D. Upjohn, 'Forty years of surgery at the Royal Melbourne Hospital' in *Royal Melbourne Hospital Clinical Reports, Centenary Volume,* vol. 14, 1948, pp. 6-7.

4 Sir Charles Bickerton Blackburn, 'The growth of specialism in Australia during fifty years and its significance for the future' in *Medical Journal of Australia,* 6 January 1951, p. 21; Sir Victor Hurley, 'The development and practice of surgery in Australia during fifty years' in *Medical Journal of Australia,* 6 January 1951, p. 6.

5 John Blandy and J. P. Williams, *The History of the British Association of Urological Surgeons 1945-1995,* London, 1995, pp. 15-16; Hilary St George Saunders, *The*

Middlesex Hospital, 1745-1948, London, 1949; H. Campbell Thomson, *The Story of the Middlesex Hospital Medical School 1835-1935,* London, 1935, p. 168; A. E. Webb-Johnson was Surgeon in the Department of Urology in 1935 and E. W. Riches was his assistant. *The Royal Hospital of Saint Bartholomew 1123-1973,* London, 1974.

H. C. Cameron, *Mr Guy's Hospital, 1726-1948,* London, 1954; Hujohn A. Ripman (ed), *Guy's Hospital 1725-1948,* London, 1951. The first orthopaedic surgeon at Guy's was appointed in 1913 and according to the hospital histories, but not the history of the BAUS, the first urologist was appointed in 1936. Perhaps the 1910 appointment was an assistant surgeon. There was a department for Genito-urinary surgery from 1908.

Robert Marshall, *The Royal Victoria Hospital, Belfast,* Belfast, 1955. William Brockbank, *Portrait of a Hospital 1752-1948, the Royal Infirmary, Manchester,* London, 1952. *The Leicester Royal Infirmary 1771-1971,* Leicester, 1971. James A. Ross, *The Edinburgh School of Surgery after Lister,* Edinburgh, 1928.

6 D. Sclater Lewis, *The Royal Victoria Hospital, Montreal, 1887-1947,* Montreal, 1969; Bertram M. Bernheim, *The Story of the Johns Hopkins,* Kingswood, 1949; Nathaniel W. Faxon, *The Massachusetts General Hospital 1935-1955,* Cambridge, Massachusetts, 1959; Peter Lawson, 'Origins of the Urological Society of Australasia' in *Australia and New Zealand Journal of Surgery,* 60, 1990, pp. 385-91; archives of the Urological Society of Australasia, hereafter USA archives.

7 USA archives; Prof. P. W. Boer, Dr J. Felderhof, Prof. Dr W. A. Moonen, Drs L. M. H. Schreinemachers (eds), *Nederlandse Vereniging voor Urologie 1908-1983;* Daniel de Moulin, *A History of Surgery with Emphasis on the Netherlands,* Dordrecht, 1988.

8 A. S. Roe, 'Reminiscences of medical Brisbane, early twentieth century' in *Medical Journal of Australia,* 15 April 1961, p. 548.

9 Interview with Stuart Gowland, 11 November 1996.

10 USA archives.

11 Peter Lawson, 'Prostatic obstruction—a personal account from 1925' in *Prospectives,* no. 1, 1992.

12 Leonard J. Murphy, 'Harry Harris and his contribution to suprapubic prostatectomy' in *Australia and New Zealand Journal of Surgery,* 54, 1984, pp.579-88 and *The History of Urology,* Springfield, 1972.

13 A. Eisdell Moore, 'Eight to eighty-eight a surgeon looks back' in David Scott (ed), *The Story of Auckland Hospital 1847-1977,* Auckland, pp. 32-3.

CHAPTER 2

1 Tape made by Alex Inglis and sent to Charles Roe, no date, RACS archives; Clifford Morson, ed., St Peter's Hospital for Stone, London, 1960, p. 61.

2 Julian Ormond Smith, *The History of the Royal Australasian College of Surgeons from 1920 to 1935,* Melbourne; Colin Smith 'The Shaping of the RACS 1920-1960', *Royal Australasian College of Surgeons Handbook 1995.*

3 Obituary of John Joseph Power, *Medical Journal of Australia,* 16 April 1966, p. 689.

4 Peter Lawson, letter to Sally Wilde, 9 December 1996.

5 Arthur E. Brown, 'The Development of Australian Hospitals in the Last Fifty Years', in *Medical Journal of Australia,* 6 January 1951, p. 41; T. S. Pensabene, *The Rise of the Medical Practitioner in Victoria,* Canberra, 1980, especially chapter X; M. A. Jones, *The Australian Welfare State, Origins, Control & Choices,* Sydney, 1980; *Ninth Report of the Charities Board of Victoria, Year ending 30 June 1932,* Melbourne.

6 See, for instance, David Evans, '"Abusing Charity". Hospitalization and the care of the sick in 20th century Victoria' in John Pearn & Catherine O'Carrigan, eds, *Australia's Quest for Colonial Health,* Brisbane; *Ninth Report of the Charities Board of Victoria,* p. 5.

7 *Official Year Book of the Commonwealth of Australia,* 1909, 1916, 1927, 1937; A. E. Brown, op. cit., pp. 41-2.

8 Iain Hay, *The Caring Commodity: The Provision of Health Care in New Zealand,* Auckland, 1989, p. 57.

9 Ibid.; Douglas Robb, *Health Services, or Doctors and Hospitals,* Wellington, 1941, p. 10.

10 Milton I. Roemer, *National Health Systems of the World,* vol. 1, *The Countries,* New York, 1991, pp. 205-8.
11 Thomas Carlyle, *On Heroes and Hero Worship. The Hero as Divinity;*
12 The notable exceptions are Leonard Murphy, *The History of Urology,* Springfield, 1972, and Peter Lawson, 'Origins of the Urological Society of Australasia', *Australia and New Zealand Journal of Surgery,* 1990, 60, pp. 385-91.

Bruce Pearson made a substantial collection of curricula vitae when working on the history of the Society, see RACS archives; the USA archives also contain many obituaries and c.v.s.

Other publications include: Keith Kirkland, 'The Progress of Urology in Australasia', *Proceedings of the Urological Society of Australasia,* 1948; Frank Breslin, 'The History of Urology in New South Wales', *Newsletter, Urological Society of Australasia,* 1995; Don Urquhart-Hay, 'The beginnings of urology in New Zealand', *Newsletter, Urological Society of Australasia,* Summer, 1996; Charles Roe, 'The beginnings of urology in Queensland', *Prospectives,* no. 2, 1992; E. J. England, 'A History of Urology in Western Australia', *Prospectives,* no. 3, 1993; Peter Lawson, 'History of Urology in Victoria—the first thirty years', *Prospectives,* no. 4, 1993.
13 *J. Coll. Surg. Aust,* 1, 65-7, 1928; Bruce Pearson to Frank Gardiner, Lawson collection; Leonard J. Murphy, 'Harry Harris and his contribution to supra-pubic prostatectomy', *Australia and New Zealand Journal of Surgery,* 1984, 54, pp. 579-88; Warwick Macky, Harry Harris Oration, 1989, revised notes 1994, USA archives.
14 A. W. Beasley, programme note, The Cowlishaw Symposium, 26 October 1996, RACS; Frank Breslin, 'The History of Urology in New South Wales,' *Newsletter, Urological Society of Australasia,* 1996; M. S. S. Earlam, 'Robert Gordon Craig', *Proceedings of the Urological Society of Australasia,* 1957; E. H. Stokes, *Sydney Hospital Clinical School,* Sydney, 1960, p. 93; Dennis Arnold to Frank Breslin, 6 February 1995, information courtesy of Frank Breslin; D. G. Hamilton, *Hand in Hand: The Story of the Royal Alexandra Hospital for Children, Sydney,* Sydney, 1979, pp. 138, 314-15.
15 Charles Roe, 'The beginnings of urology in Queensland', *Prospectives,* no. 2, 1992.
16 Charles Roe to Peter Lawson, 21 April 1987, Lawson collection; Obituaries, *Medical Journal of Australia,* 26 November 1966.
17 I. R. Vanderfield to Peter Lawson, 13 May 1987, USA archives.
18 R. J. Silverton, 'Spinal Analgesia in Urinary Surgery', *Medical Journal of Australia,* vol. 1, no. 24, 11 June 1921; Annual Reports of Royal North Shore Hospital, 1921, 1922, 1923.
19 Medical Directories of Australia; Clifford Morson, ed., *St Peter's Hospital for Stone 1860-1960,* London, 1960, p. 62.
20 Colin Edwards and Douglas Anderson, obituary of Robert Joseph Silverton, *Medical Journal of Australia,* 23 September 1967; Douglas Keller to Peter Lawson, 13 November 1987, USA archives.
21 *Report of the Director-General of Public Health, New South Wales, for the year 1935,* Sydney, 1937, Section III, 1, The Prince Henry Hospital, Sydney.
22 Alban Gee, obituary of Richard Guy Septimus Harris, *Medical Journal of Australia,* 31 August 1963; Sister M. Jeanne Hyland, LCM, letter to Peter Lawson, 8 July 1987, USA archives.
23 Sister M. Jeanne Hyland, LCM, letter to Peter Lawson, 20 April 1987, USA archives.
24 Don Urquhart-Hay, 'The beginnings of urology in New Zealand' in *Newsletter, Urological Society of Australasia,* Summer, 1996; R. Campbell-Begg, *The Secret of the Knife,* Norwich, c. 1965.
25 Rowan Webb, address to Urological Society dinner, Melbourne, 10 August 1991, USA archives; John Bowie Somerset, obituary, USA archives.
26 Obituaries, *Medical Journal of Australia,* 16 April 1966. Charles Roe, The beginnings of urology in Queensland; various press cuttings, USA archives.
27 John Blackman to Frank Breslin, 13 March 1995, information courtesy of Frank Breslin; E. H. Stokes, *Sydney Hospital Clinical School,* Sydney, 1960.
28 Extracts from diaries kept by Laidley and Earlam, 1936-38. They are bound together with a covering letter from Earlam, Urological Society collection, RACS

archives; Frank Breslin, 'The History of Urology in New South Wales', *Newsletter, Urological Society of Australasia,* 1995; *British Journal of Urology,* 1929, 'Urological Surgeons Abroad', Lawson collection; M. S. S. Earlam, obituary of J. W. S. Laidley, *Medical Journal of Australia,* 12 May 1956.

29 Obituary of Edgar Robert Reay, *New Zealand Medical Journal,* September 1969.

30 Warwick Macky, Adaptation of Harry Harris Oration, 1994, Lawson collection; Warwick Macky, biographical note on Frank Macky, MBBS, FRACS, in USA files, RACS archives.

31 Records of admission of the early Fellows, RACS archives; Warwick Macky, biographical note on Frank Macky, MBBS, FRACS, in USA files, RACS archives; Warwick Macky, Harry Harris Oration, 1989; Minutes of the Sydney Urological Association, March 1936 and Minutes of the Urological Society of Australasia, 7th Annual Meeting, Brisbane, 15 July 1946, RACS archives.

32 Henry Mortensen, *Medical Journal of Australia,* vol. II, no. 11, 12 September 1931.

33 Mortensen to Murphy to Lawson, USA archives.

34 Sir Charles Hercus & Sir Gordon Bell, *The Otago Medical School Under the First Three Deans,* Edinburgh, 1964, pp. 298, 311-12; Don Urquhart-Hay 'The Beginnings of Urology in New Zealand'; various papers, USA archives.

35 Obituary, *Medical Journal of Australia,* 14 July 1979.

36 John Jose to Peter Lawson, 16 April 1987, Lawson collection; Minutes of the Sydney Urological Association and the Urological Society of Australasia, RACS archives; Noel Bonnin to Peter Lawson, 5 May 1987; J. P. Maddern 'Both and Bonnin, Innovators', USA archives.

37 D. I. Roberts, letter to Sally Wilde, 28 July 1997.

38 Tony Low, communication to Peter Lawson, 24 July 1997; E. J. England, 'A History of Urology in Western Australia', *Prospectives,* no. 3, 1993.

CHAPTER 3

1 Julian Ormond Smith, *The History of the Royal Australasian College of Surgeons from 1920 to 1935,* Melbourne; Colin Smith 'The shaping of the RACS 1920-1960', *Royal Australasian College of Surgeons Handbook 1995.*

2 *Medical Journal of Australia,* 1937, vol. 2, 10 and 24 April 1937.

3 Programs of RACS Annual General and Scientific Meetings, 1928-1938, RACS archives.

4 Sydney Urological Association, Kirkland's letter and minutes, RACS archives.

5 Minutes of the Sydney Urological Association, inaugural meeting, RACS archives.

6 Minutes of the Sydney Urological Association, July 1935, RACS archives.

7 Moore of Melbourne, Roe of Brisbane and Mortensen of Melbourne later became Members; Lennon of Wagga, Burnell of Adelaide and Macky of Auckland later became Associate Members; Jose of Adelaide was a general surgeon with an interest in urology; Jenkins of Dunedin was the general surgeon in charge of the urology department; Collier of Newcastle was the ninth urologist to become a Fellow of the RACS, in 1931, but he later went to England and was at Paddington Hospital by 1947, see *Urological Correspondence Club Letters 1947-48,* 21 December 1947, Hugh Pearson, RACS archives and records of the early Fellows, RACS archives; Sutton of Brisbane was a urologist in Power's team at the Brisbane General; Lazarus of Melbourne was RSO at St Peter's 1930-31 and an Honorary Surgical Assistant at St Vincent's, *Knox's Medical Directory for Australia 1936-37,* Sydney, 1936.

8 Minutes of the Sydney Urological Association, March 1936, RACS archives.

9 Minutes of the Sydney Urological Association, RACS archives.

10 Keith Kirkland, 'The Progress of Urology in Australasia', *Proceedings of the Urological Society of Australasia,* no. 2, 9th Annual Meeting, Melbourne and Ballarat, 1948, pp. 5-10. Obituary Keith Lindsay Hugh Kirkland, *Medical Journal of Australia,* 5 August 1972.

11 *Urological Correspondence Club Letters 1945-46,* hereafter UCC, April 1945, Colin Edwards, RACS archives; Urological Society of Australasia, Minutes and Annual Reports, RACS archives.

12 The RACS had a longer break during the war, suspending Annual General Scientific and Ceremonial Meetings in 1940. A full program resumed in 1946. Minutes of the RACS Council, April 1940 and December 1945, RACS archives; list of RACS AGMs, RACS archives; USA Minutes and Annual Reports, RACS archives.
13 *Medical Journal of Australia,* 8 January 1938.
14 Program of the AGM and Scientific Meeting 1938, RACS archives.
15 USA, Annual Reports, RACS archives.
16 USA, 1945 Annual Report, RACS archives.
17 Ibid.
18 H. B. Devine, typed note on Annual Meetings, Specialist Surgeons and the Journal, 1946, RACS archives.
19 UCC 1947-48, February 1948, Colin Edwards, p. 166, RACS archives.
20 UCC 1947-48, Richard Harris, p. 172; John Power, p. 176, RACS archives.
21 *Memorandum and Articles of Association of the Urological Society of Australasia,* under the Companies Act 1936, Company Limited by Guarantee and Not Having a Share Capital, Certificate of Incorporation, 23 February 1948.
22 USA Minutes, RACS archives.
23 UCC 1945-46, January 1945, Henry Mortensen, p. 1, RACS archives.
24 Interviews with Jim Peters, David Webb, Mohamed Khadra, Helen O'Connell, 11 November 1996; Peter Bruce, 14 November 1996; Lorna Sisely, 22 November 1996.
25 UCC 1945-46, RACS archives.
26 USA Minutes, Annual Reports and Membership Book, RACS archives.
27 'Memorandum on the relationship of the College of Surgeons and various special sections of surgery' by George Bell, President, Harold Dew, Vice-President, 1 July 1949. The Executive disagreed with Bell and Dew and produced a 'Memorandum from the Executive re memorandum submitted by the President and Professor Dew', in which, according to Colin Smith, Searby played a major role. RACS archives.

CHAPTER 4

1 This chapter is based on information contained in the Minutes of the Executive of the Urological Society, programs of the Annual Scientific Meetings of the Society, Annual Reports, Minutes of the Annual General Meetings and Newsletters, all in the Urological Society files in the RACS archives.
2 While a Melbourne-based president, for instance, would typically attend two or three executive meetings as vice-president, three or four executive meetings as president and one or two executive meetings as past president, the Sydney men would typically attend most of the twenty to thirty executive meetings during their three years. The Sydney men were also much more likely to be elected vice-president after already spending time on the Executive, and therefore did not have to spend their vice-presidential year learning how the Executive operated. No exhaustive survey of attendance has been conducted but in 1959-60, Murphy (past president, Vic.) attended 1 out of 9 meetings, Hogg and Inglis (presidents, Qld) attended 4 out of 9, Gee (vice-president, NSW) 6 out of 9; in 1967-68, Craven (NSW past pres.) attended 8 out of 9, Jacobs (NSW pres) 9 out of 9, Mortensen (vice-pres ,Vic.) 2 out of 9. These figures do not appear to be atypical.
3 Interview with Warwick Macky, 27 February 1997.
4 Interview with Jim Peters, 11 November 1996.
5 Edgar Reay, letter to Llew Wheeler, 10 July 1957, Urological Society correspondence files, RACS archives.
6 Bill Utley, letter to Llew Wheeler, 17 October 1957, Urological Society correspondence files, RACS archives.
7 Talk given in front of the Archives Poster at the 1995 Annual Scientific Meeting, Peter Lawson.
8 Interview with John Maddern, 11 November 1996.
9 *Newsletter,* September 1971, RACS archives.

10 Interview with Dennis Arnold, 12 March 1997.
11 Dennis Arnold, letter to Peter Lawson, 25 March 1997, USA archives.
12 Interview with Geof Hirst, 27 May 1997; interview with Graham Holmes, 4 July 1997.
13 Before 1952, the Executive changed at the beginning of the annual meeting, so that the incoming president was theoretically in the chair during the meeting. Telfer was ill and did not attend the 1951 meeting. He resigned as President at the next Executive meeting, but continued to attend Executive meetings as the past President. Moore took over and was thus President for the first meeting under the new system where the incoming president took over at the end of the annual meeting—and thus had twelve months to plan the next one, generally held in his home town. Archie Telfer died early in 1953.
14 Hogg died in the winter of 1959 and Inglis replaced him as President.
15 Interview with David Golovsky, 14 November 1996.

Chapter 5

1 Rivkah Mathews, 'On Stepping Twice into the Same River: The Wet Feet of Dr. Fell', *Journal of Australian Studies,* no. 22- 5, 1988-89, pp. 16-28; Clarissa Cook and Gary Easthope, 'Symptoms of a crisis? Trust, risk and medicine: review essay', *Australia and New Zealand Journal of Sociology,* vol. 32, no. 3, Nov. 1996; John Germov, 'Medi-fraud, managerialism and the decline of medical autonomy: deprofessionalisation and proletarianisation reconsidered', *Australia and New Zealand Journal of Sociology,* vol. 31, no. 3, Nov. 1995; Diane Mary Mackay, Politics of reaction: The Australian Medical Association as a pressure group, MA thesis, La Trobe University, 1985; Patricia Moynihan, Australian Health Insurance Policy 1972-74: A study in the reproduction of capitalist medical structures, MA thesis, La Trobe University, 1981; John Nieuwenhuyse & Marina Williams-Wynn, *Professions in the Market-place: An Australian study of doctors, accountants and dentists,* MUP, 1982; Milton Lewis and Roy MacLeod, 'Medical Politics and the Professionalisation of Medicine in New South Wales, 1850-1901', *Journal of Australian Studies,* no. 22-5, 1988-89, pp. 69-82; Urological Society Correspondence files, especially 'Hospital Appointments—Problems', RACS archives.
2 Memorandum and Articles of Association, 1948, p. 4, RACS archives.
3 Keith Kirkland to the Secretary of the Section of Urology of the NSW Branch of the BMA, 5 November 1951, in Minutes of the Section, RACS archives.
4 Copy of special resolution, 16 April 1951, Minutes of Executive Meetings, RACS archives.
5 Correspondence files, Urological Society, including Noel Bonnin, Adelaide, to Hugh Pearson, 25 July 1960, A. B. Holmes, Launceston, to John Blackman, 13 February 1961, notice of special meeting of the Executive, 24 February 1961 and enclosures, RACS archives.
6 Harry Learoyd to Messrs Seymour Office Services, re minutes of Executive Meeting, 13 April 1975, p. 4 of minutes, Correspondence files, Urological Society, RACS archives.
7 The early sequence of changes in the RACS examinations in the specialities has been outlined by Colin Smith, see his letters: to Mr Carter, 10 September 1996; to Pauline in New Zealand office, 20 September 1994; to Mr Mooney, 13 February 1997; RACS archives.
8 Minutes of the Sixth AGM, Surfers Paradise, 23 April 1953; further detail is given in the Minutes of the Executive, 20 and 22 April 1953; Urological Society Sixth Annual Report, 1953-54.
9 Colin Smith letters; Minutes of the Executive, 31 July and 5 November 1953, 18 March, 1 June, 10 August, 8 October and 10 December 1954, 11 February 1955, and 22 June 1956; Urological Society, Seventh Annual Report, 1954-55. The changes during the 1960s are also discussed in the Executive Minutes of 19 January and 6 April 1962, 6 August 1963, Minutes of Special meeting, 9 August 1963, 14 October 1963, 8 March 1965, 25 March 1966.

10 Howard Hanley to Joe Murnaghan, 16 October 1967, Training file, Urological Society, RACS archives.
11 Donald Macdonald to Harold Thomas, 20 February 1972, Training file, Urological Society, RACS archives.
12 C. M. Maxwell to the Secretary, Urological Society, 14 December 1965; Minutes of the Executive, 25 March 1966.
13 'Post Graduate Training—Report of Subcommittee of Executive of the Urological Society of Australasia', originally presented to Executive on 6 May 1966 and amended by the full Executive on that date.
14 Ibid.
15 Minutes of the 'Seminar on Specialist Surgical Training and Accreditation held on 13/7/69, in the Board Room of the Royal Melbourne Hospital, Melbourne, Vic., at 11.00 a.m.', Training file, Urological Society, RACS archives; interview with Durham Smith, 5 May 1997.
16 Minutes of 'Second Seminar on Specialist Surgical training and Accreditation, held on 14th December, 1969, in the Board Room of the Royal Melbourne Hospital, Viv, at 11.00 a.m.' Training file, Urological Society, RACS archives.
17 Minutes of 23rd AGM; Urological Society *Newsletter,* April 1970; Minutes of the Executive, 1 May 1970; 'Urological Society of Australasia Training and Accreditation, Basic Proposals for Specialist Urological Training for FRACS', 24 July 1970; Joe Murnaghan to Australasian Departments of Surgery, survey of staffing structure, beds and the possibilities for training posts, 23 September 1970; Minutes of the Executive, 21 and 25 March 1971; Minutes of the Meeting of the Standing Sub-committee on Standards of Training and Accreditation, held in the Wentworth Hotel, Sydney, on Tuesday, 23 March 1971; Minutes of the Executive, 20 November 1971; President's newsletter, November 1971.
18 'The Urological Society of Australasia, Training and Accreditation Memorandum, to the Executive of the Society, from Professor G. F. Murnaghan', 5 October 1979.
19 'The Urological Society of Australasia, Proposals for the Organisation of Training, Accreditation and Education by the Urological Society of Australasia', by Joe Murnaghan, Ian Nunn, Bob Wines and Peter Maher, 28 February 1980; 'Discussion Document, The Relation of Specialist Societies and the College', E. Durham Smith, July 1979; both in Training files, Urological Society, RACS archives; interview with Durham Smith, 5 May 1997.
20 G. D. Tracy to the President of the Urological Society, 16 August 1979, Training files, Urological Society, RACS archives; interview with Durham Smith, 5 May 1997.
21 Interview with John Maddern, 11 November 1996.
22 Interview with Don Moss, 27 May 1997.
23 Minutes of the Executive, 14 October 1948; Minutes of the Executive, February 1950.
24 T. S. Pensabene, *The Rise of the Medical Practitioner in Victoria,* ANU, Canberra, 1980, pp. 171-2.
25 Minutes of the Executive, 8 March 1965; see also 31 July 1953, 1 June, 10 August, 8 October 1954, 8 December 1961, 18 June, 14 October, 26 November 1963, 14 April 1967, and 1 March 1970.
26 Minutes of the Executive, 6 May 1966; see also 16 December 1953, 11 January 1954, 2 September, 2 December 1955, 24 February 1956, 8 December 1961, 6 April, 8 May 1962, 15 January 1968, 19 and 20 March 1969.
27 T. Fox, 'The Antipodes. Private Practice Publically Supported', the *Lancet,* 20 April 1963, p. 875, quoted in Pensabene, p. 172; Minutes of the Executive, 8 November 1957; the sub-committee on fees and anomalies was set up at the 21st AGM; 1973 relative value study.
28 Minutes of the AGM, Wellington, 21 March 1973.
29 *Newsletter,* August 1971.
30 *Newsletter,* August 1974; Pensabene, pp. 172-4.
31 Minutes of the Extraordinary General Meeting, 8 November 1974; H. Thomas (Secretary of the Urological Society) to Dr G. Repin (Secretary-General of the AMA), 29 November 1974, includes a copy of the Memorandum of Association of the Australian Association of Urological Surgeons, Correspondence files, AMA.

32 Minutes of the Executive, 4 June 1976.
33 Harry Learoyd to Bob Farnsworth and Ian Nunn, 24 April 1978, Urological Society Correspondence files, BPBAC, RACS archives.
34 Allan Passmore, Assistant Secretary-General, AMA, to Stuart Taylor, Convenor, Fees and Anomalies Sub-committee, Urological Society, 31 October 1983, Urological Society Correspondence files, fees and anomalies, RACS archives.
35 Report of Australian Association of Surgeons, 18 June 1983, Urological Society Correspondence files, AAS, RACS archives.
36 Richard Colban to Ros Parisi, 14 July 1983, Report of Australian Association of Surgeons, June 1983, Urological Society Correspondence files, AAS, RACS archives.
37 Stuart Taylor to John Jose, 15 December 1984, Urological Society Correspondence files, ANZAUS, RACS archives.
38 Report from the Chairman of the Fees and Anomalies Sub-committee of the Australian and New Zealand Association of Urological Surgeons, 12 November 1985, Urological Society Correspondence files, ANZAUS, RACS archives.
39 Report from Stuart Taylor on behalf of the Australian and New Zealand Association of Urological Surgeons, 22 January 1985, Urological Society Correspondence files, ANZAUS, RACS archives.
40 Tony Low, letter to Peter Lawson, 19 December 1996.
41 Interview with Stuart Taylor, 24 June 1997; interview with Geof Hirst, 27 May 1997.
42 Interview with Gail Hill, 12 March 1997.
43 Minutes of the Third Annual Meeting of the Urological Society of Australasia, 26 March 1940; Gwynne Brockis, letter to Sally Wilde, 19 May 1997; interview with Geof Hirst, 27 May 1997; eulogy delivered by Dennis Arnold for Bruce Pearson, 11 April 1992; interview with David Golovsky, 14 November 1996; *Newsletters* of the Urological Society, 1994-1997.

CHAPTER 6

1 Interview with Dennis Arnold, 12 March 1997.
2 Interview with Llew Wheeler, 11 March 1997; interview with Dennis Arnold, 12 March 1997; interview with Glen Coorey, 26 May 1997; Mohamed Khadra 'A Urological Life—Robert Gordon Craig', typescript, 1995.
3 Interview with Llew Wheeler, 11 March 1997; Dennis Arnold, Eulogy for Bruce Pearson, delivered in the Chapel at Royal Prince Alfred Hospital, Sydney, 11 April 1992; Minutes of the Sydney Urological Association and the Urological Society of Australasia, RACS archives.
4 Interview with Llew Wheeler, 11 March 1997; Minutes of the Executive of the Urological Society, RACS archives.
5 Interview with Llew Wheeler, 11 March 1997; interview with John Rogers, 27 May 1997; John Rogers, letter to Sally Wilde, 2 June 1997; membership records of the Urological Society.
6 Frank Breslin, 'The History of Urology in New South Wales, the First 35 Years' in *Newsletter,* Urological Society of Australasia.
7 Interview with John Blackman, 10 March 1997.
8 Ian Potts, A short history of the Urology Department at Sydney Hospital, undated.
9 John Blackman, letter to Frank Breslin, 13 March 1995. re the beginnings of urology at Sydney Hospital.
10 Ibid.; Ian Potts, A short history; interview with Lionel Jacobs, 10 March 1997.
11 John Blackman, letter to Frank Breslin.
12 Ian Potts, A short history; interview with Lionel Jacobs, 10 March 1997.
13 Ian Potts, A short history.
14 John Blackman, 'The Australian Kidney Foundation: some early history,' in *Prospectives,* no. 7, 1995.
15 Interview with Joe Murnaghan, 12 March 1997; interview with Frank Breslin, 9 March 1997.
16 Interview with Lionel Jacobs, 10 March 1997.

17 Ibid.
18 Joe Murnaghan, letter to Sally Wilde, 12 August 1997.
19 Interview with Stuart Gowland, 11 November 1996; interview with Joe Murnaghan, 12 March 1997.
20 Interview with Richard Millard, 29 May 1997; interview with Ted Arnold, Richard Millard and Peter Lawson, 14 November 1996; interview with Frank Breslin, 9 March 1997.
21 Interview with John Blackman, 10 March 1997.
22 Interview with Doug Keller, 11 March 1997; minutes of the Executive of the Urological Society, RACS archives.
23 Obituary of Alban Harvey Gee by Frank Breslin, *Medical Journal of Australia*, January 1987; interview with Doug Keller, 11 March 1997.
24 Douglas Miller, *Development of Surgery in an Australian Hospital 1857-1975, St Vincent's Hospital, Sydney*, Singapore, 1977.
25 Interview with Frank Breslin, 9 March 1997.
26 Interview with Llew Wheeler, 11 March 1997.
27 Interview with Peter Maher, 14 November 1996.
28 Interview with John Blackman, 10 March 1997; interview with Dennis Arnold, 12 March 1997. interview with Michael Rochford, 29 May 1997.
29 Interview with Bill Lucas, 26 May 1997; interview with Chris Farrell, 29 May 1997.
30 P. D. Hughes 'A History of Urology in Canberra', *Newsletter*, Urological Society, Autumn 1996.
31 Stuart Taylor, notes on the history of urology in Newcastle, June 1997.
32 M. Rosen, 'A Simple Artificial Implantable Sphincter', Abstracts of the Proceedings of the Urological Society of Australasia, 28th AGM, Sydney, 1975, *British Journal of Urology* (1976) 48, 675-80.
33 Interview with Peter Maher, 14 Novermber 1996; correspondence files, Urological Society, RACS archives.
34 *Newsletter*, Urological Society, August 1955, RACS archives.
35 Minutes of the Executive of the Urological Society and *Newsletters*, RACS archives.

Chapter 7

1 Curriculum vitae and obituaries of urologists, RACS archives; R. E. Wright-St Clair, *A History of the New Zealand Medical Association, the First 100 Years*, Wellington, 1987; interview with Colin McRae, 5 December 1996; interview with Stuart Gowland, 11 November 1996; Don Urquhart-Hay, 'The beginnings of urology in New Zealand' in *Newsletter, Urological Society of Australasia*, Summer 1996, pp. 15-18.
2 See chapter 4 above; minutes of the Executive of the Urological Society of Australasia, RACS archives.
3 Marie Wild and Nancy Wright, 'Department of Urology' in Alice Silverson, ed., *The Last Thirty Years 1963-1993, The History of the Canterbury Area Health Board*, p. 236.
4 Bill Utley, 'The history of the investigation of vesico-ureteric reflux at Christchurch Hospital', typescript, June 1997; interview with Colin McRae, 5 December 1996; interview with Ted Arnold, 14 November 1996.
5 Interview with Warwick Macky, 27 February 1997.
6 Ibid.
7 Interview with Stuart Gowland, 11 November 1996.
8 A. Eisdell Moore, 'Eight to Eighty-eight: a Surgeon looks back' in David Scott, ed., *The Story of Auckland Hospital 1847-1977*, pp. 32-3.
9 Don Urquhart-Hay, 'The beginnings of urology in New Zealand'.
10 Curriculum vitae and obituaries, RACS archives.
11 Interview with Russell McIlroy and Roger Chambers, 26 February 1997; membership records, Urological Society of Australasia, RACS archives.
12 Interview with Russell McIlroy and Roger Chambers, 26 February 1997.
13 Interview with Don Urquhart-Hay, 28 February 1997; R. E. Wright-St Clair, *A History of the New Zealand Medical Association*; interview with Roy Towers, 2 March 1997.

14 Roy Towers.
15 Don Urquhart-Hay; New Zealand Medical Registers.
16 Interview with Jim Gray, 27 February 1997.
17 Interview with Pat Bary, 26 May 1997.
18 Interview with Peter Meffan, 19 May 1997; Jo Kellaway and Mike Maryan, *A Century of Care—Palmerston North Hospital 1893-1993*, pp. 96, 118.
19 Interview with Jim Gray, 27 February 1997; Don Urquhart-Hay, 'The beginnings of urology in New Zealand' in *Newsletter,* Urological Society of Australasia, Summer 1996.
20 Interview with Don Urquhart-Hay, 28 February 1997.
21 Interview with Stuart Gowland, 11 November 1996.
22 Interview with Roger Chambers and Russell McIlroy, 26 February 1997.
23 Interview with Jim Gray, 27 February 1997.
24 STUF booking form, August 1987.

Chapter 8

1 Charles Roe, 'A History of Roe's Kamp, South Stradbroke Island, 1882-1991', p. 48.
2 Interview with John Phillips, 29 May 1997; Jeff Watson, letter to Charles Roe, 20 August 1991.
3 Obituary of Francis William Rennick Lukin, *Medical Journal of Australia,* 29 June 1974.
4 Jeff Watson, letter to Charles Roe, 20 August 1991.
5 Interview with John Phillips, 29 May 1997; Charles Roe, 'Some notes on the beginnings of Urology as a Specialty in Queensland'.
6 Interview with John Phillips, 29 May 1997.
7 'Notes on our Urological Predecessors at Royal Brisbane Hospital', typescript c. 1992.
8 Phone conversation with Graham Holmes, 4 July 1997.
9 Ibid.; Medical Registers of Australia; interview with Stephen Stening, 27 May 1997;
10 Geof Hirst, letter to Sally Wilde, 2 July 1997; Jeff Watson, letter to Charles Roe, 20 August 1991.
11 John Lynch, letter to Charles Roe, 24 September 1991.
12 Interview with Geof Hirst, 27 May 1997.
13 Ray Que Hee, letter to Charles Roe, undated.
14 Ibid.
15 Steve Ferguson, letter to Peter Lawson, August 1997.
16 Paul Hopkins, letter to Jeff Watson, 13 November 1989; Ros Parisi, notes on urology in North Queensland; John Sander, letter to Charles Roe, 14 August 1991; David Splatt, letter to Charles Roe, 27 August 1991; Stephen Stening, letter to Charles Roe, 14 January 1992; membership records of the Urological Society; Medical Registers of Australia.
17 Phone conversation with Graham Holmes, 4 July 1997; interview with Philip McDougall, 26 May 1997; minutes of the Executive of the Urological Society, especially 1958, 1961, 1975; Annual Reports of the Urological Society.

Chapter 9

1 Noel Bonnin, letter to Peter Lawson, 5 May 1987, USA archives.
2 Interview with John Jose, 14 November 1996.
3 Interview with Graham Sinclair, 14 November 1996.
4 Peter Harbison, 'Urology in South Australia and the Northern Territory', *Newsletter,* Urological Society of Australasia, Autumn 1996.
5 Interview with Geoffrey Burfield, 29 May 1997.
6 Interview with Terry Morgan, 27 June 1997; citation for presentation of the Fellowship of the Urological Society of Australasia to Professor Villis Marshall, Auckland, 13 March 1995.
7 Interview with Adrian Porter, 27 June 1997.

8 Graham Sinclair, letter to Peter Lawson, 22 May 1997; interview with Adrian Porter, 27 June 1997.
9 Urological Society, Annual Report, 1983, RACS archives.

CHAPTER 10

1 Interview with Alan Holmes conducted by Terry Morgan, January 1997; Medical Registers of Australia; membership records of the Urological Society.
2 D. I. Roberts, letters to Sally Wilde, 28 July 1997 and 5 August 1997.
3 Ibid.
4 Interview with Alan Holmes conducted by Terry Morgan, January 1997; interview with Douglas Stephens, 6 February 1997.
5 Medical Registers of Australia.
6 Interview with Alan Holmes conducted by Terry Morgan, January 1997.
7 Interview with Terry Morgan, 27 June 1997.

CHAPTER 11

1 *Victorian Year Books,* 1962, 1966, 1971, 1976, 1981, 1986, 1994; survey of Victorian members of the Urological Society conducted by Peter Lawson, 1997. The great majority of respondents recorded significant, and complex, change in their practice patterns. Few practised exclusively in the eastern suburbs, but there was a tendency over time to add one or more eastern suburbs hospitals and one or more eastern suburbs private practices to their appointments at Melbourne's major teaching hospitals. Between them the respondents appear to have broadly covered the whole of Melbourne with the exception of the north-west. They listed practice sites in Williamstown, Preston, Lilydale, Berwick, Frankston and even Phillip Island. This huge coverage was achieved by a group of men who lived almost exclusively in Melbourne's inner and inner southern and eastern suburbs. In 1997, they may have moved their consulting rooms from Collins Street, but they had not yet moved their principal residences from Kew and Malvern and Brighton.
2 Interview with David Webb, 11 November 1996.
3 Warren Johnson, notes on the history of the Royal Melbourne Hospital, manuscript, May 1997; Alex Wood, letter to Peter Lawson, 8 February 1994, USA archives.
4 Obituary of Harold Moore, *Medical Journal of Australia,* 3/10 January 1976; note on William Harold James Moore, typescript, undated, from David Webb; Rowan Webb, William Moore of Moore House, typescript of talk given at Carey Grammar School, undated, from David Webb.
5 Warren Johnson, manuscript.
6 Somerset gave up his appointment at Prince Henry's Hospital when he became head of the Royal Melbourne unit.
7 Peter Bruce, letter to David Webb, 4 February 1997.
8 Peter Lawson, 'History of Urology in Victoria—the first thirty years', *Prospectives,* no. 4, 1993; Rowan Webb, typescript of notes on Douglas Duffy, undated, from David Webb; Warren Johnson, manuscript.
9 Interview with Laurence Harewood, 26 May 1997; Warren Johnson, manuscript.
10 Interview with Laurence Harewood, 26 May 1997; interview with David Webb, 11 November 1996; interview with Peter Bruce, 14 November 1996; interview with Warren Johnson, 27 May 1997; interview with Rod Syme, 27 May 1997.
11 Interview with Harold Story, 26 November 1996.
12 Dan Lenaghan,'History of Urology at St Vincent's Hospital, Melbourne', typescript, March 1990, p. 6.
13 Ibid.; interview with Mrs Murphy, 3 February 1997; J. Gerard Joyce, 'Leonard James Thomas Murphy born 30th November 1914—died 2nd July 1994', *Newsletter,* Urological Society, Spring 1994.
14 J. Gerard Joyce, 'Daniel Lenaghan', *Newsletter,* Urological Society, Winter 1994.
15 Interview with Gerry Joyce, 17 April 1997.

16 *Year Book of Victoria,* 1963, p. 265.
17 *Alfred Hospital Faces and Places,* 1996, p. 102.
18 David Gunter, Kennedy Burnside and the Alfred Hospital Urology Unit, undated typescript.
19 Ibid.
20 David Kennedy, History of the Urology Unit at Alfred Hospital, undated typescript, Lawson collection; *Alfred Hospital Faces and Places,* 1996, p. 43.
21 Alex Wood, letter to Sally Wilde, 20 August 1997.
22 David Gunter, typescript; David Kennedy, typescript.
23 *Victorian Year Book,* 1964, pp. 286-7.
24 Interview with Jim Peters, 11 November 1996.
25 W. G. E. Straffon, History of Urology in Australasia, Prince Henry's Hospital, typescript, 1989.
26 Interview with Jim Peters, 11 November 1996.
27 W. G. E. Straffon, typescript.
28 *Victorian Year Book,* 1966.
29 Interview with Harold Story, 26 November 1996; Harold Story, Austin Hospital, Heidelberg: The Development of the Urology Unit, typescript, 1990.
30 Interview with Rod Syme, 27 May 1997.
31 David Ellis, letter to Sally Wilde, 5 December 1996; Harold Story, typescript; interview with Rod Syme, 27 May 1997.
32 *Victorian Year Book,* 1967; interview with Gerry Joyce, 17 April 1997.
33 Interviews with Lorna Sisely, 20 and 22 November 1996.
34 Interview with Peter Bruce, 14 November 1996; 'The History of the Urology Unit at the Queen Victoria Hospital, Victoria Medical Centre and the Monash Medical Centre', undated, unsigned typescript, Lawson collection, c. 1988; R. A. McMahon, letter to Durham Smith, 8 December 1989; Emma Russell, *Bricks or Spirit? The Queen Victoria Hospital Melbourne,* Melbourne, 1997.
35 *Victorian Year Book,* 1964, p. 284.
36 Interview with Douglas Stephens, 6 February 1997.
37 Ibid.; Durham Smith, 'Paediatric Urology at Royal Children's Hospital, Melbourne,' typescript, 1989.
38 Alan Woodward, letter to David Golovsky, 25 June 1986, correspondence files, Urological Society, RACS archives; interview with Durham Smith, 5 May 1997; Peter Lawson, 'History of Urology in Victoria—the first thirty years,' *Prospectives,* no. 4, 1993; Durham Smith, Douglas Stephens Banquet, Chicago, 16 October 1986, typescript of speech.
39 James Mortensen, letter to Geoff Watson, 16 September 1971, RACS archives; interview with Alan Crosthwaite, 11 June 1997.
40 David Ellis, letter to Sally Wilde, 5 December 1996.
41 Australian Medical Workforce Advisory Committee, The Urology Workforce in Australia 1995-2006, May 1996.
42 Ian Gordon, Forty Years of Urology in Country Victoria, typescript of talk to the Victorian Branch of the Urological Society of Australasia given at the country meeting held at Bendigo, 1995.
43 Membership records of the Urological Society; Australian Medical Workforce Advisory Committee, The Urology Workforce in Australia 1995-2006, May 1996, p. 15.
44 Interview with Gerry Joyce, 17 April 1997; Kennedy Burnside, letter to Geoff Gibson, 29 July 1970, RACS archives.
45 Urological Society Annual Report, 1983, RACS archives.

Chapter 12

1 *Western Australia Year Books*; E. J. England, 'A History of Urology in Western Australia', *Prospectives,* 1993; a longer version of the same paper was sent to Bruce Pearson in April 1991, RACS archives.
2 W. P. Harris, Director (Medical Services) Repatriation Department, Western Australian Branch, letter to W. E. E. Langford, Chief Director (Medical Services)

Repatriation Department Central Office, Victoria, 21 April 1965, in response to a query from the Urological Society re general surgeons performing urological procedures, RACS archives; Medical Directories of Australia.

3 Alex Cato, letter to Stan Wisniewski, 29 April 1993; obituary, Ralph Jackson Cato, *Newsletter,* Urological Society, Winter 1993.

4 Medical Directories of Australia; interview with Stan Wisniewski, 29 May 1997.

5 Ernie England, 1991; interview with Stan Wisniewski, 29 May 1997.

6 Gwynne Brockis, letter to Sally Wilde, 19 May 1997; John Gwynne Brockis, An autobiography, typescript, c. 1988, courtesy of Tony Taylor.

7 Medical Directories of Australia; *Royal Australasian College of Surgeons Handbook, 1995,* p. 7.

8 Urological Society: minutes of the meeting of the standing sub-committee on standards of training and accreditation, 23 March 1971, RACS archives.

9 Interviews with Keith Kaye, 11 November 1996, Tony Low and Tony Taylor, 14 November 1996, Pat Bary, 26 May 1997, Alastair Tulloch, 27 May 1997, Stan Wisniewski, 29 May 1997; 'Spend a Penny', August 1993; The Urological Research Centre Incorporated, Annual Report, 1996.

10 Interviews with Alastair Tulloch, 27 May 1997, Stan Wisniewski, 29 May 1997.

11 Minutes of the Executive of the Urological Society, 1957-60; interview with Tony Low and Tony Taylor, 14 November 1996; Urological Society, Annual Report, 1983; program of Western Australian Branch Annual Scientific Meeting, Rottnest Island, 3-4 September 1988, RACS archives.

Appendix
Past Officers

~

Presidents

1937	R. H. Bridge
1938	J. J. Power
1939	J. Thomson-Tait
1940	R. J. Silverton
1941	A.S. Roe
1942	H. N. Mortensen
1944–45	H. N. Mortensen
1945–46	M. S. S. Earlam
1946–47	J. J. Power
1947–48	K. L. H. Kirkland
1948–49	H. N. Mortensen
1949–50	R. G. S. Harris
1950–51	F. W. R. Lukin
1951	A. C. Telfer
1951–52	W. H. J. Moore
1952–53	J. J. Power
1953–54	C. M. Edwards
1954–55	J. B. Somerset
1955–56	E. P. Row
1956–57	M. S. S. Earlam
1957–58	E. H. Reay
1958–59	L. J. Murphy
1959–60	G. C. Hogg
1960	A. Inglis
1960–61	A. H. Gee
1961–62	J. S. Peters
1962–63	H. H. Pearson
1963–64	L. D. Wheeler
1964–65	D. B. Duffy
1965–66	J. W. F. Macky
1966–67	R. A. Craven
1967–68	L. A. Jacobs
1968–69	P. J. Mortensen
1969–70	J. P. Maddern
1970–71	J. E. Blackman
1971–72	J. G. Watson
1972–73	H. W. Gowland
1973–74	K. B. Burnside
1974–75	B. S. Pearson
1975–76	I. F. Potts
1976–77	S. H. Watson
1977–78	P. A. Harbison
1978–79	I. N. Nunn
1979–80	W. L. Utley
1980–81	G. F. Murnaghan
1981–82	D. D. Arnold
1982–83	R. Parisi
1983–84	D. Lenaghan
1984–85	J. S. Jose
1985–86	E. J. England
1986–87	J. M. Gray
1987–88	H. M. Learoyd
1988–89	R. B. Brown
1989–90	P. O. Maher
1990–91	E. G. Holmes
1991–92	V. R. Marshall
1992–93	W. F. Johnson
1993–94	J. S. Taylor
1994–95	E. P. Arnold
1995–96	J. H. Rogers
1996–97	A. I. Low
1997–98	D. Golovsky
1998–99	D. I. Moss

Chairmen

AUSTRALIA AND NEW ZEALAND ASSOCIATION OF UROLOGIC SURGEONS

1974–77 B. S. Pearson
1977–78 H. M. Learoyd
1978–80 J. H. Rogers
1980–83 A. P. Tynan
1983–88 J. S. Taylor
1988–91 G. H. Hirst
1991–94 L. K. Cleeve
1994–97 B. W. McGregor
1997–98 D. G. Travis

Chairmen

TRAINING ACCREDITATION AND EDUCATION COMMITTEE

1981–86 J. P. Maddern
1986–88 R. B. Brown
1988–91 V. R. Marshall
1991–93 E. P. Arnold
1994–97 D. I. Moss
1997–98 R. J. Millard

Honorary Secretaries

1937–46 K. L. H. Kirkland
1946–52 A. H. Gee
1952–55 H. H. Pearson
1955–58 L. D. Wheeler
1958–61 J. E. Blackman
1961–63 J. A. Blackwood
1964–66 I. F. Potts
1966–69 D. D. Arnold
1969–72 G. R. Gibson
1972–75 H. Thomas
1975–78 H. M. Learoyd
1978–81 P. O. Maher
1981–84 R. D. Wines
1984–87 D. Golovsky
1987–90 J. Boulas
1990–93 C. R. Farrell
1993–96 P. J. Langdon
1996–98 A. B. Grant

Honorary Treasurers

1937–45 K. L. H. Kirkland
1945–50 A. L. Carrodus
1950–53 K. L. H. Kirkland
1953–55 J. W. S. Laidley
1955–57 C. M. Edwards
1957–61 R. A. Craven
1961–63 B. S. Pearson
1964–66 L. A. Jacobs
1966–68 J. E. Blackman
1968–71 F. H. Breslin
1971–74 G. Schnitzler
1974–77 R. H. Farnsworth
1977–80 J. H. Rogers
1980–83 B. G. Storey
1983–88 M. J. Rochford
1988–91 E. I. Korbel
1991–94 A. Lalak
1994–97 K. J. Vaux
1997–98 L. J. Hayden

Annual Scientific Meeting Conveners

1993–94 A. I. Low
1994–95 R. F. McIlroy
1995–96 R. D. Wines
1996–97 M. R. Spork
1997–98 D. E. Yoffa

Keith Kirkland Prize Winners

1983	Z. S. Wisniewski
1984	L. C. Thompson
	D. R. Eisinger
1985	B. Blythe
1986	G. L. Russell
1987	P. M. Katelaris
1988	J. M. B. Chrisp
	M. J. Monsour
1989	D. G. Travis
1990	M. Frydenberg
1991	D. M. Bolton
1992	N. G. Redgrave
1993	Hin-wai Yap
1994	D. B. Sillar
1995	P. Cozzi
1996	M. Holmes
1997	J. Kourambas

INDEX

~

The use of italics for page numbers indicates an illustration.

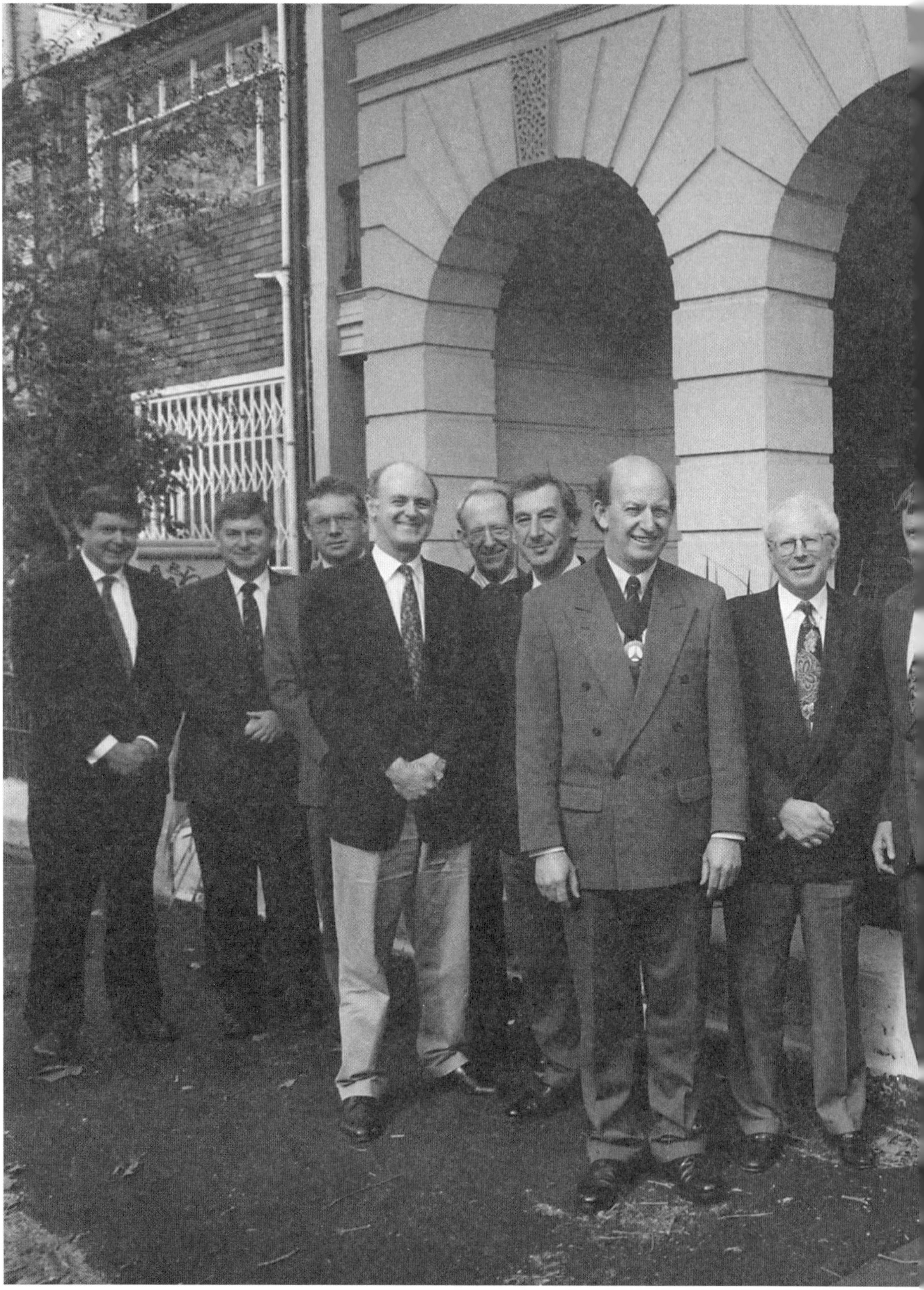